PHYSICIANS' GUIDE TO
OCULOSYSTEMIC DISEASES

Ophthalmoscopic Physical Diagnosis

William V. Delaney Jr., M.D.

MEDICAL ECONOMICS BOOKS
Oradell, New Jersey 07649

X
LRO
NMJ
GH

Library of Congress Cataloging in Publication Data

Delaney, William V.
 Physicians' guide to oculosystemic diseases.

 Includes bibliographical references and index.
 1. Ophthalmoscope and ophthalmoscopy.   2. Ocular
manifestations of general diseases.   I. Title.
[DNLM: 1. Diagnosis, Differential.   2. Eye
manifestations.   3. Ophthalmoscopy.   WW 475 D337p]
RE78.D44   617.7'1   81-81301
ISBN 0-87489-250-3   AACR2

Design by Elaine Kilcullen

ISBN 0-87489-250-3

Medical Economics Company Inc.
Oradell, New Jersey 07649

Printed in the United States of America

To Gloria, Susan, and Lori.
They never once mentioned that the time
I devoted to this effort
was time I could have spent with them —
although I know it is so.

CONTENTS

PUBLISHER'S
NOTES

This unusual volume describes in words and pictures the ophthalmoscopic findings that can play an integral part in physical diagnosis. The author's emphasis on systemic disease, his uncluttered text, and the 588 illustrations —160 of them in color—make this book a valuable reference and practical clinical tool for medical students and non-ophthalmologist physicians, who constitute the majority of users of the monocular, hand-held ophthalmoscope.

William V. Delaney Jr., M.D., is assistant clinical professor of ophthalmology, Upstate Medical Center, State University of New York, Syracuse. He is medical director of the Eye Research Institute of Central New York and a member of the board of directors of the Eye Defect and Vision Research Foundation. He also conducts a private medical practice in Syracuse.

PREFACE

This book deals principally with examination of the interior of the eye and those structures best viewed through the monocular, hand-held ophthalmoscope, an instrument that most physicians have. It's a technique that is noninvasive, comfortable for the patient, easy to do, and provides a magnified view of living tissue.

Customarily, the eyes, because of their anatomical position, are an early part of the physical examination of the patient. But ritualistic examination from top to bottom is not necessarily good medicine. Nor is there any law in diagnosis that requires a single organ to be examined in toto before the examiner moves on to the next. I would suggest the examiner first carry out a functional examination of visual acuity and ocular movements to the extent of his interest and capability. Then he can examine the exterior of the eye, determining in the process whether the pupil can be safely dilated. By the time the remainder of the physical examination is complete, an instilled mydriatic drop will have effected dilation, which greatly facilitates internal ocular examination.

My experience has shown that during physical examination of patients, many doctors observe eye findings they do not understand, make their clinical diagnosis on the basis of other findings, and, if they are curious, go to a textbook to see if the eye findings substantiate their opinion. I've written this text to help them include the eye findings in the decision-making process. I believe it will improve the accuracy of their diagnoses, and therefore improve patient care. Even though this is not a sit-down-to-read textbook, the good physician will want to leaf through it to look at the photographs and store them in his memory for recall when the patient sits in front of him.

I've organized this text then, not by diagnosis, but by physical finding. My intent is to provide the differential diagnosis of the physical findings encountered. This is a large task. Many diseases have similar findings. I have tried to sort out the overlapping information as clearly as possible.

Because the findings overlap, the reader is in many places referred to other parts of the book. An explanation of the method of referring is necessary. I've organized the book in outline form, with the principal headings in each chapter designated by Roman numerals. The next level is designated by capital letters. The following subordinate levels are keyed, respectively, to Arabic numerals, lower-case letters with close parentheses, and Arabic numerals enclosed in parentheses.

I've used these designations to make the cross references. Thus, for example, in Chapter 2, Red Reflection, I note a finding that may be seen in choroidal melanoma. The reader is referred, then, to the formal treatment of choroidal melanoma in this way: see Chapter 7:VIA. That is, part VI, subsection A, of Chapter 7.

Recognizing that most physicians who use the ophthalmoscope are not ophthalmologists, I've placed emphasis on ophthalmoscopic findings in systemic disease. For the sake of completeness, I've included many strictly ocular diseases as well. These, too, may be presently unrecognized manifestations of generalized disease. I've chosen to limit the references to texts and journals likely to be available in medical libraries or in the office of an ophthalmologist colleague. I have selected them also for their quality.

Undoubtedly, this book has omissions, and new or presently unrecognized ocular findings will have to be included. But it's a beginning. I hope that corrections and additions will be made by a new generation of physicians stimulated by it.

ACKNOWLEDGMENTS

This book is the result of a course in ophthalmoscopic physical diagnosis I've given for sophomore medical students since 1964. The idea of teaching this kind of course to a large group originated with William Havener, professor and chairman of the Department of Ophthalmology at Ohio State University College of Medicine. It is a delight to teach. The students are eager, they are surprised by what they see and they leave the three-hour session with a sense of accomplishment. I'm reminded yearly of Dr. Havener's ingenuity and I try to pass on his enthusiasm.

A fine clinician and an accomplished eye pathologist, Torrence Makley, professor of ophthalmology, Ohio State University College of Medicine, based my ophthalmoscopic observations in microscopic facts.

The support of these two patient and skillful men encouraged me to start the eye pathology laboratory and retina clinic at the State University of New York Upstate Medical Center. Both of these men have contributed photographs to this book.

I have called on many other colleagues for illustrations. Each is acknowledged with thanks. J. Donald Gass, Robert Ellsworth, and Paul Torrisi have been especially generous supplying photographs or criticism of the text.

Jacqueline Lombardo and Kathleen DiFulvio took most of the photographs, patiently searched for just the right ones, and typed from my impossible hand-written manuscript. Paula Dewey assisted with these tasks. Delilah R. Cohn did the illustrations. Elaine Hester provided the organization to bring all the various aspects of this endeavor together.

It was only 100 years ago that doctors used a mirror ophthalmoscope to examine the interior of the eye in the reflected, flickering light of a candle. Since then, there have been many researchers whose skill, patience, and plain hard work have provided us with a base of published information that we blithely accept. I must acknowledge them as joint authors.

COMMONLY USED OPHTHALMIC ABBREVIATIONS

AC	anterior chamber (from back of the cornea to the iris and pupil)
AS	arteriosclerosis
AT	applanation tension
A/V	artery-to-vein ratio
AVZ	avascular zone (same as CFZ)
BDR	background diabetic retinopathy
BP	blood pressure
BRAO	branch retinal artery occlusion
BRVO	branch retinal vein occlusion
CF	counting fingers (refers to visual acuity)
CFZ	capillary-free zone (same as AVZ)
CL	contact lens
CME	cystoid macular edema
CRA	central retinal artery
CRAO	central retinal artery occlusion
CRD	chorioretinal degeneration
CRV	central retinal vein
CRVO	central retinal vein occlusion
CT or CAT	computerized axial tomography
CW	cotton wool (same as SE)
D	diopter
DM	diabetes mellitus
DR	diabetic retinopathy
DX	diagnosis
E	esophoric on distant viewing

E^1	esophoric on near viewing
EOM	extraocular movements
E(T)	intermittent esotropia
ET	constant esotropia
FVD	fibrovascular tissue on the disc
FVE	fibrovascular tissue elsewhere in the retina
HE	hard exudate
HM	hand motion (visual acuity less than counting fingers—moving form vision only)
INA	inferior nasal artery
INQ	inferior nasal quadrant
INV	inferior nasal vein
IOL	intraocular lens
IOP	intraocular pressure
IRH	intraretinal hemorrhage
IRMA	intraretinal microvascular abnormalities
ITA	inferior temporal artery
ITQ	inferior temporal quadrant
ITV	inferior temporal vein
IVB	intravitreal blood
LC	light coagulation (photocoagulation)
MA	microaneurysms
ME	macular edema
NS	nuclear sclerosis of lens
NSR	neurosensory retina
NVD	neovascularization on the disc
NVE	neovascularization elsewhere in the retina
O	orthophoric on distant viewing
OD	oculus dexter (right eye)

OKN	optokinetic nystagmus
ON	optic nerve
OS	oculus sinister (left eye)
OU	oculus uterque (each eye)
PC	posterior chamber (from pupil to the front of the vitreous)
PDR	proliferative diabetic retinopathy
PMB	papillomacular bundle
PRH	preretinal hemorrhage
PRP	panretinal photocoagulation
PSC	posterior subcapsular cataract
PVD	posterior vitreous detachment
RBC	red blood cells
RD	retinal detachment
RLF	retrolental fibroplasia
RPE	retinal pigment epithelium
RX	treatment
SE	soft exudate (same as CW)
SMD	senile macular degeneration
SNA	superior nasal artery
SNQ	superior nasal quadrant
SNV	superior nasal vein
SRNV	subretinal neovascularization
STA	superior temporal artery
STQ	superior temporal quadrant
STV	superior temporal vein
TA	tension, applanation
VA	visual acuity or visual axis
WBC	white blood cells
X	exophoric on distant viewing
X^1	exophoric on near viewing
X(T)	intermittent exotropia
XT	constant exotropia
6/6 (20/20)	letter or test object subtending 5-minute arc is seen at a distance of 6 meters (20 feet)

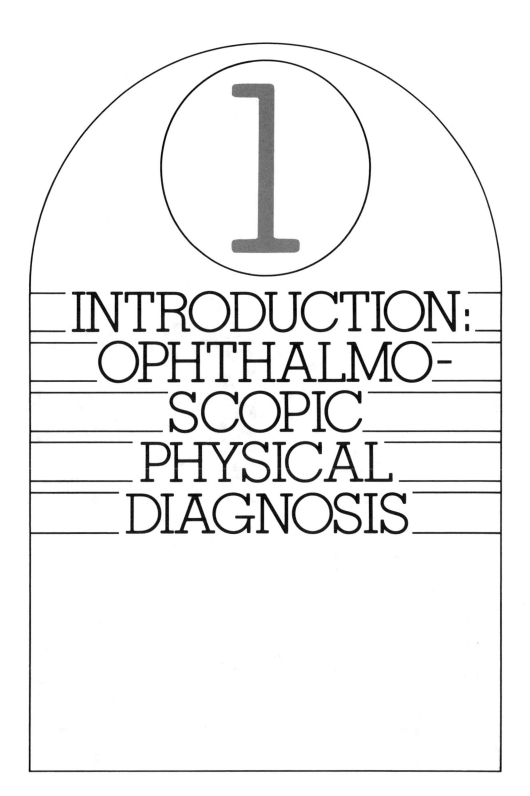

INTRODUCTION: OPHTHALMO-SCOPIC PHYSICAL DIAGNOSIS

In ophthalmoscopy, the light passes through the cornea, the anterior chamber, the pupil, the lens, and the vitreous until it finally reaches the retina. In order for you to view these structures, the light must return by the same route (Fig. 1.1). The cornea, lens, and vitreous are essentially transparent, unless there is pathology, and are, therefore, in their normal state difficult to see in detail with the hand ophthalmoscope. The slit lamp microscope is valuable for viewing transparent structures.

The photographs illustrating the text have been taken with a camera that has a larger field of view than the hand-held ophthalmoscope. The examiner sees an area of about 2 disc diameters (3mm), while the camera photographs 5 disc diameters (Fig. 1.2).

Fig. 1.1 Light entering the eye must, to be seen, be reflected back to the observer.

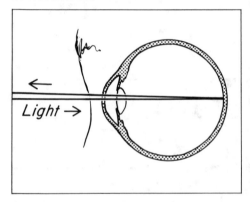

Fig. 1.2 Camera field of view is 5 disc diameters, while ophthalmoscope has a field of only 2 disc diameters (3 mm).

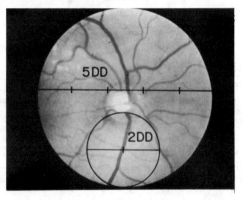

Fig. 1.3 The curved surface of the eye and the anterior limit of the retina (ora serrata) in an autopsy eye. Also shown in color section.

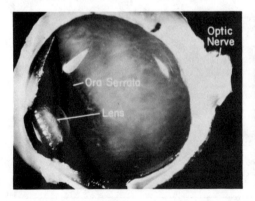

Fig. 1.4 The posterior retina at the fovea and optic disc in an autopsy eye. Also shown in color section.

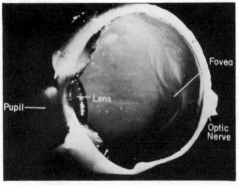

I. ANATOMICAL REVIEW

A review of the gross anatomy of the eye will help you to understand the structure, purpose, uses, and benefits of the ophthalmoscope.

The back of the eye, unlike the back of a camera, is a curved surface. The retina ends anteriorly, not far from the border of the lens, at the ora serrata (Fig. 1.3; see also in color section). Blood vessels enter and leave at the optic nerve and run forward through the retina, stopping at the ora serrata (Fig. 1.4; see also in color section). The vitreous lies against the internal limiting membrane of the retina. Light must traverse this vitreous and the whole thickness of the neurosensory retina before activating the rods and cones, which are closely opposed to the retinal pigment epithelium (Fig. 1.5)

Invagination of the developing optic cup creates the neurosensory retina from its inner layer and the retinal pigment epithelium from its outer layer (Fig. 1.6). There's a cleavage between the two layers, an important factor in some disease processes. Large blood vessels are present only in the inner layers of the retina, and capillaries from these vessels can be seen as far down in the retina as the inner plexiform layer. There are no large blood vessels in the outer layers. These layers, including the rods and cones, are supplied by the choroid through the retinal pigment epithelium (Fig. 1.7).

Since the retina is transparent, you can see the retinal pigment epithelium (Fig. 1.8; see also in color section). If it's thin or missing, you'll see the choroid (Fig. 1.9; see also in color section), and the bare sclera is visible if the choroid is absent (Fig. 1.10; see also in color section). If trauma has damaged the posterior sclera, you may see the retrobulbar tissue.

Fig. 1.5 Rods and cones are closely opposed to the retinal pigment epithelium. Entering light must pass through the retina to reach them. Note the pigmentation of the choroid is greatest near the sclera. Histologic section on the left courtesy of Torrence Makley, M.D., Ohio State University.

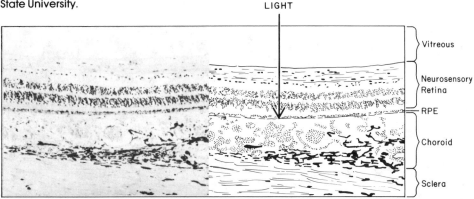

LIGHT

Vitreous

Neurosensory Retina

RPE

Choroid

Sclera

Fig. 1.6 The inner layer of the optic cup becomes the neurosensory retina and the outer layer the retinal pigment epithelium.

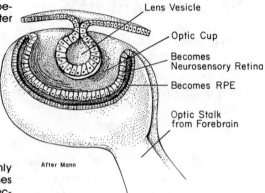

Lens Vesicle

Optic Cup

Becomes Neurosensory Retina

Becomes RPE

Optic Stalk from Forebrain

After Mann

Fig. 1.7 Large retinal blood vessels occur only in the inner retinal layers. The rods and cones are supplied from the choroid. Histologic section courtesy of Torrence Makley, M.D., Ohio State University.

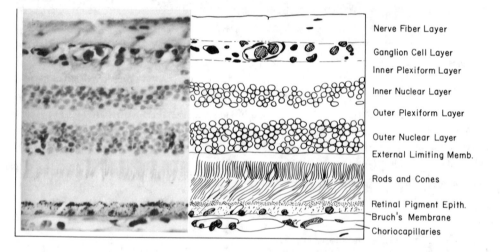

Nerve Fiber Layer

Ganglion Cell Layer

Inner Plexiform Layer

Inner Nuclear Layer

Outer Plexiform Layer

Outer Nuclear Layer

External Limiting Memb.

Rods and Cones

Retinal Pigment Epith.

Bruch's Membrane

Choriocapillaries

Fig. 1.8 Gross pathology specimen with the neurosensory retina removed, except at the disc, exposing the retinal pigment epithelium. Note the darker pigmentation at the macula. Also shown in color section.

Fig. 1.9 Gross pathology specimen with the neurosensory retina and retinal pigment epithelium removed to expose the choroid. Also shown in color section.

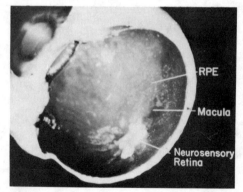

RPE

Macula

Neurosensory Retina

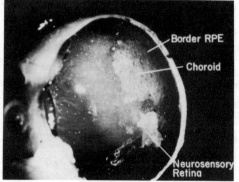

Border RPE

Choroid

Neurosensory Retina

Fig. 1.10 Gross pathology specimen with the retina, retinal pigment epithelium, and choroid removed to expose the sclera. Also shown in color section.

Fig. 1.11 Histologic section through the optic disc. The retina and retinal pigment epithelium stop as the nerve fiber layer of the retina courses through the sclera at the lamina cribrosa. Courtesy of Torrence Makley, M.D., Ohio State University.

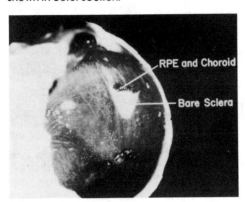

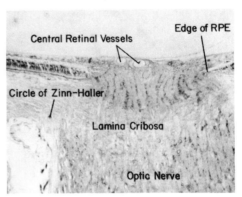

The nerve fibers from the retina course posteriorly and leave the globe through the lamina cribrosa, an opening in the sclera. Because the neurosensory elements, the rods and cones, stop at the borders of the optic nerve (Fig. 1.11), the optic nerve is insensitive to light. The retinal pigment epithelium also stops at the border of the optic nerve. The retinal pigment epithelium may contain more melanin at the border of the optic nerve and be more readily visible (see Fig. 3.3 in color section).

If the nerve fibers coursing from the globe cover the whole lamina cribrosa, the lamina will be hidden from your view. Frequently, however, you'll see it at the bottom of the normal physiologic depression in the optic nerve. The lamina has a sieve-like appearance, with the open spots in the sieve slightly gray in appearance. Usually, the central retinal artery and vein are present in the lamina and spread out into the retina from that point.

Immediately behind the sclera and thus hidden from your view, a ring of blood vessels, called the circle of Zinn-Haller, surrounds the optic nerve. Variations in vasculature of the eye may result in the retina's nourishment by blood vessels from the circle of Zinn-Haller entering the eye over the edge of the optic disc rather than from the central retinal vessels (see Fig. 3.6). These so-called cilioretinal arteries are common. In some disease processes, there is visible anastomosis between retinal blood vessels and the circle of Zinn-Haller.

As they synapse with the rods, cones, and the ganglion cells, the bipolar cells have a vertical orientation (see Fig. 1.7) that prevents horizontal dispersion. Therefore, hemorrhage or other extravasations at this level, when seen with the ophthalmoscope, appear round or oval. The horizontal orientation

Fig. 1.12 Histologic section through the fovea. Direction of incoming light is indicated by arrows. Light reflected at the foveal depression creates the classic foveal light reflex. Courtesy of Torrence Makley, M.D., Ohio State University.

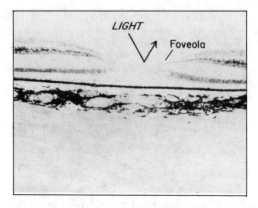

Fig. 1.13 Composite rendering of the left eye of a normal patient with the approximate densities of rods and cones noted (a, left); composite rendering of the same patient with visual acuity noted (b, right).

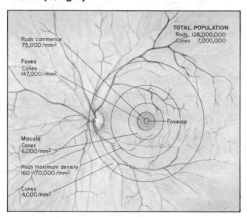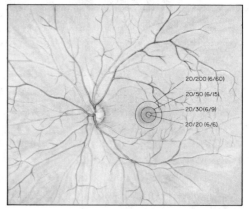

Fig. 1.14 Composite rendering with the direction of the retinal nerve fibers shown.

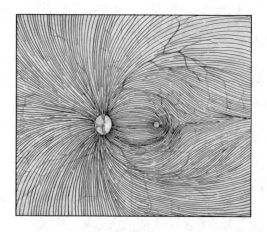

of the nerve fiber layer is also important, since hemorrhage in this area will take a horizontal aspect and appear flame-shaped.

The macula is about 3,000 microns (2 disc diameters) in size. The fovea is an area about half that size and is centered in the macula. Its central area, where rods and cones are concentrated, is called the foveola. Almost every cone in the foveola synapses with a nerve fiber. As a result, the nerve fibers pile up around the margins of the foveola, as Henle's layer, forming a pit. The pit often reflects light (foveal light reflection) from its depth (Fig. 1.12). The retinal pigment epithelium contains a larger amount of pigment in the macula, and the cells there are taller. In addition, yellow pigment (macula lutea) is present in the retina. The retinal pigment epithelium and neuro-sensory retina work at a high metabolic rate. Visual recovery after light exposure is almost instantaneous in the healthy eye.

No retinal blood vessels are present in the foveola. Their absence and the sloping of Henle's layer at the foveola allow even greater light transmission to the neurosensory elements in this area of maximum visual acuity. The density of rods and cones is related to visual acuity (Fig. 1.13a). Visual acuity decreases dramatically just a few degrees from the foveola, a phenomenon underscoring the importance of this area (Fig. 1.13b). This can be demonstrated by first looking directly at an eye chart and then trying to read it while looking a few degrees to either side.

Nerve fibers from the whole retina course toward and compose the optic nerve (Fig. 1.14). The astute examiner, using the red-free light of the ophthalmoscope, will be able to see the nerve fiber layer near the optic nerve (see Fig. 1.33; see also in color section). Knowing the direction in which the nerve fibers course helps in understanding patients' visual symptoms. A horizontal raphe separates the superior and inferior nerve fiber layers.

The macula, with its fovea and foveola, provides enough nerve fibers to form the whole temporal half of the optic nerve. The rest of the nerve fibers from the periphery of the eye must course to the nasal side. This accounts for the thicker and less distinct nasal disc margin.

II. PRINCIPLES OF OPHTHALMOSCOPY

There are two basic methods of ophthalmoscopy, indirect and direct. Of the indirect methods, binocular has largely replaced monocular ophthalmoscopy. Indirect is more difficult to master than direct, because the image is inverted and the hand-held lens needs to be accurately placed. Advantages of indirect ophthalmoscopy include a more detailed view of the peripheral aspects of the eye and a stereoscopic image of a larger field. You see a virtual and aerial image of the interior of the eye formed at the focal point of the hand-held lens, a point between your eyes and the lens.

Fig. 1.15 Light cast into the eye by the ophthalmoscope is viewed by the observer as it is reflected (a, left). Concave and convex lenses before the eye (b, right) illustrate how refractive error is corrected by ophthalmoscope's lens wheel.

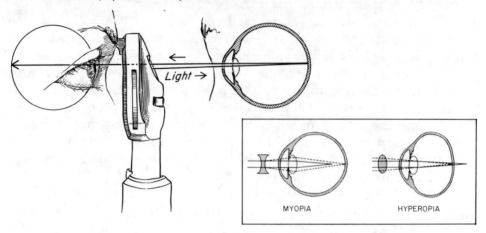

In direct monocular ophthalmoscopy (Fig. 1.15a), light entering the eye must be reflected from the interior so that you can focus it on your own retina. The lens wheel compensates for both the patient's and your refractive error (Fig. 1.15b). If the patient is emmetropic, you can employ a lens on the wheel to compensate for the working distance and a tendency to accommodate during the examination. Divergent rays in the farsighted patient require a plus lens; convergent reflected light from the myopic eye requires a minus lens. In most ophthalmoscopes, the black numbers on the lens wheel represent the plus lenses, and the red numbers represent the minus lenses (Fig. 1.16).

Light directed into the eye may be reflected, absorbed, or transmitted. Any or all of these effects may occur to some degree at any of the interfaces met by the light as it enters or leaves the eye. To some degree, all of these effects occur in the normal eye (Fig. 1.17). You must be continually aware of the fact that the observed light is returning from the interior of the eye. It's critical that you take account of the effects of reflection, absorption, and transmission.

Although the eye can be illuminated, it may be difficult to observe the interior of the eye due to opacities that obstruct the returning light (Fig. 1.18). You can sometimes determine the location of opacities by the manner in which they obstruct the returning light. Whether they are anterior or posterior to the nodal point of the eye makes a difference in the direction they move relative to you. If the opacity is anterior to the nodal point of the eye (slightly posterior to the lens), it appears to move in the same direction as you shift your point of observation (Fig. 1.19). If the opacity is posterior to the nodal point, it appears to move in the opposite direction as you move your head. If

PHYSICIANS' GUIDE TO OCULOSYSTEMIC DISEASES

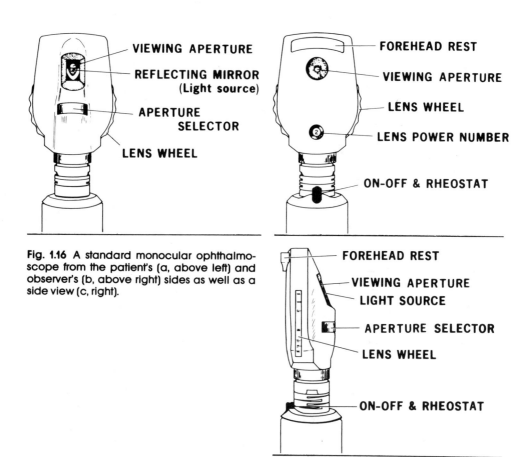

Fig. 1.16 A standard monocular ophthalmoscope from the patient's (a, above left) and observer's (b, above right) sides as well as a side view (c, right).

Fig. 1.17 Light entering the eye is reflected, absorbed, refracted, or transmitted.

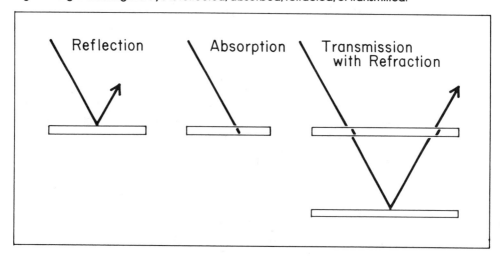

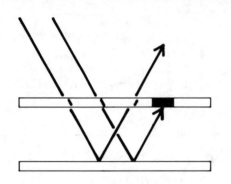

Fig. 1.18 Light may enter around an opacity but be blocked from returning to the observer.

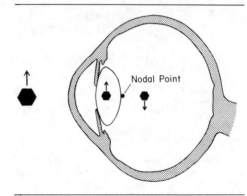

Fig. 1.19 Anterior objects seem to move in the direction of the observer's movement, while posterior objects seem to move in the opposite direction.

Nodal Point

the opacity is so large that it prevents light from entering the eye, you'll have no view at all.

You may find reflections from the surfaces of the eye bothersome, but they can also be helpful (Fig. 1.20). You can see reflections of the filament of the light source on the front and back surfaces of the cornea and the front and back surfaces of the lens. To illustrate this phenomenon, shine a penlight on a simple lens. Reflections will come from both the front and back surfaces. By moving and tilting the lens, you can superimpose the reflections at the optical center.

III. TECHNIQUE USED IN OPHTHALMOSCOPY

A. ENLARGING THE PUPIL (MYDRIASIS)

Dilating the pupil with a mydriatic solution facilitates examination of the interior of the eye. In rare cases, dilating the pupils of patients prone to the disease may actually precipitate acute glaucoma. Mydriasis under controlled circumstances is sometimes used as a provocative test for acute, narrow-angle glaucoma. Office precipitation of glaucoma is an accepted procedure and preferable to undetected angle-closure glaucoma ignored by the patient until the eye is blind.

Most individuals predisposed to acute glaucoma are farsighted. The farsighted patient's anterior chamber is likely to be very shallow. If you find plus lenses in the patient's glasses, you can suspect such a predisposition. When you move glasses with plus lenses side to side, objects appear to move in the opposite direction. The stronger the lens, the more pronounced the movement. The reverse occurs with minus lenses (Fig. 1.21). Myopic patients usually have deep anterior chambers.

When you view the eye from the side, you can see the distance between the cornea and the iris plane, especially if you use a small flashlight or the light of the ophthalmoscope. If you shine the light from the side of the eye, and if the anterior chamber is deep, the whole iris plane will be illuminated. If the iris bows forward so that the distance between it and the back of the cornea is very narrow, light coming from the side won't illuminate the complete iris, and you'll see a shadow. Although it's intended primarily for other purposes, the slit aperture on the hand ophthalmoscope is useful in determining the depth of the anterior chamber. The amount of displacement of the vertical slit as it crosses the cornea and illuminates the iris indicates the depth of the anterior chamber. The amount of displacement of the vertical slit is directly proportional to the depth of the chamber (Fig. 1.22).

B. SELECTING THE PROPER OPHTHALMOSCOPE APERTURE
(Fig. 1.23)

You might think that if the patient's pupil is small, you should use the small aperture. Using the larger aperture in such cases results in corneal reflections that interfere with the view. However, the closer you are to the patient's eye, the more light you can direct through the pupil, and so, at close range, a larger aperture may be used, even with a small pupil. It's advantageous to use the large aperture, because you can direct most of the light to the interior of the eye, thereby increasing the field of view.

Fig. 1.20 Light reflections can be cast aside by slightly tilting the ophthalmoscope. When you superimpose the light reflections from the front and back surface of a lens, you have found the optical axis of the lens.

Fig. 1.21 If you move glasses with plus lenses for farsightedness side to side, objects you see through them seem to move in the opposite direction; they appear to move in the same direction as the movement of the glasses with minus lenses (for nearsightedness).

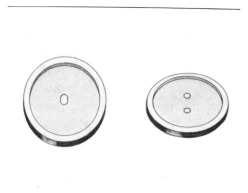

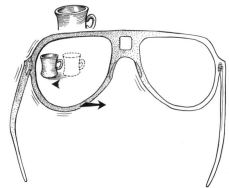

Fig. 1.22 Light entering one side of a shallow anterior chamber does not reach the opposite side.

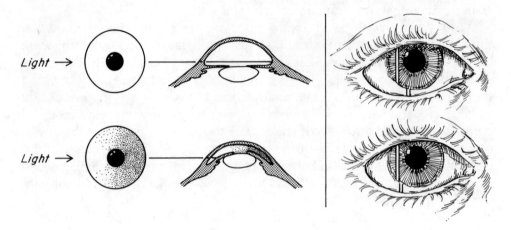

Fig. 1.23 Most available ophthalmoscopes have a large and a small aperture and a red-free light source. Some have a light slit and cross hairs or circles and lines to project on the patient's retina.

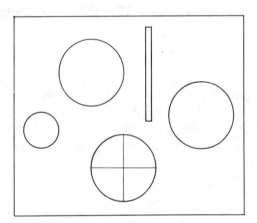

Some ophthalmoscopes have a slit aperture whose purpose is to emphasize light displacement and aid in determining elevation or depression. But the slit aperture simply displays the presence of an elevation or depression. It doesn't accurately measure the magnitude of these changes.

Some ophthalmoscopes have a measuring device that can be projected on the patient's retina. It's of limited use in lesions larger than a single ophthalmoscopic field, but it does make possible measurement of eccentric fixation. Some patients with strabismus or retinal pathology fixate with areas outside of the fovea. If you project the grid on the retina and ask the patient to look at its center, the foveal light reflection may be a few degrees from the point of the patient's fixation. The other eye must be covered during this test.

Most monocular ophthalmoscopes have a red-free filter to increase contrast between interior eye structures that are red and those that reflect light

Fig. 1.24 The ophthalmoscope is held in the right hand for the right eye (a, left) and left hand for the left eye (b, right). It is braced against the patient's forehead and the handle is tilted outward 45°. The index finger is on the lens wheel for rapid focusing.

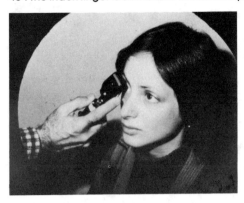 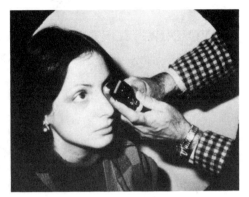

of different colors. Structures that reflect only red light, of course, appear black with the filter (see Fig. 1.33; see also in color section).

C. SIGHTING THROUGH THE OPHTHALMOSCOPE

Unless you have substantial astigmatism, don't wear corrective lenses while using the hand-held ophthalmoscope. The lens wheel compensates for your own refractive error as well as the patient's. Brace the ophthalmoscope against your forehead in such a way that the aperture for viewing is steady in front of your eye. Use your right eye for the patient's right eye, your left for the patient's left. If, however, you have a monocular disability, use your better eye at all times.

Hold the ophthalmoscope with your right hand when you're looking at the patient's right eye, and with your left hand when looking at the patient's left eye (Fig. 1.24). Hold the ophthalmoscope at an angle of approximately 45°. This angle permits you to get closer to the patient's eye and, therefore, to have a better view. Brace the ophthalmoscope against your forehead and the forehead of the patient, and keep your forefinger poised over the lens wheel to make quick changes in the lens system. Depending on the area you're observing, you may keep your thumb on the rheostat so you can increase or decrease the illumination.

D. THE RED REFLECTION

In your examination, you must direct the light from the ophthalmoscope on the patient's pupil to create a red reflection. Begin this procedure from approximately an arm's length away. Keep the red reflection in view as you move toward the patient's forehead. If you lose the red reflection during this maneuver, move back and start again. With practice, you'll be able to find the red reflection at a closer distance. The purpose of this procedure is to note defects in the red reflection.

E. AVOIDING LIGHT REFLECTIONS

You can avoid most of the bothersome light reflections from the cornea and lens by keeping the ophthalmoscope close to the patient. As noted above, it should be so close that the patient's forehead touches the instrument. Occasionally, it's necessary to tilt the ophthalmoscope slightly to cast light reflections aside.

F. FINDING THE DISC

Once you've found the red reflection and have moved close to the patient, turn the lens wheel until the retina comes into sharp focus. The first view may be that of a peripheral retinal blood vessel. Bifurcations of the retinal blood vessels act as arrows pointing the way to the optic disc (Fig. 1.25). As you move the light on the patient's retina, you must keep the ophthalmoscope braced firmly against your forehead. The movements needed to change direction of the light are small and in a direction opposite from the area to be viewed (Fig. 1.26). Encourage the patient to maintain steady fixation with the other eye; this steadies the eye being examined.

G. FINDING THE FOVEA

The fovea with its central foveola is approximately 1½ disc diameters temporal to the temporal border of the optic disc (Fig. 1.27). Although often

Fig. 1.25 One's first view of the interior of an eye is usually of retinal blood vessels out of focus (photograph purposely out of focus to illustrate). Once blood vessels are brought into focus with the lens wheel, their bifurcations point the way to the optic disc (arrows).

Fig. 1.26 Moving the ophthalmoscope's light along the blood vessels to the disc requires the observer to move in the opposite direction from the area to be viewed.

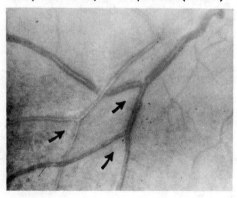

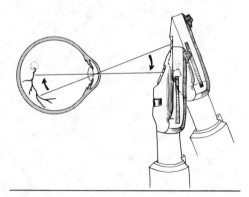

directly on the median raphe, it may be slightly below horizontal. Because of the patient's sensitivity to light in this area, it may be necessary to reduce the illumination. If you have difficulty finding the fovea, it will help to have the patient look into the light of the ophthalmoscope.

H. SEEING THE PERIPHERY

Systematically follow each retinal blood vessel into the periphery. Observe all the structures in this pathway as far into the periphery as you can comfortably and clearly see. For a more extensive peripheral examination, you must have the patient look in the direction of the area to be examined. At the same time, you should move in the opposite direction (Fig. 1.28a). As the patient looks aside, you must look through the patient's lens obliquely, which induces astigmatism and makes a clear view more difficult to obtain (Fig. 1.28b). This is one limitation of the ophthalmoscope in examining the

Fig. 1.27 The fovea is approximately 1½ disc diameters temporal to the disc on the horizontal meridian.

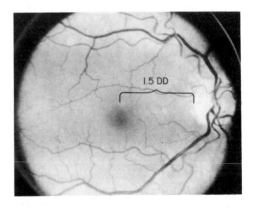

Fig. 1.28 To examine peripheral parts of the eye, move the ophthalmoscope in a direction opposite to the patient's gaze (a, left). This changes the distance the returning light must travel, and refocusing may be necessary to correct this and the astigmatism created by looking through the patient's lens obliquely (b, right).

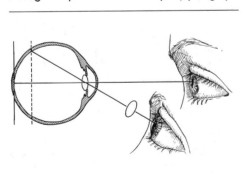 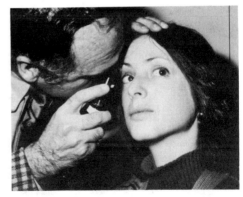

far peripheral parts of the eye. The pupil, which appears round in the straight-on view, becomes elliptical, reducing illumination and pupil size. Once again, to avoid difficulty in light alignment and decreasing illumination, it's essential that you brace the ophthalmoscope against your forehead and remain close to the patient (Fig. 1.29).

Fig. 1.29 Peripheral examination involves looking through an increasingly oval and therefore smaller pupil. The illumination needs to be increased. Careful alignment and bracing of the ophthalmoscope are essential.

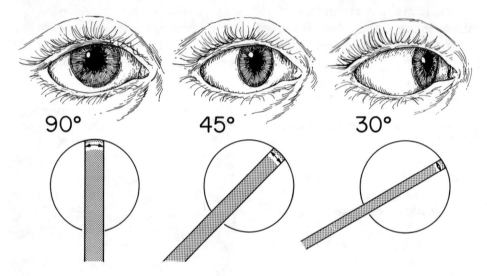

Fig. 1.30 Light reflections from the retina around the fovea and the foveal pit. At the higher magnification of the ophthalmoscope, the retinal surface may have thousands of fine scintillations called Gunn's dots. Yellow luteal pigment at the foveola is seen in Fig. 5.3.

Fig. 1.31 The width of the light reflection from the surface of the retinal arteriole and vein give an indication of the thickness of their walls. Note the vessels just below the disc.

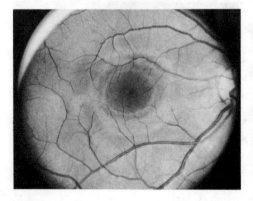

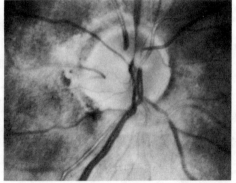

I. USING LIGHT REFLECTIONS

You can use light reflections to determine the distance of a structure from the point of observation. For example, with regard to the fovea, the slight depression and the internal limiting membrane of the retina cause light to be reflected back to the observer, giving the typical foveal light reflection (Fig. 1.30). You should note the presence or absence of light reflections. Some tissues are more reflective than others. For example, you'll often see Gunn's dots in the relatively thick retinas of young patients. In addition, reflections may appear as rings around the optic disc and the fovea. These reflections are due to flat spots in the retinal surface that mirror the light.

Such reflections are often absent in older patients and others are more evident. For example, the widening of the arteriolar light reflex can be equated with the thickness of the blood vessel wall in older patients (Fig. 1.31).

J. PROXIMAL ILLUMINATION

Not all of the light entering the eye is reflected. Some is absorbed by the tissues, and some is internally reflected before being absorbed or reflected. You should observe not only the area illuminated by the ophthalmoscope, but also the darker surrounding areas. As illumination scatters light through the tissues, internally reflected light gives clues to the nature of lesions there may be within the tissue. For example, an opaque substance blocks internally reflected light so that in proximal illumination or retroillumination, it appears black in relief. On the other hand, a cystic lesion that has its own internal reflection tends to enhance the light (Fig. 1.32).

Fig. 1.32 Proximal illumination differentiates an opaque lesion, such as a blood clot, from a retinal hole or cyst. The internal reflection of a cyst (lower diagram) enhances the reflected light.

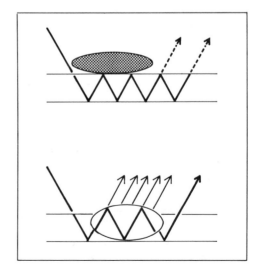

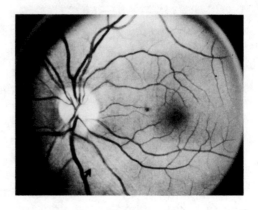

Fig. 1.33 Red-free light enhances the view of structures that reflect other wavelengths, such as the nerve fiber layer of the retina (arrow). Note the blood vessels are black. Also shown in color section.

K. RED-FREE ILLUMINATION

When red-free light illumines the interior of the eye, those structures that principally reflect red light appear black. This increases the contrast between totally red structures and those that reflect other colors, as seen in the nerve fiber layer (Fig. 1.33; see also in color section). It should be emphasized that when you use the red-free filter, you aren't seeing only one color. In other words, the view is not monochromatic. It's a view with a light from which one color, red, has been removed. Structures that reflect all other colors, or structures that partially reflect other colors, remain visible.

L. MEASURING ELEVATIONS AND DEPRESSIONS

The slit aperture on the ophthalmoscope is helpful for discerning elevation or depression. You can get further clues about elevation or depression by observing the convergence of lines. However, due to the short distances involved in the interior eye, these lines may provide only limited information concerning depth. When you focus the monocular ophthalmoscope sharply on a structure at 15 times magnification, any elevated or depressed areas will be out of focus. This is one of the best monocular clues to depth within the eye. Shadow casting is also an important factor.

You can measure the magnitude of elevation or depression by turning the lens wheel (Fig. 1.34). Note the difference in diopter power required to focus an object at the normal plane compared to the elevated or depressed plane. Approximately 3 diopters are equivalent to 1 mm of change. Fine blood vessels of equal size at both levels are usually used for this comparison.

M. MEASURING SIZE AND POSITION

Use the disc as a reference to estimate the size and position of objects within the interior of the eye. The average disc diameter is approximately 1.5 mm in a horizontal direction (Fig. 1.35). Estimate the size of objects relative to the number of disc diameters that would be required to cover them. You can describe the size of a lesion in disc diameters in both the horizontal and vertical plane.

For the position of a lesion, estimate the number of disc diameters between the lesion and the disc. One purpose of estimating the position and size of a lesion is to make it easier to find it again for re-evaluation (Fig. 1.36). A typical estimate might describe a nevus as 1½ disc diameters in size and 4 disc diameters from the optic nerve in the superior nasal quadrant. Keep in mind that the measurements of elevation or depression, size, and position are approximations.

Fig. 1.34 Focusing with the lens wheel on small blood vessels (arrows), one near the disc (a, left) and one in the depth of a large cup (b, right) and recalling the number of clicks of the lens wheel give an indication of depth. About 3 diopters (clicks) equals 1 mm.

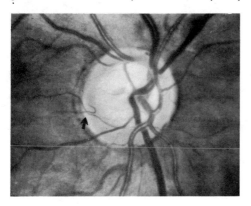
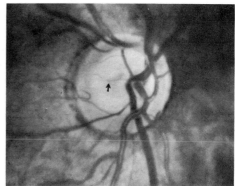

Fig. 1.35 The average optic disc is 1.5 mm in horizontal diameter.

Fig. 1.36 The pigmented lesion 1½ disc diameters from the disc margin in the 1:30 o'clock meridian fits within a circle that is approximately 1 disc diameter in size.

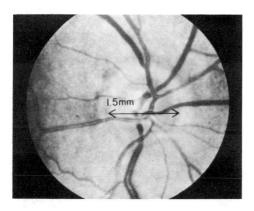
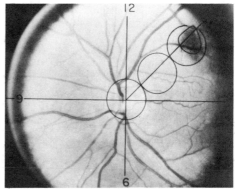

N. FOCUSING OFF THE RETINAL PLANE

Examination of the vitreous is best accomplished as your last maneuver. More plus (or less minus) power in the lens wheel will focus your view off the retinal plane into the vitreous. Gradually increasing plus lens power brings the focal plane forward until you see the iris. To view the vitreous at the outset of the examination is less systematic. You don't know at the start what lens you'll need and therefore in which direction to turn the lens wheel. To emphasize this point, the last chapter considers the vitreous.

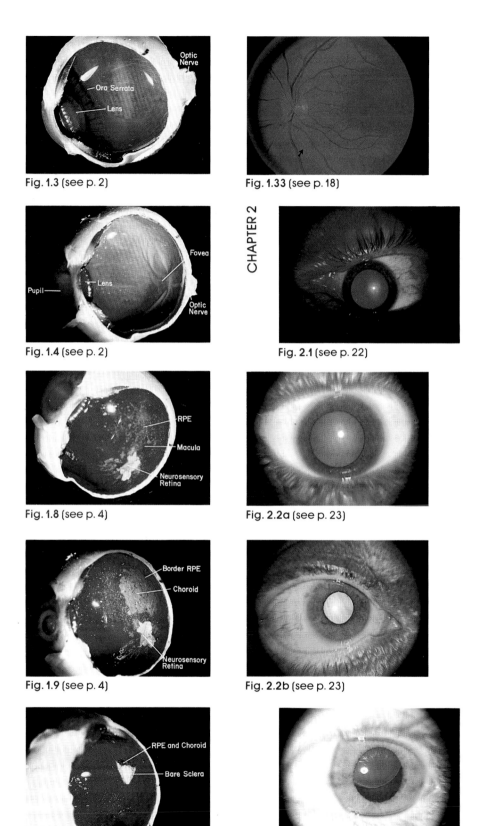

Fig. 1.3 (see p. 2)

Fig. 1.33 (see p. 18)

Fig. 1.4 (see p. 2)

Fig. 2.1 (see p. 22)

Fig. 1.8 (see p. 4)

Fig. 2.2a (see p. 23)

Fig. 1.9 (see p. 4)

Fig. 2.2b (see p. 23)

Fig. 1.10 (see p. 5)

Fig. 2.3 (see p. 23)

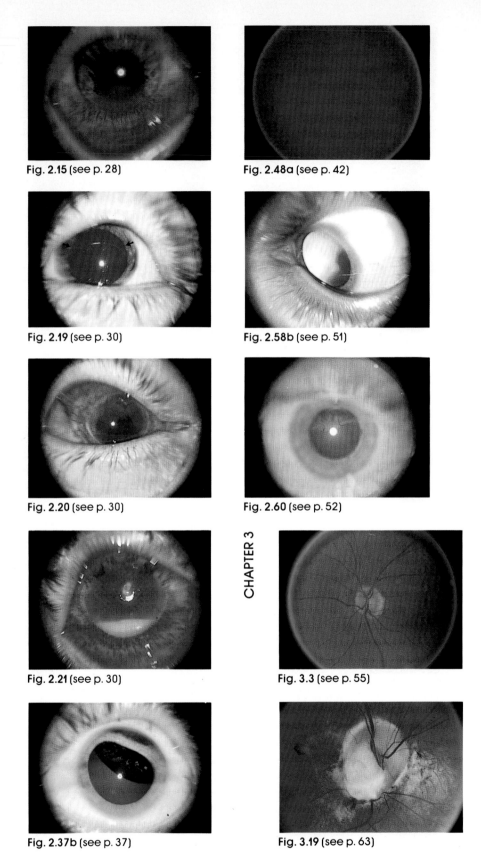

Fig. 2.15 (see p. 28)

Fig. 2.48a (see p. 42)

Fig. 2.19 (see p. 30)

Fig. 2.58b (see p. 51)

Fig. 2.20 (see p. 30)

Fig. 2.60 (see p. 52)

Fig. 2.21 (see p. 30)

Fig. 3.3 (see p. 55)

Fig. 2.37b (see p. 37)

Fig. 3.19 (see p. 63)

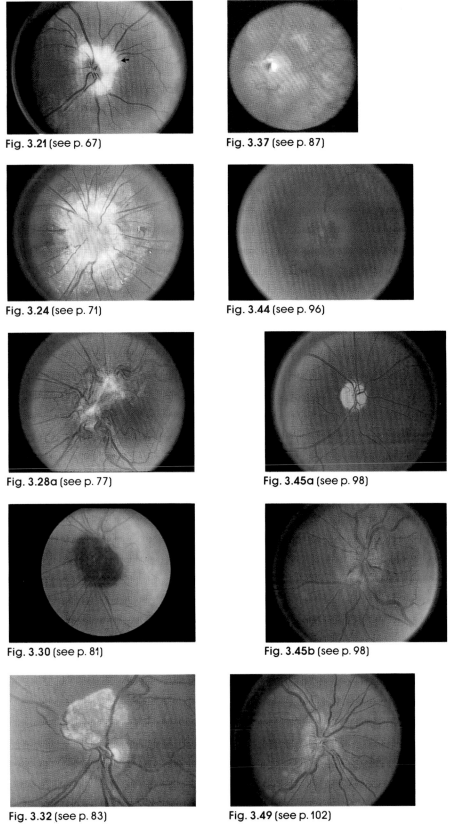

Fig. 3.21 (see p. 67)

Fig. 3.37 (see p. 87)

Fig. 3.24 (see p. 71)

Fig. 3.44 (see p. 96)

Fig. 3.28a (see p. 77)

Fig. 3.45a (see p. 98)

Fig. 3.30 (see p. 81)

Fig. 3.45b (see p. 98)

Fig. 3.32 (see p. 83)

Fig. 3.49 (see p. 102)

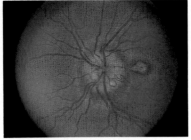

Fig. 3.52a (see p. 106)

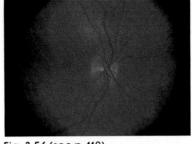

Fig. 3.56 (see p. 110)

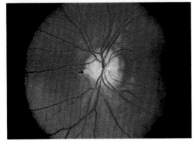

Fig. 3.52c (see p. 106)

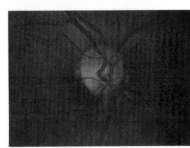

Fig. 3.59a (see p. 115)

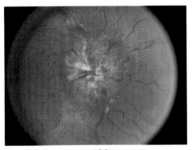

Fig. 3.54a (see p. 109)

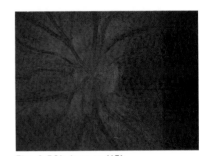

Fig. 3.59b (see p. 115)

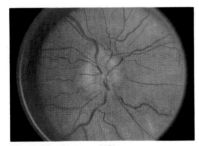

Fig. 3.55a (see p. 110)

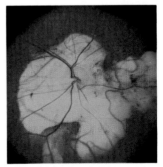

Fig. 3.60 (see p. 116)

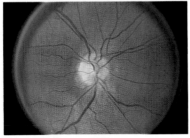

Fig. 3.55b (see p. 110)

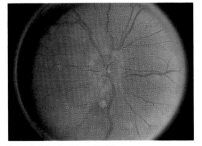

Fig. 3.61a (see p. 116)

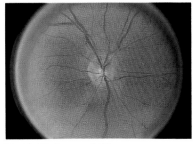

Fig. 3.61b (see p. 116)

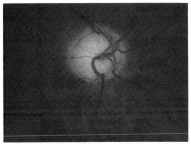

Fig. 3.65 (see p. 123)

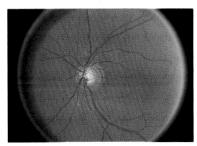

Fig. 3.66a (see p. 124)

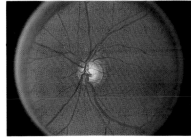

Fig. 3.66b (see p. 124)

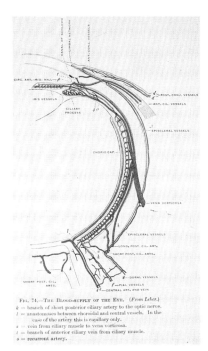

FIG. 74.—THE BLOOD-SUPPLY OF THE EYE. (From Leber.)
k = branch of short posterior ciliary artery to the optic nerve.
l = anastomoses between choroidal and central vessels. In the
    case of the artery this is capillary only.
s = vein from ciliary muscle to vena vorticosa.
t = branch of anterior ciliary vein from ciliary muscle.
o = recurrent artery.

Fig. 4.1 (see p. 128)

Fig. 4.6b (see p. 131)

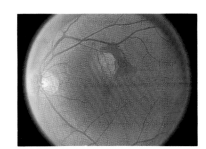

Fig. 4.12 (see p. 135)

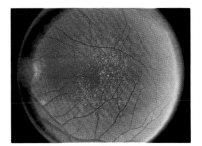

Fig. 4.25 (see p. 145)

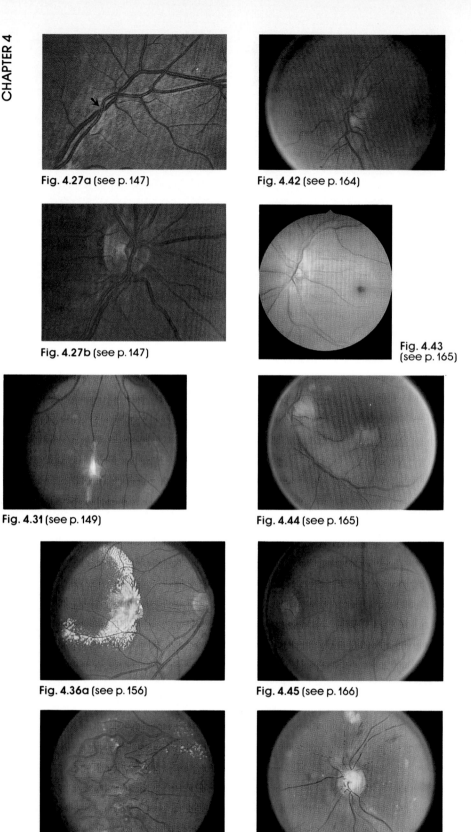

Fig. **4.27a** (see p. 147)

Fig. **4.42** (see p. 164)

Fig. **4.27b** (see p. 147)

Fig. **4.43**
(see p. 165)

Fig. **4.31** (see p. 149)

Fig. **4.44** (see p. 165)

Fig. **4.36a** (see p. 156)

Fig. **4.45** (see p. 166)

Fig. **4.36b** (see p. 156)

Fig. **4.47** (see p. 166)

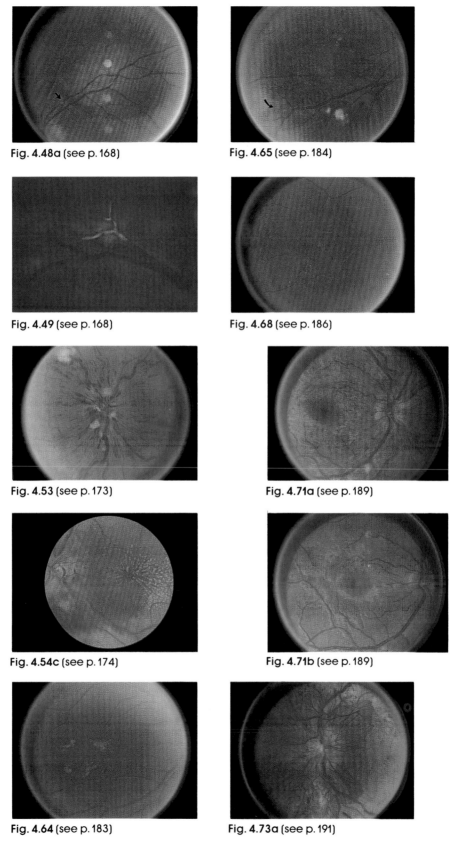

Fig. **4.48a** (see p. 168)

Fig. **4.65** (see p. 184)

Fig. **4.49** (see p. 168)

Fig. **4.68** (see p. 186)

Fig. **4.53** (see p. 173)

Fig. **4.71a** (see p. 189)

Fig. **4.54c** (see p. 174)

Fig. **4.71b** (see p. 189)

Fig. **4.64** (see p. 183)

Fig. **4.73a** (see p. 191)

Fig. **4.74** (see p. 192)

Fig. **5.5** (see p. 226)

Fig. **4.78a** (see p. 194)

Fig. **5.6** (see p. 229)

Fig. **4.78b** (see p. 194)

Fig. **5.10** (see p. 232)

Fig. **4.85** (see p. 200)

Fig. **5.14** (see p. 238)

Fig. **4.93** (see p. 219)

Fig. **5.15** (see p. 238)

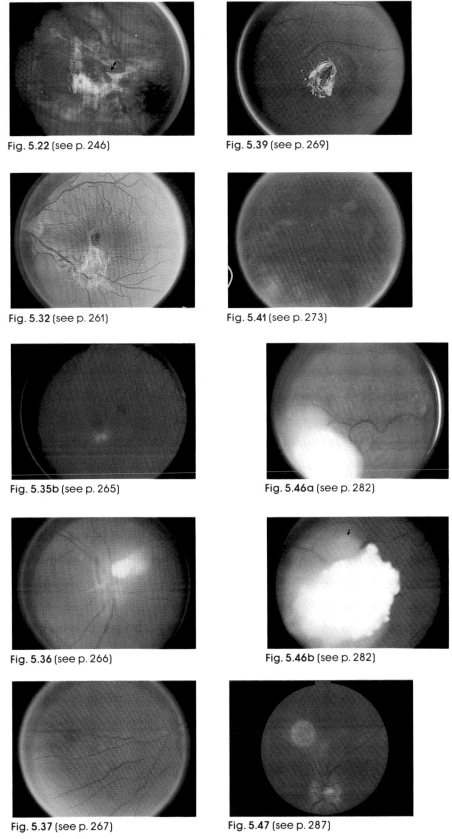

Fig. 5.22 (see p. 246)

Fig. 5.39 (see p. 269)

Fig. 5.32 (see p. 261)

Fig. 5.41 (see p. 273)

Fig. 5.35b (see p. 265)

Fig. 5.46a (see p. 282)

Fig. 5.36 (see p. 266)

Fig. 5.46b (see p. 282)

Fig. 5.37 (see p. 267)

Fig. 5.47 (see p. 287)

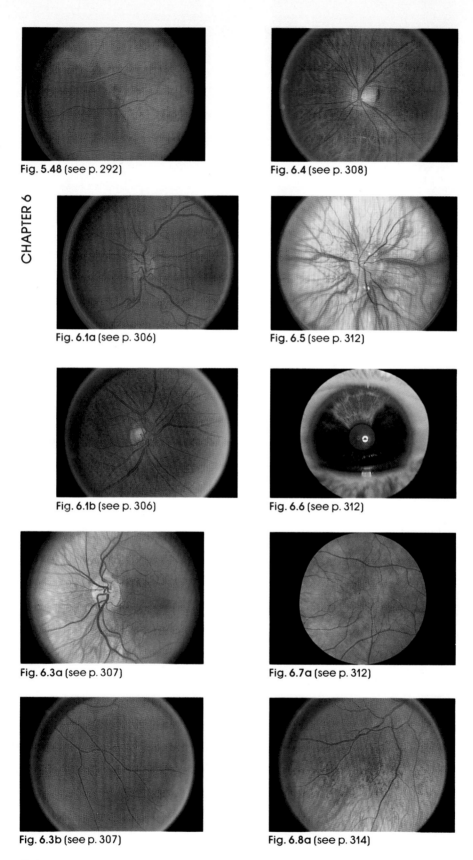

Fig. 5.48 (see p. 292)

Fig. 6.4 (see p. 308)

Fig. 6.1a (see p. 306)

Fig. 6.5 (see p. 312)

Fig. 6.1b (see p. 306)

Fig. 6.6 (see p. 312)

Fig. 6.3a (see p. 307)

Fig. 6.7a (see p. 312)

Fig. 6.3b (see p. 307)

Fig. 6.8a (see p. 314)

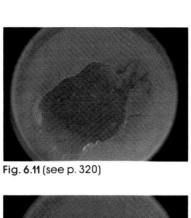

Fig. 6.11 (see p. 320)

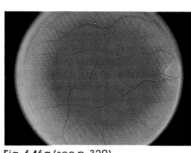

Fig. 6.16a (see p. 329)

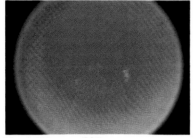

Fig. 6.12 (see p. 321)

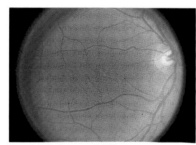

Fig. 6.16b (see p. 329)

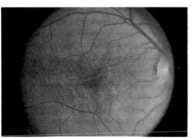

Fig. 6.13b (see p. 324)

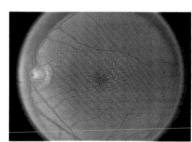

Fig. 6.17a (see p. 333)

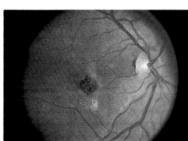
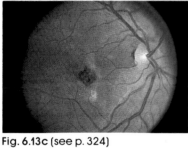

Fig. 6.13c (see p. 324)

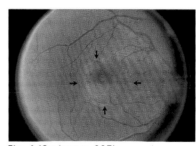

Fig. 6.19a (see p. 337)

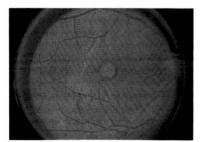

Fig. 6.14a (see p. 325)

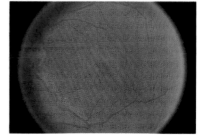

Fig. 6.19b (see p. 337)

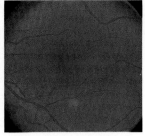

Fig. **6.20b** (see p. 340)

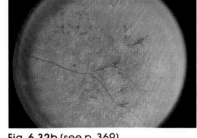

Fig. **6.32b** (see p. 369)

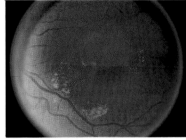

Fig. **6.20d** (see p. 340)

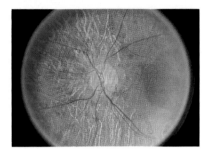

Fig. **6.33a** (see p. 375)

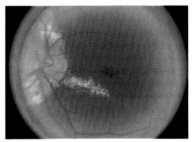

Fig. **6.23a** (see p. 344)

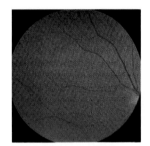

Fig. **6.38** (see p. 383)

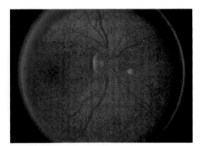

Fig. **6.25** (see p. 348)

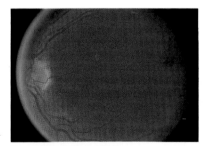

Fig. **6.43a** (see p. 392)

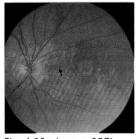

Fig. **6.28a** (see p. 357)

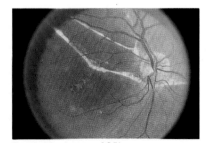

Fig. **6.46a** (see p. 395)

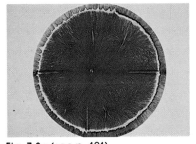

Fig. 7.3a (see p. 401)

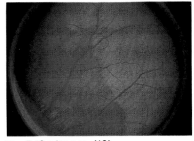

Fig. 7.10a (see p. 413)

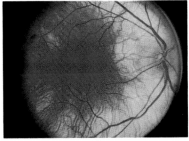

Fig. 7.8a (see p. 408)

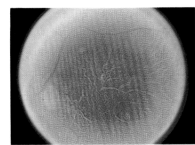

Fig. 7.11 (see p. 417)

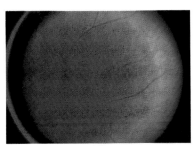

Fig. 7.8d (see p. 408)

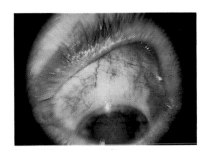

Fig. 7.12a (see p. 419)

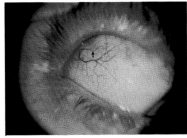

Fig. 7.9a (see p. 410)

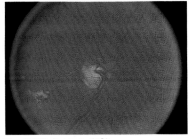

Fig. 7.12b (see p. 419)

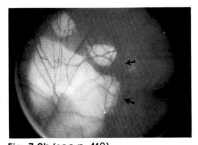

Fig. 7.9b (see p. 410)

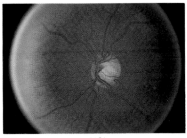

Fig. 7.12c (see p. 419)

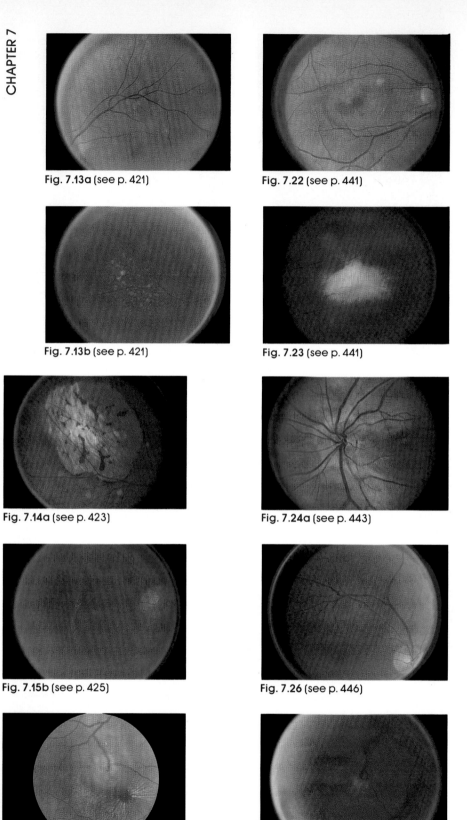

Fig. 7.13a (see p. 421)

Fig. 7.22 (see p. 441)

Fig. 7.13b (see p. 421)

Fig. 7.23 (see p. 441)

Fig. 7.14a (see p. 423)

Fig. 7.24a (see p. 443)

Fig. 7.15b (see p. 425)

Fig. 7.26 (see p. 446)

Fig. 7.17b (see p. 430)

Fig. 7.27 (see p. 446)

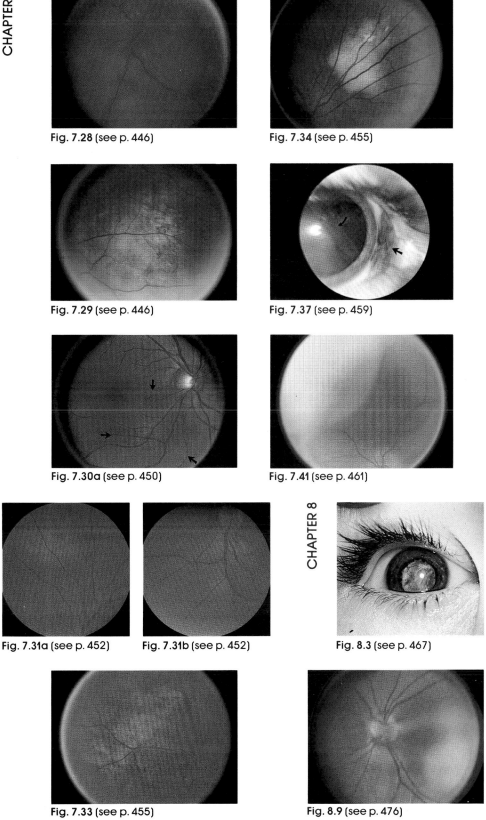

Fig. 7.28 (see p. 446)

Fig. 7.34 (see p. 455)

Fig. 7.29 (see p. 446)

Fig. 7.37 (see p. 459)

Fig. 7.30a (see p. 450)

Fig. 7.41 (see p. 461)

Fig. 7.31a (see p. 452)

Fig. 7.31b (see p. 452)

Fig. 8.3 (see p. 467)

Fig. 7.33 (see p. 455)

Fig. 8.9 (see p. 476)

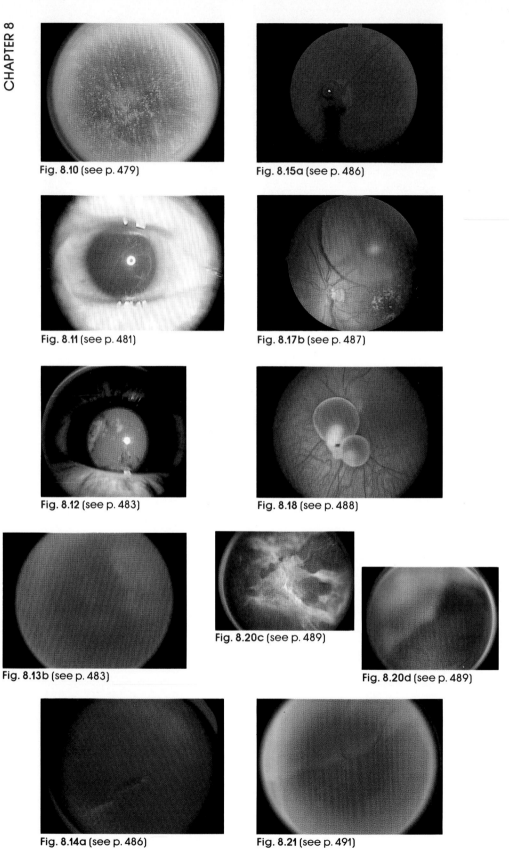

Fig. 8.10 (see p. 479)

Fig. 8.15a (see p. 486)

Fig. 8.11 (see p. 481)

Fig. 8.17b (see p. 487)

Fig. 8.12 (see p. 483)

Fig. 8.18 (see p. 488)

Fig. 8.13b (see p. 483)

Fig. 8.20c (see p. 489)

Fig. 8.20d (see p. 489)

Fig. 8.14a (see p. 486)

Fig. 8.21 (see p. 491)

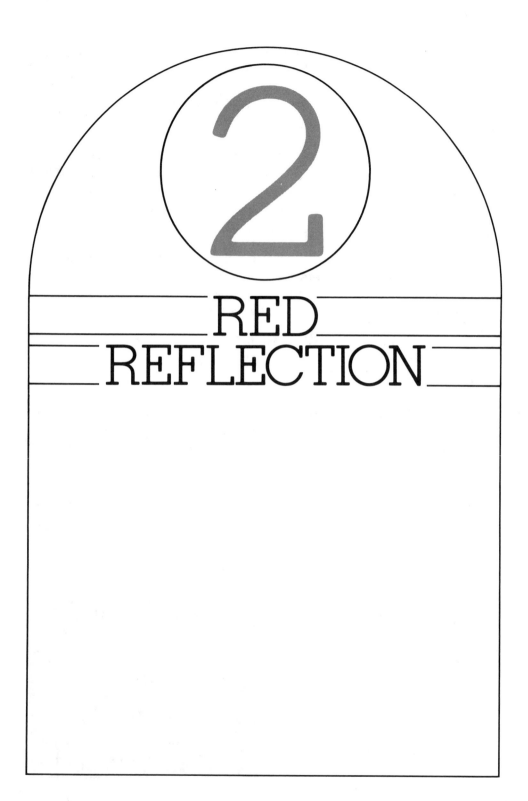

2

RED
REFLECTION

We've all seen the reflection of light from the interior of the eye. We've seen it as the beam from a flashlight or the headlights of an automobile strike an animal's eyes. The eyes of nocturnal animals reflect a greenish-yellow light because of a light-gathering tapetum in the retina. Humans, as daytime animals, don't have a tapetum, and the light reflected from ocular blood vessels is red.

This chapter describes the red reflection, its normal variations, and diseases that alter its appearance. Examination of the red reflection is the first step in ophthalmoscopy. The first principle to keep in mind is that light must enter the eye to be reflected. A defect may alter part or all of the entering or reflected light.

Using a bright light in a dark room enhances the red reflection, making observation easier. Some disturbances of the reflection may be seen only with a dilated pupil, and others may be transient, changing as the patient blinks or moves the eye. Different positions of gaze may disclose variations in the reflection and, accordingly, examination of all quadrants should be routine.

I. VARIATIONS OF NORMAL

The red reflection fills the whole pupil (Fig. 2.1; see also in color section), whether it is large or small. With a small pupil, reflections from the cornea and lens may mask much of the red color. These reflections may be cast aside by positioning. Light reflected from the eye before entering appears white to the observer, as seen by the light reflections from the cornea in the photographs. Light returning from the interior is normally red. Obstruction to the returning light appears black or a dark shade, depending on its light transmission.

Fig. 2.1 The normal red reflection fills the whole pupil. When the pupil is small, reflections from the cornea and lens hide much of the red reflection. Also shown in color section.

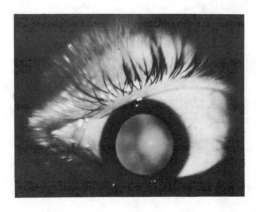

The returning light is not always a homogeneous red, but shades of red as the reflection or absorption varies with different tissues. The red reflection from black patients has a deeper color (Fig. 2.2a; see also in color section), and poorly pigmented eyes have a white reflection (Fig. 2.2b; see also in color section).

The brightness of the reflection is also variable. Most observers interpret red as brighter than blue, even when the luminosity is equal.

The quality of the reflection varies with the focus of the light. Light returning through the aphakic part of the pupil in a patient with a subluxated lens looks different from that returning through the lens (Fig. 2.3; see also in color section). In patients with large astigmatic errors, shadows in the red reflection may appear as a scissors opening and closing as you sweep the light across the pupil.

Fig. 2.2 The normal reflection in a black patient is deeper red (a, left). In poorly pigmented eyes, as in patients with albinism or high myopia, the reflection may be very light (b, right). Also shown in color section.

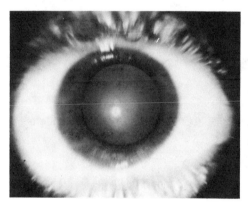 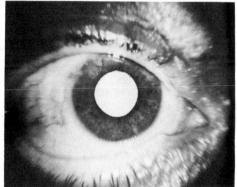

Fig. 2.3 In this patient with a subluxated lens, the light is returning through the lens in the upper part of the pupil and beneath the lens in the lower part. This shows how the focus of light alters the red reflection. Also shown in color section.

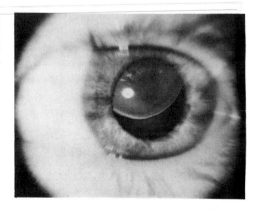

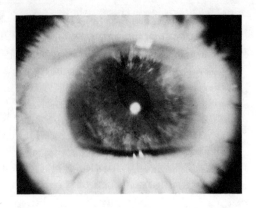

Fig. 2.4 Eccentrically placed pupil. This condition is due to developmental variation, but more often to disease.

The field stop, or margins of the red reflection, are the pupillary borders. The pupil may be eccentrically placed (Fig. 2.4). If the iris is missing, the field stop becomes the scleral ring or the ciliary body.

II. INTERRUPTION OF THE RED REFLECTION AT THE CORNEA

(Figs. 2.5 - 2.18; see 2.15 also in color section)

The cornea is the first ocular tissue to affect light entering the eye. This air-to-tissue passage of light accounts for 50 of the approximately 65 diopters refracting (light-bending) power of the eye. Slight alterations of the corneal surface have a marked visual significance for the patient.

Ophthalmoscopic findings

o   Light transmission by the cornea may be dull or absent, depending on the size and number of defects. Small and scattered opacities allow some light to pass.

o   Superficial opacities due to mucous, epithelial filaments, or particles in the tear film move with blinking.

o   Fluid-filled spaces (blebs) in the cornea have a water-drop lens appearance.

o   Fine deposits on the back of the cornea (endothelium) occur in inflammatory disease, after trauma, in specific corneal diseases, and associated with glaucoma, as in Krukenberg's spindle.

Fig. 2.5 Cloudy lower cornea with irregularity of the iris and anterior capsular cataract due to corneal infection.

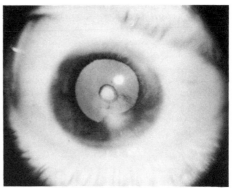

Fig. 2.6 Corneal blood vessels with hemorrhage in a 65-year-old white male who wore a poorly fitting soft contact lens for six months without removal. Courtesy of Leslie Woodcock, M.D., Syracuse, New York.

Fig. 2.7 Fatty corneal degeneration of unknown cause.

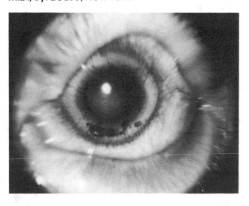

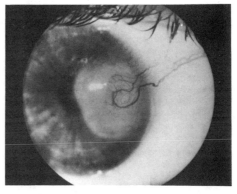

Fig. 2.8 Corneal laceration in an infant that healed spontaneously, leaving a vertical scar (below light reflection). The mother thought the child had "pink eye."

Fig. 2.9 Fine corneal epithelial filaments in a patient with a dry eye from overwearing contact lens. Note blood vessels entering the corneal periphery (arrow).

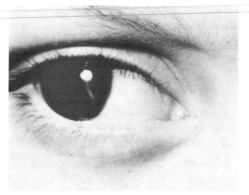

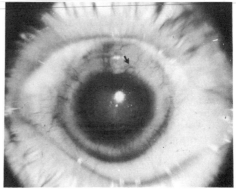

Fig. 2.10 Hereditary corneal dystrophy in a 74-year-old female.

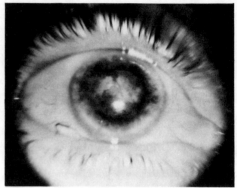

Fig. 2.11 Copper deposited in the peripheral cornea in a patient with hepatolenticular degeneration (Wilson's disease). Similar deposits are seen in the lens. From Donaldson D: Kayser-Fleischer ring in hepatolenticular degeneration (Wilson's disease). **Arch Ophthalmol** 72:116, 1964, Copyright © 1964, American Medical Association. Used with permission.

Fig. 2.12 Watery filtering bleb created surgically for glaucoma control hangs over the upper cornea.

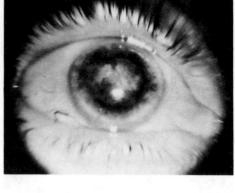

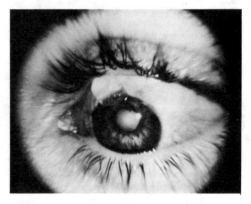

Symptoms and signs

o Opacities of the central cornea affect vision according to degree of light transmission, reflection, or scattering.

o Pain is common in infection, trauma, or bullous edema of the cornea.

Other confirmed findings

o History of hereditary ocular disease, trauma, infection, surgery, and drug exposure need to be reviewed. A partial list of diseases and treatments associated with corneal opacities is given in Table 2.1.

o Physical examinations of eye, including biomicroscopy.

Table 2.1

SYSTEMIC DISEASES AND TREATMENTS
ASSOCIATED WITH CORNEAL OPACITIES, PARTIAL LIST

Deposits

Cystinosis
Fabry's disease
Gout
Hurler's disease and other mucopolysaccharidoses
Juvenile rheumatoid arthritis (band keratopathy)
Multiple myeloma
Uremia

Increased visibility of corneal nerves

Hyperparathyroidism
Ichthyosis
Indomethacin, chloroquine, thioridazine
Leprosy
Neurofibromatosis
Pemphigus
Refsum's disease

Pigmentation

Bismuth
Chlorpromazine
Copper (Wilson's disease; Kayser-Fleischer ring)
Gold
Iron
Silver

Infectious and inflammatory disease

Bacterial, viral, and fungal infections
Herpes simplex
Herpes zoster
Rosacea
Sarcoidosis
Syphilis (interstitial keratitis)
Tuberculosis
Vaccinia

Fig. 2.13 Membrane and blood vessels (epithelial downgrowth) on the inside of the cornea (arrow) following glaucoma surgery. Note the cataract.

Fig. 2.14 Foreign body on cornea.

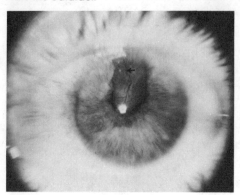

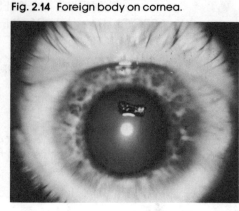

Fig. 2.15 Fluorescein-stained corneal abrasion from permanent-wave solution and rubbing. Also shown in color section.

Fig. 2.16 Herpetic corneal ulcers have a characteristic dendritic appearance. Courtesy of Paul Torrisi, M.D., Syracuse, New York.

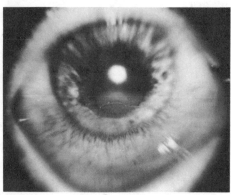

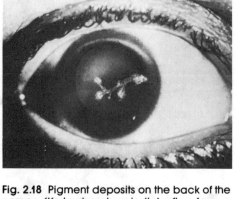

Fig. 2.17 Band keratopathy in a nine-year-old rheumatoid arthritis patient. Note the iris synechiae to the lens from anterior uveitis.

Fig. 2.18 Pigment deposits on the back of the cornea (Krukenberg's spindle) often form a vertical line in patients disposed to pigmentary glaucoma.

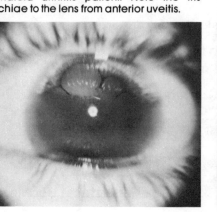

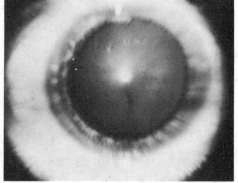

o   General medical evaluation for related diseases.

o   Laboratory, radiologic, and other studies as indicated.

Main differential diagnosis

o   Trauma

o   Infection or inflammation

o   Dystrophy

o   Deposits from disease or treatment

References

Abrahamson IA: Color Atlas of Anterior Segment Eye Diseases. Oradell, NJ: Medical Economics, 1974.

Berliner ML: Biomicroscopy of the Eye. New York: Hoeber, 1949.

Duke-Elder S, Jay B: System of Ophthalmology, vol 8. St. Louis: Mosby, 1969.

Grant WM: Toxicology of the Eye. Springfield, Ill: Thomas, 1974.

King JH Jr, McTigue JW: The Cornea. Washington: Butterworths, 1965.

Waring GO 3rd, Rodrigues MM, Laibson PR: Corneal dystrophies: 1. Dystrophies of the epithelium, Bowman's layer and stroma. Surv Ophthalmol 23:71, 1978.

III. ANTERIOR CHAMBER INTERRUPTION OF THE RED REFLECTION
(Figs. 2.19-2.26; see 2.19-2.21 also in color section)

Disease or foreign materials may cloud the otherwise normally clear aqueous of the anterior chamber.

Ophthalmoscopic findings

o   Blood, fibrin, and protein dull the red reflection in the anterior chamber. This is particularly apparent in comparison with the normal other eye.

o   Foreign bodies in the anterior chamber may be of many sizes and forms. These include such materials as tumor particles and white blood cells accumulated in the presence of infection. All obscure the red reflection.

Symptoms & signs

o   Loss of vision if the pupil aperture is obscured or if internal ocular injury occurred.

o   Pain if corneal injury or iritis is present.

Fig. 2.19 Round blood clot (arrows) in the anterior chamber has the appearance of a red reflection at first glance, but the red reflection was completely obscured. The patient sustained a blunt injury. The source of the hemorrhage at the periphery of the iris could be seen. Also shown in color section.

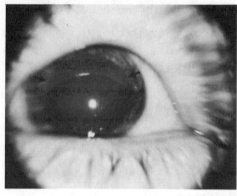

Fig. 2.20 Hemorrhage in the anterior chamber from diabetic neovascularization of the iris. Note the flat fluid level that the unclotted blood forms in the lower anterior chamber. Also shown in color section.

Fig. 2.21 Hypopyon (pus cells) in the anterior chamber due to infection after cataract surgery. The cloudy aqueous and swollen cornea obscure the red reflection. Also shown in color section.

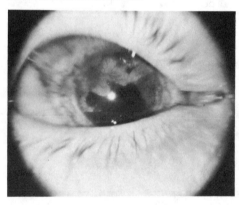

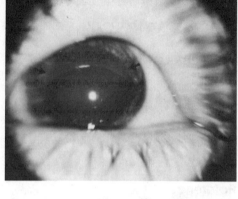

Fig. 2.22 Lens nucleus floating freely in the eye after unsuccessful cataract surgery. It came through the pupil into the anterior chamber.

Fig. 2.23 Hypermature cataract spontaneously ruptured, spilling the calcified nucleus of the lens into the anterior chamber. Glaucoma resulted and destroyed vision.

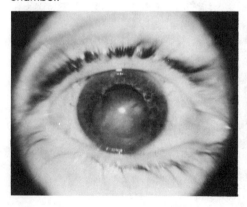

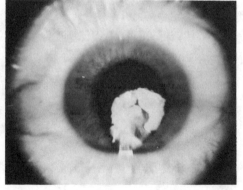

Fig. 2.24 Ointment placed in an eye following cataract surgery found its way into the anterior chamber (arrow). Note the irregular, updrawn pupil.

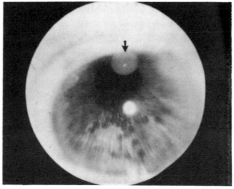

Fig. 2.25 Cysts in the anterior chamber of a patient with a ciliary body tumor (diktyoma). Courtesy of Torrence Makley, M.D., Ohio State University.

Fig. 2.26 Artificial lens in the pupil to optically correct the eye after removal of a cataract. The red reflection is dull because of a retinal detachment. Note the two surgically created peripheral iridectomies that are present in the upper iris.

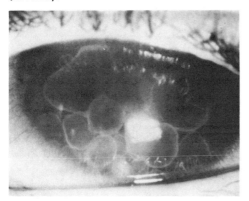

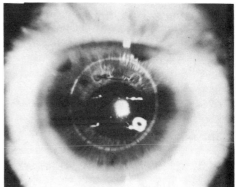

Other confirming findings

o   History of ocular disease, trauma, or systemic disease with metastatic tendencies.

o   Physical examination for evidence of generalized disease and eye examination to include slit lamp biomicroscopy.

o   Cultures, radiologic study, biopsies, laboratory testing where appropriate.

Main differential diagnosis

o   Trauma

o   Infection

o   Cataract complications

o   Inflammatory disease unrelated to infection or trauma

References

Duke-Elder S, Ashton N, Smith RJH, et al: Systems of Ophthalmology, vol 7. St. Louis: Mosby, 1963.

IV. THE RED REFLECTION AND IRIS ABNORMALITIES
(Figs. 2.27 - 2.36)

As the field stop for light reflected from the interior of the eye, iris abnormalities alter the red reflection by their contour and light transmission.

A. MISSING IRIS

Ophthalmoscopic findings

o   Reflected light comes back to the observer through defects in the iris.

o   The defects may be single or multiple, large or tiny. Some are surgically created (see Fig. 2.24).

o   Near total absence of the iris (aniridia) is occasionally seen at birth.

Symptoms & signs

o   Children born with aniridia and patients with large iris defects or poorly pigmented irides are often photophobic.

o   Visual acuity is usually normal, unless other pathology is present.

Other confirming findings

o   History of ocular disease, trauma, or surgery is usually available. Essential iris atrophy is more common in women.

o   Biomicroscopic, gonioscopic, ophthalmoscopic, and radiologic findings help confirm the reasons for iris absence or the presence of an intraocular foreign body.

o   Aniridia, an autosomal, dominantly inherited condition, is sometimes associated with Wilms's tumor, which may be inherited as an autosomal recessive disease. Poor vision due to foveal hypoplasia, nystagmus, cataract, and glaucoma are common in aniridia.

o   Pediatric evaluation with appropriate laboratory and radiologic studies is indicated.

Fig. 2.27 Congenital coloboma of the iris due to incomplete closure of the fetal fissure. The lens, choroid, and retina also have a coloboma. The patient has a cataract.

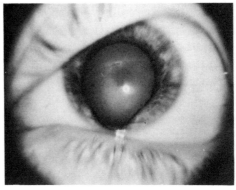

Fig. 2.28 A large part of the upper iris had to be removed surgically because it prolapsed when the eye was lacerated.

Fig. 2.29 A tiny red reflection (arrow) through the iris gave a clue to the presence of a metallic chip in the vitreous. The patient had been pounding with a hammer, felt something hit his eye, but was asymptomatic within a few hours.

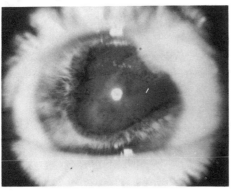

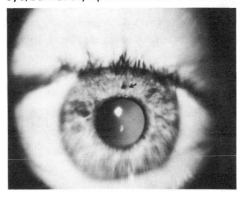

Fig. 2.31 Red reflection through the poorly pigmented peripheral iris of a patient with Waardenburg's syndrome. From Bard LA: Heterogeneity in Waardenburg's syndrome. **Arch Ophthalmol** 96:1193, 1978. Copyright © 1978, American Medical Association. Used with permission.

Fig. 2.30 Disinsertion of the iris periphery by a severe contusion. Note the flattening, or "squaring off," of the normally round pupil.

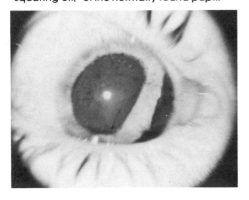

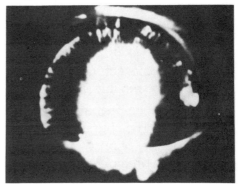

o   Electroretinography is helpful in foveal hypoplasia and metallic foreign-body evaluation.

o   Radiology and ultrasonography may aid foreign-body localization.

Main differential diagnosis

o   Congenital abnormalities of iris

o   Trauma

o   Surgical iris removal

o   Anterior uveitis

References

Abrahamson IA: Color Atlas of Anterior Segment Eye Diseases. Oradell, NJ: Medical Economics, 1974.

Freeman HM, ed: Ocular Trauma. New York: Appleton-Century-Crofts, 1979.

Havener WH, Gloeckner SL: Atlas of Diagnostic Techniques and Treatment of Intraocular Foreign Bodies. St. Louis: Mosby, 1969.

Miller RW, Fraumeni JF, Manning MD: Association of Wilms's tumor with aniridia, hemi-hypertrophy, and other congenital malformations. N Engl J Med 270:922, 1964.

B. PUPIL MARGIN ABNORMALITIES

Ophthalmoscopic findings

o   Pupil margin is an important indicator of disease. It should be observed for peaking or distortion, flattening (Fig. 2.33), accentuation of the pigmented iris frill, eccentricity, and vascular tufts.

o   Forward position of the iris may cause shallowing of the anterior chamber.

Symptoms & signs

o   Visual acuity may be affected if iris abnormalities prevent light from entering the eye.

o   Photophobia, aching pain, and redness are common in inflammatory, traumatic, and infectious diseases involving the iris.

o   Acute glaucoma may be very painful or associated with multiple mild episodes. The characteristic symptoms are aching pain in or around the eye, steamy or misty vision, and nausea with severe pain. Sitting in the dark may precipitate an attack. As the pupil constricts in sleep, an attack may cease.

Fig. 2.32 Slight peaking of the pupil toward 12 o'clock, the gray discoloration of the lens, and a shallow anterior chamber suggested the patient's complaints of intermittent eye pain were due to acute glaucoma attacks.

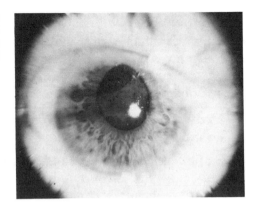

Fig. 2.33 This iris cyst was only suggested by a slight flattening of the pupil margin when the pupil was undilated.

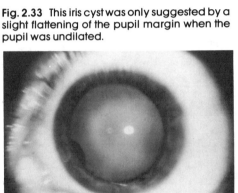

Fig. 2.34 These iris cysts could be seen only by examining the red reflection at an angle.

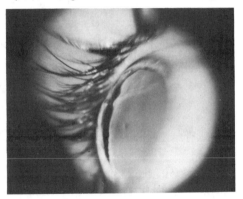

Fig. 2.35 Neovascularization of the iris (arrow) has distorted the pupil margin in this 35-year-old diabetic patient with hemorrhagic glaucoma.

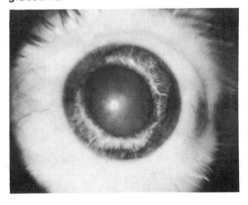

Fig. 2.36 Ectropion uveae. The pigmented back of the iris has been pulled around onto the front surface by inflammation.

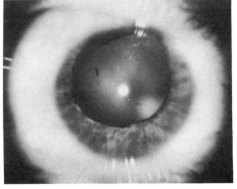

o   Many glaucoma patients have a constricted field.

o   Patients with myotonic dystrophy may have vascular tufts of pupil margin.

Other confirming findings

o   History of ocular or systemic disease should include symptoms related to poor blood supply to the head, as with carotid stenosis.

o   Pediatric or medical evaluation with appropriate laboratory, radiologic, and other studies to evaluate the patient for such conditions as metastatic tumor, inflammatory disease, diabetes mellitus, cardiovascular disease, myotonic dystrophy.

o   Biomicroscopic, gonioscopic, and indirect ophthalmoscopic examination.

o   Tonometry and visual field examination.

o   Fluorescein angiography for tumors and vascular tufts.

Main differential diagnosis

o   Acute or subacute glaucoma

o   Anterior synechiae due to iris inflammatory disease (anterior uveitis)

o   Primary or metastatic iris tumor

o   Benign iris cysts

o   Ciliary body tumor

o   Rubeosis iridis (multiple causes)

o   Nevoxanthoendothelioma

References

Cobb B, Shilling JS, Chisholm IH: Vascular tufts at the pupillary margin in myotonic dystrophy. Am J Ophthalmol 69:573, 1970.

Ferry AP, Font RL: Carcinoma metastatic to the eye and orbit: 1. A clinicopathologic study of 227 cases. Arch Ophthalmol 92:276, 1974.

Kolker AE, Hetherington J: Becker-Shaffer's Diagnosis and Therapy of the Glaucomas. St. Louis: Mosby, 1970.

Rodrigues M, Shields JA: Iris metastasis from a bronchial carcinoid tumor. Arch Ophthalmol 96:77, 1978.

Schulze RR: Rubeosis iridis. Am J Ophthalmol 63:487, 1967.

C. IRIS COLOR (see Chapter 6: II)

V. THE RED REFLECTION AND THE CILIARY BODY
(Figs. 2.37 - 2.40; see 2.37b also in color section)

Hidden by the iris, abnormalities in the ciliary body are difficult to see until they displace adjacent structures. It takes a high level of suspicion to detect them early.

Ophthalmoscopic findings

o   Interruption of the red reflection originates behind the iris.

o   Margins of the interruption may be smooth, multilobular, or serrated.

o   Lens opacification or iris distortion are often associated and, when they occur, are localized to the area of the ciliary body affected.

Symptoms & signs

o   Visual acuity is affected only if the visual pathway, the central pupil, is covered, the lens is cataractous or subluxated, or the retina has been elevated by posterior extension of the disease.

o   Painful or nonpainful glaucoma usually means the ciliary body disease has blocked aqueous movement through the pupil or damaged more than two-thirds of the trabecular meshwork at the iris root.

Other confirming findings

o   History of trauma, ocular surgery, and system review essential.

o   Physical examination, with emphasis on neoplastic disease.

Fig. 2.37 Melanoma of the ciliary body (arrow) is seen at the iris periphery (a, left). Note the slight flattening of the pupil margin in that quadrant. When the pupil was dilated, the true size of the tumor was revealed (b, right). Fig. 2.37b also shown in color section.

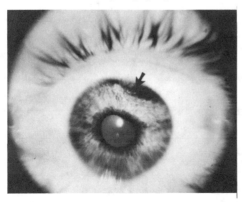 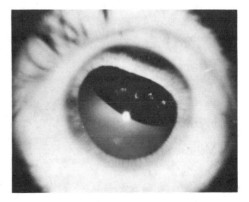

Fig. 2.38 Melanoma of the ciliary body has flattened the pupil margins and caused a localized cataract (arrow).

Fig. 2.39 Hemorrhage from the ciliary body streams from the impact site behind the iris and over the back of the lens.

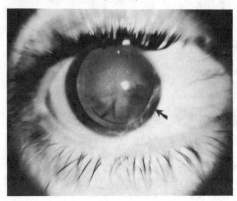 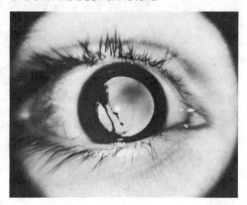

Fig. 2.40 Undetected scleral rupture at the ciliary body, caused by a Frisbee, led to the growth of a fibrovascular sheet of tissue over the back of the lens (a, left). Because the tissue reflects light, it appears white. The fine blood vessels are confirmed by fluorescein angiogram (b, right).

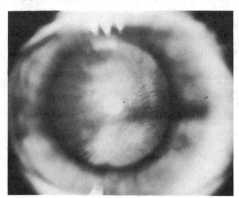 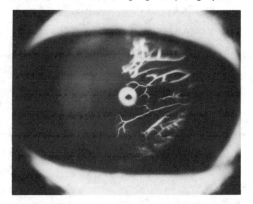

o   Indirect ophthalmoscopy, biomicroscopy, gonioscopy define ocular disease.

o   Fluorescein angiography.

o   Ultrasonography.

o   Computerized axial tomography.

Main differential diagnosis

o   Melanoma, medulloepithelioma, and other malignant primary tumors of the ciliary body

o   Benign ciliary body cyst (epitheliomas)

o   Metastatic tumor

o   Trauma

o   Persistent hyperplastic primary vitreous

o   Retrolental fibroplasia

References

Duke-Elder S, Jay B: System of Ophthalmology, vol 9. St. Louis: Mosby, 1969.

Freeman HM: Ocular Trauma. New York: Appleton-Century-Crofts, 1979, p 141.

Reese AB: Tumors of the Eye. Hagerstown, Md: Harper & Row, 1976.

VI. THE RED REFLECTION AND THE LENS

This section concentrates on specific types of light interruptions by the lens. The ophthalmoscope is helpful, but inferior to the slit lamp biomicroscope in the diagnosis of lens disease.

A. CATARACT (Figs. 2.41 - 2.52)

Any opacity of the crystalline lens or its capsule is called a cataract. The lens gains new layers throughout life. The layers of some opacities roughly date the onset of a cataract.

Ophthalmoscopic findings

o   The opacities may be small or involve the whole lens.

o   They may be localized to a small part of the lens or involve multiple sites within the lens.

o   You may be able to look around the opacity if it is small. The view is often better with the pupil dilated, especially in central opacities.

o   Small opacities sometimes can be localized by observing their position relative to light reflections from the front and back of the lens.

o   The cataract may discolor the appearance of the interior of the eye, depending on the wavelength of light admitted. Red discoloration is common with nuclear sclerosis (see Fig. 2.48a in color section).

Symptoms & signs

o   Visual acuity varies with reflection and scattering of entering light.

o   Central lens opacities interfere with vision more than peripheral ones, especially as the pupil constricts in bright light or with accommodation.

Fig. 2.42 Congenital cataract with three components: a small, white, anterior capsule opacity, embryonal nucleus abnormality, and riders that arch around the equator of the lens. Visual acuity unobtainable because the patient is mentally retarded.

Fig. 2.41 Embryonal nuclear cataract of a patient whose mother had rubella late in gestation.

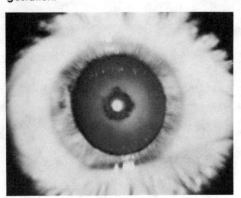

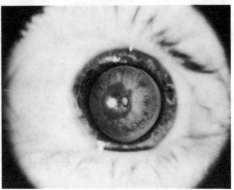

Fig. 2.43 Anterior subcapsular cataract. Similar cataracts may be seen in children with galactosemia.

Fig. 2.44 Beginning posterior subcapsular cataract in a 22-year-old male on prolonged oral steroids for juvenile rheumatoid arthritis. Visual acuity was 6/7.5 (20/25).

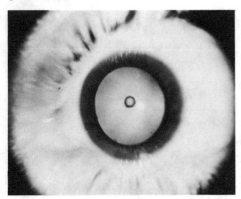

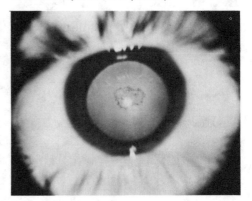

Only a small clear central area is required for good vision when ocular tissues and central nervous system functions are normal.

o Reduction of entering light by a cataract causes complaints of dimness and of poor vision at dusk. Night vision is impaired. In bright light, reflection and scattering of light by the cataract dazzle the patient. The patient with nuclear cataracts may say vision is best when the days are not too bright or too dark. Patients with posterior subcapsular cataracts have particular difficulty with reading.

o A white-out of vision after exposure to bright outdoor light may last hours to days.

- Patient may be unable to perceive colors whose wavelengths are reflected by the cataract.
- Some opacities split the pupil and give monocular double or triple vision.
- Cataracts often cause false scotomata on field testing.

Other confirming findings

- Cataracts are associated with many diseases, conditions, and treatments. Table 2.2 is a partial list.
- Slit lamp biomicroscopy aids definition of cataract type.
- Ultrasonography helps determine calcification and rupture of lens.
- Appropriate laboratory, radiologic, and other studies are necessary for determination of related systemic disease.

Fig. 2.45 Rapidly developing cataract in a 21-year-old diabetic patient. Visual acuity was 6/18 (20/60).

Fig. 2.46 Cortical spoke cataract. Visual acuity was 6/6 (20/20). Compare with the riders in congenital cataract in Fig. 2.42.

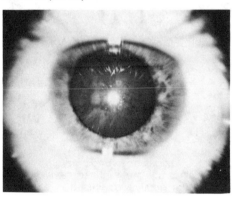

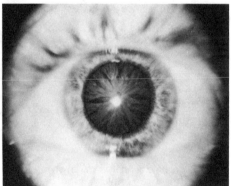

Fig. 2.47 Nuclear sclerosis and posterior sub-capsular cataract in an adult. A family history of adult-onset cataracts was present. Note the cortical spokes in the common inferior location. Visual acuity was 6/60 (20/200).

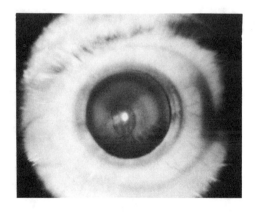

Fig. 2.48 Nuclear sclerosis gives a ruby red color to the fundus (a, left). The other eye had less nuclear sclerosis (b, right). Compare these photographs with Figs. 7.10, 7.30. Fig. 2.48a also shown in color section.

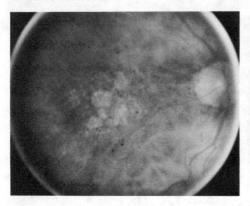
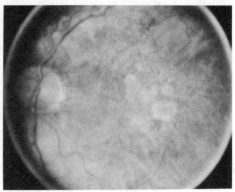

Fig. 2.49 Advanced nuclear, posterior subcapsular, and cortical spoke cataract in an adult. Visual acuity was limited to counting fingers.

Fig. 2.50 Mature cataract involving the whole lens in an adult with a family history of the disease. Visual acuity was limited to seeing hand motion.

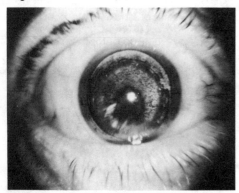
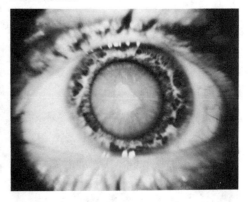

Fig. 2.51 Traumatic cataract, involving glass, localized to the site of injury. Visual acuity was 6/18 (20/60).

Fig. 2.52 Partially absorbed cataract after an injury with a nail that ruptured the lens capsule. Visual acuity was limited to counting fingers at 1 meter.

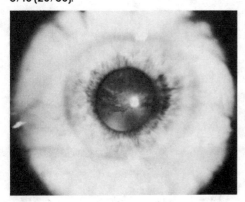
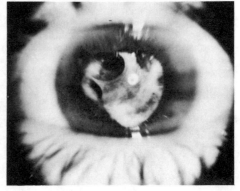

Table 2.2

DISEASES, TREATMENTS, AND CONDITIONS
ASSOCIATED WITH CATARACT, PARTIAL LIST

Anorexia nervosa	Mucopolysaccharidoses
Atopic dermatitis	Myotonic dystrophy
Carotid stenosis	Ocular neoplasms
Congenital ichthyosis	Osteitis deformans
Congenital syphilis	Parasitic infection
Craniofacial dysostosis	Phospholine iodide
Diabetes mellitus	Pulseless disease
Dinitrophenol	Retinal detachment
Direct trauma	Retinitis pigmentosa
Electric shock	Rubella
Endophthalmitis	Senility
Fabry's disease	Steroid treatment
Galactosemia	Toxoplasmosis
Glaucoma	Turner's syndrome
Heredity	Uveitis
Hypercholesterolemia	Wagner's vitreoretinal degeneration
Hypothyroidism	Werner's syndrome
Incontinentia pigmenti	Wilson's disease

Main differential diagnosis

o Persistent posterior hyperplastic primary vitreous

o Retrolental fibroplasia

o Retinoblastoma

o Coats's disease

o Retinal detachment

o Intravitreal hemorrhage (all causes)

References

Bellows JG: Cataract and Abnormalities of the Lens. New York: Grune & Stratton, 1975.

Duke-Elder S, Jay B: System of Ophthalmology, vol 11. St. Louis: Mosby, 1969, p 63.

Francois J: Congenital Cataracts. Springfield, Ill: Thomas, 1963.

Grant WM: Toxicology of the Eye. Springfield, Ill: Thomas, 1974.

Harley RD, ed: Pediatric Ophthalmology. Philadelphia: Saunders, 1975.

B. DEPOSITS ON THE LENS (Figs. 2.53 - 2.57)

Fine particles deposited on the lens are seen with difficulty with the ophthal-moscope, but larger particles are easily visible against the red reflection.

Ophthalmoscopic findings

o   Pigment on the anterior lens capsule may be present congenitally in the form of fine star-shaped deposits or iridocapsular lines. When the pupil is dilated, inflammatory iris adhesions to the lens may break, resulting in a partial or complete circle of pigment. A severe contusion may cause a similar pigment (Vossius' ring) on the lens capsule. Pigment similar to deposits on the corneal endothelium (Krukenberg's spindle) may also be seen on the equator of the lens. The equator of the lens has to be viewed with a dilated pupil (Fig. 2.55).

o   Blood and hemosiderin on or in the lens appear black in the red reflection.

o   Foreign bodies may lodge in the lens, and copper is deposited in hepatolenticular degeneration in a typical sunflower cataract.

o   Pseudoexfoliation deposits on the lens occur mostly in the pupil. With the pupil dilated, these deposits may be seen as a fine ragged circle against the red reflection.

o   Endophthalmitis or severe noninfectious inflammatory disease may lead to purulent material on the lens.

Symptoms & signs

o   Visual acuity will be reduced if light cannot enter or is diffused as it enters the lens. Small pigment or other deposits rarely affect vision.

o   The patient may describe streaks made by light, photophobia, or dimness of lights.

o   Monocular diplopia or triplopia is unlikely. Usually, the patient also has a cataract.

o   Color perception may be faulty.

Other confirming findings

o   A review of systems and family history is necessary, including specific ocular trauma, surgery, and vascular and liver disease.

o   Slit lamp biomicroscopy is essential.

o   Laboratory, radiologic, radionuclear, and specialty consultation will be indicated by the history and physical examination.

Fig. 2.53 Fine congenital deposits on the anterior lens capsule often appear as a cluster of pigmented stars (arrow). They are a normal variant.

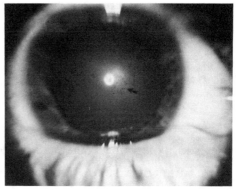

Fig. 2.54 Pigment on the anterior capsule from iris adhesions in a 56-year-old female with necrotizing angiitis. Hemosiderin has stained the posterior lens capsule and the vitreous a dull orange (ochre) color.

Fig. 2.55 Pigment deposit on the equator of the lens in a patient with pigmentary glaucoma and retinal detachment.

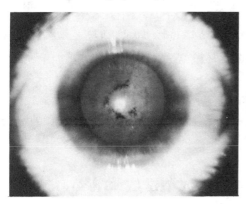

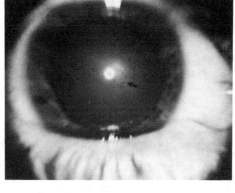

Fig. 2.56 Foreign body can be seen in the lens just below and to the left of the circular light reflection. Courtesy of William Havener, M.D., Ohio State University.

Fig. 2.57 Pseudoexfoliation seen against the red reflection. Fine, fluffy deposits can be seen on the lens and in the iris angle.

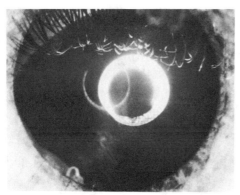

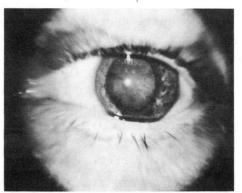

o   Patients who have or will later develop chronic glaucoma and some who are predisposed to retinal detachment may have pigment deposits on the lens.

Main differential diagnosis

o   Trauma, including intraocular foreign bodies

o   Anterior uveitis (iritis) from multiple causes

o   Pseudoexfoliation of lens and glaucoma

o   Pigment deposition, glaucoma, and vitreoretinal degeneration

o   Hepatolenticular degeneration (Wilson's disease)

o   Hemosiderosis and hemorrhage

References

Delaney, WV Jr: Equatorial lens pigmentation, myopia, and retinal detachment. Am J Ophthalmol 79:194, 1975.

Freeman HM, ed: Ocular Trauma. New York: Appleton-Century-Crofts, 1979.

Havener WH, Gloeckner SL: Atlas of Diagnostic Techniques and Treatment of Intraocular Foreign Bodies. St. Louis: Mosby, 1969.

Kolker AE, Hetherington J: Becker-Shaffer's Diagnosis and Therapy of the Glaucomas. St. Louis: Mosby, 1970.

Mitchell AM, Heller GL: Changes in Kayser-Fleischer ring during treatment of hepato-lenticular degeneration. Arch Ophthalmol 80:622, 1968.

C. SUBLUXATION AND DISLOCATION OF THE LENS (see Fig. 2.3)

Partial displacement of the lens from its proper location is termed subluxation. Dislocation refers to total displacement.

Ophthalmoscopic findings

o   The lens equator appears in the red reflection as a curvilinear border across the pupil. If the lens is cataractous, the red reflection is dulled or absent through the lens but visible around its margin. Artificially implanted lenses out of position have a similar effect on the red reflection. The splitting of the red reflection by the equator of the subluxated lens varies with the direction of displacement. The lens subluxates in a characteristic direction in some diseases.

o   To view the disc and retina, you need different lens powers in the ophthalmoscope for looking through and looking around the subluxated lens. The latter requires relatively more plus lens power. The view through the aphakic part of the pupil is usually better because of astigmatism induced by the tilted lens.

o With dislocation of the lens you need a plus lens for a clear view of the disc, except in very myopic patients. The lens may lie on the retina and may float in and out of view when the patient changes position.

o With subluxation or dislocation of the lens, the iris will wobble with eye or head movements (iridodonesis). This can be observed with the ophthalmoscope used as a flashlight or in focus with a high plus lens. Loss of pigment, which allows transillumination, may be the earliest sign of Marfan's syndrome in children. It may precede lens subluxation.

o Nontraumatic lens subluxations or dislocations are nearly always bilateral, but not always equal in degree.

Symptoms & signs

o The astigmatism in a clear lens brought on by subluxation reduces visual acuity — 6/12 (20/40) to 6/120 (20/400) or less. Some correction with glasses may be possible. Visual acuity through the aphakic part of the pupil is poor but correctable with glasses, if the remainder of the visual system is intact. Dislocated lenses may float over the macula and temporarily reduce vision when the patient changes position.

o Displacement of the lens partially or completely through the pupil into the anterior chamber may cause acute painful glaucoma. Traumatic lens displacement indicates severe ocular injury. Other injuries, such as angle recession, retinal disinsertion, choroidal rupture, and blow-out orbital fracture may coexist.

o Photophobia, ciliary flush, and other evidence of iritis may accompany lens displacement.

o Marfan's syndrome patients are predisposed to retinal detachment.

Other confirming findings

o History of ocular trauma, surgery, or infection related to lens displacement can be confirmed by indirect ophthalmoscopy, biomicroscopy, and ultrasonography.

o Diseases associated with spontaneous lens subluxation or displacement are outlined in Table 2.3.

o Hyperlysinemia, porphyria, and urinary excretion of S-sulfo-L-cysteine, sulfite, and thiosulfite have also been reported with ectopia lentis.

Table 2.3

DISEASES ASSOCIATED WITH
SPONTANEOUS LENS SUBLUXATION OR DISPLACEMENT

Disease	Inheritance and age at onset	Skeletal	Ocular
Marfan's syndrome	Autosomal dominant with high penetrance Onset at birth	Tall, long arms, legs, toes, and fingers Pigeon breast or funnel breast Kyphoscoliosis High palate	Ectopia lentis (usually superior), bilateral in most patients, occurs in 70% of Marfan's syndrome patients; 70% of congenital ectopia lentis patients have Marfan's syndrome Acute glaucoma Myopia Blue sclera Retinal detachment Cloudy cornea Microphakia Heterochromia iridis
Homocystinuria	Autosomal recessive Onset at birth	Hyperreflexia Kyphoscoliosis Pigeon breast Genu valgum Loose joints Tall patients Crowding of teeth	Ectopia lentis (usually inferior), may be progressive Myopia Optic atrophy Zonular cataract Acute glaucoma Retinal detachment
Weill-Marchesani syndrome (hereditary spherophakia)	Autosomal dominant with low penetrance Possible consanguinity Onset at birth	Short stature Depressed nasal bridge Round head Short pudgy hands and feet	Ectopia lentis (usually inferior) Glaucoma Retinal detachment Optic atrophy
Ehlers-Danlos syndrome	Autosomal dominant with low penetrance Onset at birth	Hyperextensible joints Kyphoscoliosis Pseudotumors at pressure points Hip dislocation	Epicanthal folds Ectopia lentis (uncommon) Blue sclera Microcornea Glaucoma Myopia Retinal degeneration Retinal detachment
Hereditary microphakia	Autosomal dominant Onset in first decade	Normal height and stature	Ectopia lentis Retinal degeneration and retinal detachment

Table 2.3 (continued)

DISEASES ASSOCIATED WITH
SPONTANEOUS LENS SUBLUXATION OR DISPLACEMENT

Cardiovascular	Other signs	Diagnostic studies
Dilated pulmonary artery Dilated aorta Aortic regurgitation Dissection of aortic aneurysms Myxomatous aortic valve Mitral insufficiency Hypertension	Mental retardation rare	Skeletal findings by examination and radiology Cardiovascular study by electro- and echocardiography, etc. Slit lamp biomicroscopy and indirect ophthalmoscopy
Thrombosis of coronary, renal, cerebral, and other arteries Hypertension Gangrene	Mental retardation common Seizures Schizophrenia Hemiplegia Malar flush on exertion Blotchy red skin Failure to thrive as infants	Homocystine in urine distinguished from cystine by electrophoresis or chromatography
Patent ductus arteriosus	Possible mental retardation Cleft palate	Skeletal and ocular findings
Bundle branch block Dissection of aortic aneurysms	Dental abnormalities Elastic wrinkled skin Easy bleeding of skin	Blood coagulation studies (normal)
None known	Normal mentality	Aminoaciduria may be present

Main differential diagnosis

o Trauma, including ocular surgery and birth trauma

o Inflammatory disease

o Inborn errors of metabolism

o Hereditary sphero- or microphakia without apparent metabolic defect

o Aniridia with ectopia lentis

o Coloboma

References

Duke-Elder S, Jay B: System of Ophthalmology, vol 11. St. Louis: Mosby, 1969.

Geeraets WJ: Ocular Syndromes. Philadelphia: Lea & Febiger, 1976.

Laster L, Irreverre F, Mudd SH, et al: A previously unrecognized disorder of metabolism of sulfur-containing compounds — abnormal urinary excretion of S-sulfo-L-cysteine, sulfite, and thiosulfite in a severely retarded child with ectopia lentis. J Clin Invest 46:1082, 1967.

Maumenee IH: Vitreoretinal degeneration as a sign of generalized connective tissue diseases. Am J Ophthalmol 88:432, 1979.

McKusick VA: Heritable Disorders of Connective Tissue. St. Louis: Mosby, 1966.

Smith TH, Holand ME, Woody NC: Ocular manifestations of familial hyperlysinemia. Trans Am Acad Ophthalmol Otolaryngol 75:355, 1971.

VII. VITREOUS ALTERATIONS OF THE RED REFLECTION
(see Chapter 8)

VIII. RETINAL AND CHOROIDAL ALTERATIONS OF THE RED REFLECTION (Figs. 2.58 - 2.60; see 2.58b and 2.60 also in color section)

The light returning from the interior of the eye varies with the absorption and reflection by retina, retinal pigment epithelium, and choroid. It's necessary to inspect each quadrant.

Ophthalmoscopic findings

o Whitening of the red reflection is a nonspecific finding to be explained by detailed examination. Retinoblastoma, a life-threatening tumor of childhood, often is first discovered because of a "cat's eye reflection" (see Fig. 2.2b).

Fig. 2.58 Retinoblastoma in a two-and-one-half-year-old child is not seen in straight-ahead gaze (a, left), but is readily visible when he looks nasally (b, right). This may account for the parents' statement that the child's eyes looked abnormal only at certain times. Fig. 2.58b also shown in color section.

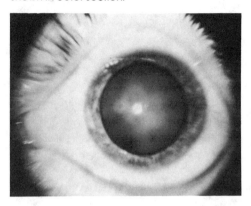 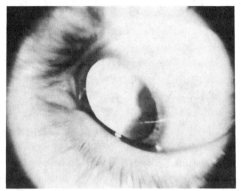

o Exposure of the sclera from the inside may also produce whitening of the reflection (see Fig. 1.10).

o Darkening of the reflection is also nonspecific and may indicate light absorption or internal reflection by an irregular surface as in choroidal melanoma, preventing the light returning to the observer (see Chapter 7: VIA).

Symptoms & signs

o No specific symptoms and signs can be attributed to an abnormal red reflection from the interior of the eye. Diagnosis is by further opthalmoscopy and study.

Other confirming findings

o Detailed systemic review is indicated. Special emphasis on the family history of tumors is important in children. Parents may overlook ocular trauma in their children.

o Indirect ophthalmoscopy and biomicroscopy, under anesthesia if necessary.

o Ultrasonography and computerized tomography.

o Fluorescein angiography.

o Other specific studies as suitable for each disease.

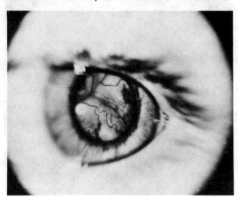

Fig. 2.59 Coats's disease causing the retina to detach and nearly reach the back of the lens.

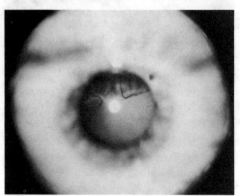

Fig. 2.60 Rhegmatogenous retinal detachment in a 61-year-old white male. He described floaters, flashes of light, and a shadow in his inferior field of vision. The superior retina hangs down almost to the mid-line. Also shown in color section.

Main differential diagnosis

o   Retinoblastoma

o   Melanoma of the choroid

o   Metastatic tumor of the choroid

o   Myopic degeneration

o   Coats's disease

o   Preretinal hemorrhage (multiple causes)

o   Cataract

o   Persistent hyperplastic primary vitreous

o   Retinal detachment

o   Coloboma of the choroid

References

Peyman GA, Sanders DR, Goldberg MF, eds: Principles and Practice of Ophthalmology. Philadelphia: Saunders, 1980.

Tasman W: Retinal Diseases in Children. New York: Harper & Row, 1971.

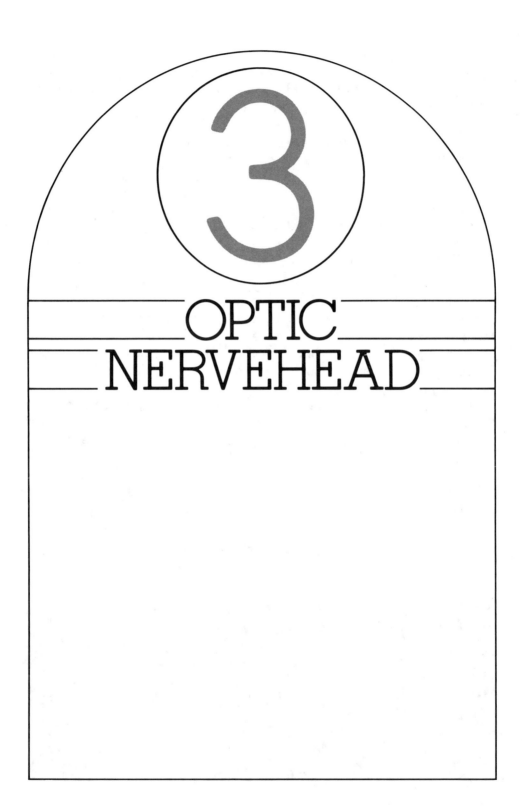

3

OPTIC
NERVEHEAD

The optic nervehead (Fig. 3.1), or disc, is the connection of the retina to the brain. Most of the nerve fibers are sensory fibers from the ganglion cells to the lateral geniculate body. Ophthalmoscopic observation shows the nerve fibers, their accompanying supportive glial elements, and vascular tissue of the optic nerve at its ocular end. The deeper layers of the disc include the lamina cribrosa — the opening in the sclera through which nerve fibers pass — and the margins of the retinal pigment epithelium and choroid where they part to allow the nerve fibers to exit through the lamina.

I. OPHTHALMOSCOPIC ANATOMY

A. MARGINS OF THE DISC

The many nerve fibers from the macular area (Fig. 3.2) take up nearly the whole temporal half of the disc, leaving only the superior, inferior, and nasal borders of the disc for the remaining nerve fibers from the whole interior of the eye. As a consequence, the nerve fibers pile up on the nasal side and frequently obscure that margin of the disc compared to the temporal border. Inexperienced observers commonly confuse this so-called blurring of the disc margin with papilledema.

The retinal pigment epithelium and the choroid stop at the disc margin. It's the absence of these two that gives the sharp contrast between the optic disc and the adjacent tissue. Occasionally, either naturally or as the result of disease, the cells at the disc margin may be hyperpigmented (Fig. 3.3; see also in color section).

The underlying choroid also stops at the optic nerve, although it sends small vessels to supply the optic nerve. In myopic patients, it's not unusual

Fig. 3.1 The optic nervehead consists of the retinal nerve fiber bundles at the opening in the sclera through which they pass.

Fig. 3.2 The fibers entering the optic nerve temporally all come from the macula. The remainder of the nerve fibers crowd into the nasal disc, obscuring the margin (arrow).

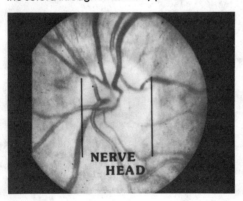

NERVE HEAD

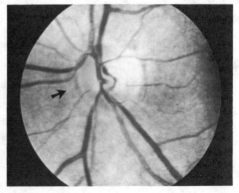

Fig. 3.3 Hyperpigmentation at the disc margin. Also shown in color section.

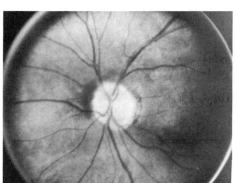

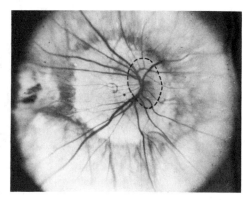

Fig. 3.5 Variations in shape of disc: Oval discs are often associated with astigmatism (a, left); triangular disc (b, right).

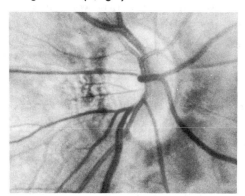

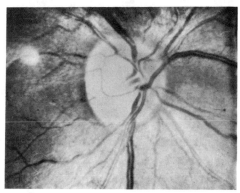

for the retinal pigment epithelium to stop some distance from the border of the optic disc, exposing the choroidal vessels to view (Fig. 3.4). If the choroidal vessels are sparse, the bare sclera is seen. Don't confuse this myopic crescent as part of the optic disc. There is considerable variation in the shape of the normal disc (Fig. 3.5).

B. SIZE

Whenever possible, you should compare the optic discs in the two eyes. Usually they are almost mirror images of each other, and differences give clues to disease. The normal disc is approximately 1½ mm in horizontal diameter. The farsighted patient usually has small optic discs, possibly as small as 1 mm in horizontal diameter. By contrast, the myopic patient may have a disc with a horizontal diameter of 2 mm. The patient's refractive error

OPTIC NERVEHEAD

may magnify or minify, accounting for some of the size difference. The disc is used as a measuring device (see Chapter 1: IIIM): It's used to estimate the size of a finding within the eye and, for easy relocation, its distance from the disc (see Fig. 1.36).

C. DISC COLOR, REFLECTIONS AROUND THE DISC, AND THE PHYSIOLOGIC DEPRESSION

Even the most experienced ophthalmoscopists find it difficult to assess disc color. The color of a disc is a factor of its blood supply (Fig. 3.6). Disc pallor may be due to poor blood supply or pale blood. Polycythemia has the opposite effect. It's important not to confuse the large physiologic depression visible in some patients (Fig. 3.7) with pallor of the optic nerve.

A thick, flat mirror-like nerve fiber layer around the disc margin causes light reflections. There is considerable variation in these reflections. In general, younger patients have more reflections than do older patients (Fig. 3.8). These reflections can be helpful in evaluating a patient who has questionable disc swelling. Swelling of the optic nerve and adjacent retina makes these reflections disappear, an important sign if the other eye is uninvolved and comparison is possible.

Fig. 3.6 The prelaminar arterial blood for the optic disc comes from the choroid and leaves by the central retinal vein. The circle of Zinn-Haller and the pial vessels are the supply posterior to the lamina.

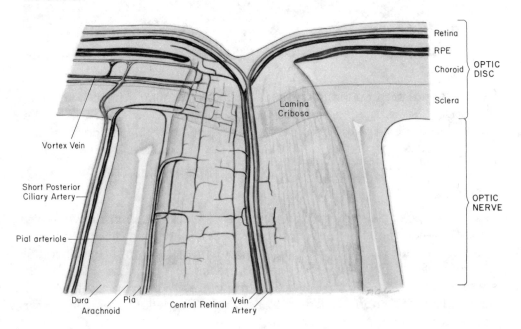

Fig. 3.7 The lamina cribrosa may be exposed normally at the bottom of the physiologic depression in the optic disc.

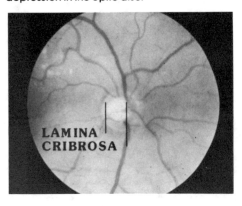

LAMINA
CRIBROSA

Fig. 3.8 Light reflections (Gunn's dots) around the disc are more visible in young patients.

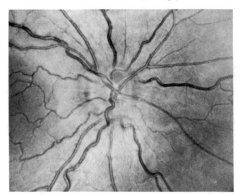

Fig. 3.9 Early branching gives the appearance of separate vessels (a, left). Late bifurcation requires they loop back down to the retinal plane (b, right).

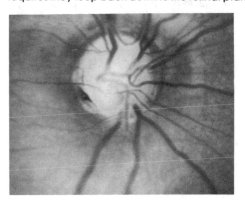
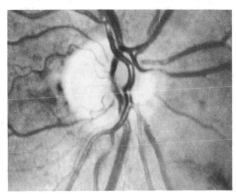

D. ARTERIES, VEINS, AND CAPILLARIES ON THE DISC

Central retinal vessels vary in branching and course on the disc. It's not uncommon for the central retinal artery or vein to divide deeply in the optic disc substance and appear as separate vessels (Fig. 3.9a). Occasionally, the opposite is true: Their branching occurs above the disc (Fig. 3.9b). Cilio-retinal vessels are common, entering the disc substance at its margin rather than centrally. They originate from the vascular plexus of Zinn-Haller around the optic nerve behind the globe (Fig. 3.10).

In some patients, the venous drainage of the retina crosses from the expected course to join the vein of another quadrant (Fig. 3.11). Most choroidal venous blood drains anteriorly to the vortex ampulae. In patients with thin retinal pigment epithelium, a large choroidal vascular ribbon may be

Fig. 3.10 Two cilioretinal arteries on the temporal disc (arrow, a, left) and a double one nasally (right side) from the circle of Zinn-Haller behind the globe (b, right). Most cilioretinal arteries are single and temporal.

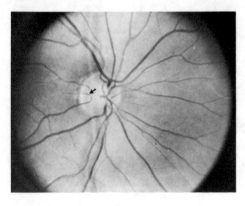

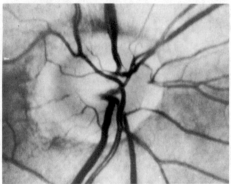

Fig. 3.11 Venous anomaly on the disc shunts blood from the inferior to the superior retinal veins (arrow).

Fig. 3.12 In a lightly pigmented patient, choroidal venous drainage to the circle of Zinn-Haller is readily visible (arrows).

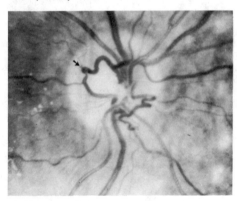

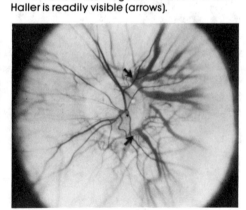

Fig. 3.13 Disc and macula of a right eye with situs inversus: The central retinal vessels pass through the temporal disc tissue. Nasal side of the disc is to the right.

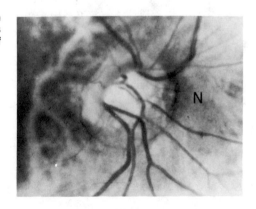

seen exiting from the globe at the disc margin (Fig. 3.12). The central retinal vessels usually pass through the nasal disc tissue. The reverse of this is called situs inversus (Fig. 3.13).

Intraocular pressure may at times, as in acute glaucoma, exceed pressure in the central retinal artery. But because corneal edema prevents a view and the eye rapidly adjusts to the pressure, pulsation of the central retinal artery usually ceases by the time the patient is seen. External pressure on the globe can collapse the central retinal artery. This maneuver is used in an estimation of ophthalmic artery pressure called ophthalmodynamometry. Comparison of the ophthalmic artery pressure in the two eyes is a useful test of carotid artery patency.

The entrance of arterial blood bolus into the closed globe is often sufficient to collapse the central retinal vein during systole. This has given rise to the inaccurate phrase "spontaneous venous pulsation." If there is no venous pulsation, you can provoke it by slight digital pressure on the globe. In the differential diagnosis of papilledema, the presence of spontaneous venous pulsation suggests other causes for a swollen disc (Fig. 3.14).

The smaller capillaries of the optic nerve substance and of the pre-papillary plexus are not visible. If the disc is swollen, however, dilation makes them distend to a visible size. Intravenous fluorescein enhances their visibility. Superficial hemorrhages from these blood vessels follow the nerve fiber layer and are linear or splinter-shaped (Fig. 3.15).

E. VITREOUS AND HYALOID ARTERY ADJACENT TO THE DISC

Remnants of the embryonic hyaloid artery system are sometimes visible over the central disc and vary from a fine glial remnant called Bergmeister's papilla (Fig. 3.16) to a complete hyaloid artery remnant extending forward

Fig. 3.14 Collapse of the blood column in the central retinal vein (arrows, a, left, and b, right) occurs with arterial pulsation in many normal eyes (so-called spontaneous venous pulsation).

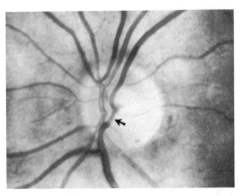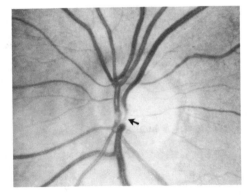

Fig. 3.15 Fluorescein angiogram of the pre-papillary capillaries that extend out from the disc. Subretinal hemorrhage around the disc and vasodilatation accentuate the vessels in a patient with Terson's syndrome.

Fig. 3.16 Bergmeister's papilla (arrow) is an embryonic remnant of the hyaloid artery system.

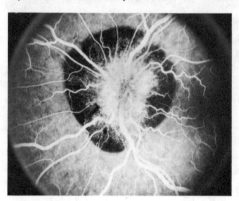

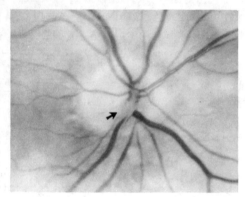

all the way to the lens (see Fig. 8.3). In most patients younger than 60, the vitreous is attached at the margins of the disc. In older patients, it's common for the vitreous to separate, completely or only partially, from the disc (see Fig. 8.7), leaving a faint ring in the vitreous that moves with the patient's eye movement.

II. THE MISSING OR INCOMPLETE DISC

An incomplete optic disc is the result of congenital or developmental abnormality. Trauma occasionally results in avulsion of the optic nerve. Be sure first to rule out hiding of the structurally complete disc by other tissues.

A. APLASIA (NONDEVELOPMENT) OF THE OPTIC NERVE
(Fig. 3.17)

Ophthalmoscopic findings

o Optic disc is missing; there is only a pit where disc should be.

o Retinal blood vessels are absent; choroid is present.

o You may see colobomas in the posterior and peripheral eye.

Symptoms & signs

o Poor fixation and/or exotropia from birth.

o No light perception.

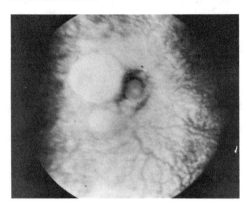

Fig. 3.17 Aplasia (nondevelopment) of the optic nerve. Note the absence of retinal blood vessels. Choroidal vessels are present. Courtesy of Paul Whitmore, M.D., Walter Reed Army Medical Center.

o Pupil larger on affected side; no response to light.

o Possible consensual response to light directed into normal eye, but not the reverse (Marcus Gunn's sign).

Other confirming findings

o Bilateral disease usually associated with severe central nervous system maldevelopment.

o Unilateral disease; other eye may be normal.

o Affected eye microphthalmic; axial length short on ultrasonography.

o Optic foramen small on radiologic study.

o Appearance elsewhere in family history.

Main differential diagnosis

o Hypoplasia of the optic nerve

o Avulsion of the optic nerve

References

Little LE, Whitmore PV, Wells TW Jr: Aplasia of the optic nerve. J Pediatr Ophthalmol 13:84, 1976.

Walsh FB, Hoyt WF: Clinical Neuro-Ophthalmology, vol 1. Baltimore: Williams & Wilkins, 1969, p 661.

Fig. 3.18 Optic nerve hypoplasia in the right eye (a, left). Left eye of the same patient is normal (b, right).

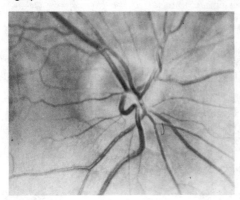 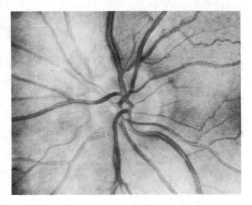

B. HYPOPLASIA (INCOMPLETE DEVELOPMENT) OF THE OPTIC NERVE (Fig. 3.18)

Ophthalmoscopic findings

o   Small disc, possibly one-third normal size.

o   Crowding of central retinal blood vessels on disc, or situs inversus.

o   Disc may be pale and appear otherwise normal, or may have normal color.

Symptoms & signs

o   Very poor vision from birth; vision rarely sufficient for more than counting fingers.

o   Pupil may react poorly to light and give a poor consensual response to the other eye (Marcus Gunn's sign).

o   Affected eye may have defective color vision.

o   Affected eye may be normal size or microphthalmic.

o   Esotropia (crossed-eye) or exotropia (wall-eye) may be present.

o   Nonprogressive.

Other confirming findings

o   Rarely bilateral.

o   Sporadic appearance elsewhere in family history.

o May be more common in children of epileptic mothers on anticonvulsant drugs.

o On radiologic study, small optic foramen on affected side in half of cases.

Main differential diagnosis

o Farsightedness

o Acquired optic atrophy

o Tilted disc (dysversion)

o Coloboma of the disc

References

Mosier MA, Lieberman MF, Green WR, et al: Hypoplasia of the optic nerve. Arch Ophthalmol 96:1437, 1978.

Peterson RA, Walton DS: Optic nerve hypoplasia with good visual acuity and visual field defects. Arch Ophthalmol 95:254, 1977.

Walsh FB, Hoyt WF: Clinical Neuro-Ophthalmology, vol 1. Baltimore: Williams & Wilkins, 1969, p 661.

C. COLOBOMA OF THE DISC (Fig. 3.19; see also in color section)

Failure of the fetal fissure to close during development of the embryonic eye leaves an inferior defect that may include the iris, lens, choroid, and optic disc. The optic disc may be at the bottom of a large excavation (coloboma), or the disc itself may have a coloboma.

Ophthalmoscopic findings

o Disc margin incomplete, excavated, or stretched out inferiorly.

o Retinal blood vessels enter over edge of defect.

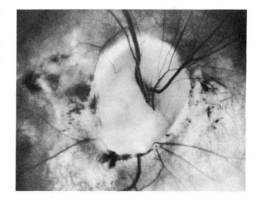

Fig. 3.19 Coloboma of the inferior disc in the right eye of a male patient who has only a lower field of vision. His left eye was blind from birth from a more extensive defect. His sister has similar findings. Also shown in the color section.

o Retinal pigment and choroid defective also.

o Disc may be within a coloboma of whole inferior eye (see Fig. 7.6).

o Colobomatous part of disc is pale.

Symptoms & signs

o Vision varies, depending on the extent of neurosensory retinal deficit. It ranges from normal vision to poor light perception. Pupil response varies with vision.

o Superior field is defective.

o Color vision is variable in the affected eye.

o Eye is usually normal size.

o With poor vision, possible esotropia or exotropia.

o Nonprogressive, except in rare cases in which subretinal neovascularization, hemorrhage, or retinal detachment may cause further loss of vision.

Other confirming findings

o Rarely bilateral.

o Occasionally inherited.

o Possible other evidence of a defect in the closure of fetal fissure (see Fig. 2.27).

Main differential diagnosis

o Persistent posterior hyperplastic primary vitreous

o Acquired juxtapapillary inflammatory scarring

o Morning glory syndrome

o Tilted disc

o Retinoblastoma

o Optic disc pit

References

Savell J, Cook JR: Optic nerve colobomas of autosomal-dominant heredity. Arch Ophthalmol 94:395, 1976.

Walsh FB, Hoyt WF: Clinical Neuro-Ophthalmology, vol 1. Baltimore: Williams & Wilkins, 1969, p 670.

Fig. 3.20 Developmental anomaly resulting in a pit of the disc (arrow). Pulsation of the gray material in the pit is sometimes present.

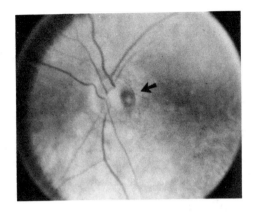

D. OPTIC PIT OR HOLE (Fig. 3.20)

A rare but distinct pit may occur in the optic nervehead. Its origin is congenital.

Ophthalmoscopic findings

o   Disc margin is complete, but an excavated pit separated from the physiologic depression is visible in the disc substance, usually on the temporal side.

o   Pit is often filled with pigmented or lacy gray tissue.

o   Tissue in pit may pulsate.

o   Possibly other developmental anomalies, such as persistent hyaloid artery or coloboma, may be present.

o   On cursory examination, pit may look like an elevation rather than a deep excavation. Slit aperture of the ophthalmoscope may help confirm the depth.

Symptoms & signs

o   Patient usually has good vision; discovery of the pit is commonly made on routine examination.

o   In some patients, a serous detachment of the neurosensory retina emanates from an optic pit and extends to the foveola, causing distortion of images and decreased vision.

o   Detailed visual field examination may reveal an arcuate or centrocecal scotoma.

Other confirming findings

o   Rarely bilateral.

o   No hereditary pattern.

o   Nonprogressive, and symptoms are rare.

Main differential diagnosis

o   Hamartomas of the retinal pigment epithelium

o   Coloboma of the disc

o   Central serous choroidopathy

o   Retinal detachment

o   Bergmeister's papilla

o   Glaucomatous cupping

References

Gass JDM: Stereoscopic Atlas of Macular Diseases. St. Louis: Mosby, 1977, p 368.

Walsh FB, Hoyt WF: Clinical Neuro-Ophthalmology, vol 1. Baltimore: Williams & Wilkins, 1969, p 669.

III. THE LARGE OR IRREGULAR DISC

The disc may appear large, or it may actually be large. You may over-estimate its dimensions if you mistakenly consider nearby pathologic processes to be part of the disc.

Following are conditions that might lead you to assume that either the disc is too large or its margins are irregular.

A. MYELINATED NERVE FIBERS (OVERGROWTH OF MYELIN SHEATHS OF THE NERVE FIBERS)

(Fig. 3.21; see also in color section)

Ophthalmoscopic findings

o   Invariably white, often with dark slits.

o   Feathery distal margin is accentuated by red-free light.

o   Always in superficial retina; always hides underlying structures.

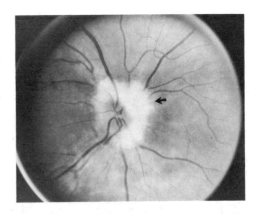

Fig. 3.21 Myelination of the nerve fibers extending into the adjacent retina. Note the feathery edges (arrow) and the superficial location at the level of the retinal blood vessels. Also shown in color section.

o Rare involvement of papillomacular bundle fibers. Usually located at the upper or lower disc margin, but can be isolated in peripheral patches in the retina. Large areas from the disc into the peripheral retina are seen occasionally.

o Course and caliber of retinal blood vessels are undisturbed.

Symptoms & signs

o No symptoms. Almost exclusively an incidental finding.

o Scotoma corresponding to the defect can be found on detailed visual field testing.

Other confirming findings

o Rarely bilateral.

o May be associated with unilateral myopia, amblyopia, and strabismus; rare association with keratoconus, coloboma, and polycoria (multiple pupils).

o Sometimes seen in patients with oxycephaly or other malformations of the skull.

o No known hereditary predisposition.

o Nonprogressive and unchanging.

Main differential diagnosis

o Juxtapapillary scars from trauma or inflammatory disease

o Myopic crescent

o Coloboma

o Papilledema

References

Straatsma BR, Heckenlively JR, Foos RY, et al: Myelinated retinal nerve fibers associated with ipsilateral myopia, amblyopia, and strabismus. Am J Ophthalmol 88:506, 1979.

Walsh FB, Hoyt WF: Clinical Neuro-Ophthalmology, vol 1. Baltimore: Williams & Wilkins, 1969, p 665.

B. RETROLENTAL FIBROPLASIA (ABNORMAL FIBROVASCULAR TISSUE GROWTH BEHIND THE LENS)
(Fig. 3.22; see Chapter 4: VIIIA)

C. JUXTAPAPILLARY SCARRING (CHORIORETINAL INJURY NEXT TO THE DISC) (Fig. 3.23)

Multiple causes include syphilis, toxoplasmosis, Toxocara canis, histoplasmosis syndrome, and serpiginous choroiditis.

Ophthalmoscopic findings

o Can surround the disc or be localized at one side.

o Pigment clumping, exposure of choroid and sclera.

o Subretinal neovascularization and hemorrhage may be present.

o Occasional retinal and choroidal vessel anastomoses.

o Neurosensory retina over scar may be cystic on proximal illumination.

o Peripheral chorioretinal scars, atrophy, or pigment clumping may be present.

o May be unilateral or bilateral.

Symptoms & signs

o Vision loss depends on the location of the chorioretinal scar and on whether it disrupts conduction in the papillomacular nerve fiber layer. Central vision is poor if the papillomacular bundle is disrupted.

o The loss of field of vision corresponds with damage to arcuate fibers from the periphery.

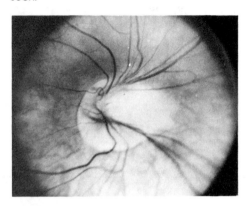

Fig. 3.22 Disc malformation in a myopic female who weighed 2 pounds at birth. Peripheral retinal abnormalities consistent with abortive retrolental fibroplasia could be seen.

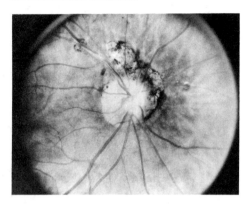

Fig. 3.23 Retinal and choroidal injury at the disc margin in a 41-year-old man involved in an automobile accident.

o   Dimness of vision in the affected eye is a common complaint.

o   Color vision (especially blue-yellow) may be defective in the involved eye.

Other confirming findings

o   History and confirming evidence of syphilis, stillborn siblings, ocular inflammation, ocular trauma, meningitis, collagen disease.

o   Chorioretinal scars elsewhere in the same or other eye.

o   Appropriate laboratory and other studies as indicated by history and examination (see Table 7.2).

Main differential diagnosis

o   Myopic crescent

o   Histoplasmosis syndrome

o   Central nervous system syphilis

o   Toxoplasmosis

o   Toxocara canis or other parasitic disease

References

Duke-Elder S: System of Ophthalmology, vol 3. St. Louis: Mosby, 1964, p 627.

Walsh FB, Hoyt WF: Clinical Neuro-Ophthalmology, vol 6. Baltimore: Williams & Wilkins, 1969, p 1577.

D. JUXTAPAPILLARY TUMORS (see VF, below)

E. MORNING GLORY SYNDROME (Fig. 3.24; see also in color section)

This rare developmental anomaly of the optic disc is associated with poor vision. Its distinct appearance is difficult to forget.

Ophthalmoscopic findings

o   Disc is deep in a funnel (morning glory).

o   Disc tissue often pink in a white halo.

o   Blood vessels loop over edge from the vascular plexus of Zinn-Haller.

o   Circumpapillary chorioretinal atrophy with gray and black pigment.

Symptoms & signs

o   Poor vision from birth.

o   Probable esotropia or exotropia.

o   Poor pupil response to light on affected side; poor consensual response to opposite eye.

Other confirming findings

o   No hereditary pattern.

o   Nearly always unilateral.

o   Other congenital anomalies may be present.

o   Optic foramen normal size on radiologic examination.

o   Ultrasonography and computerized tomography scan findings are probably abnormal (not reported as of this writing).

Main differential diagnosis

o   Juxtapapillary scarring from trauma or inflammation

o   Coloboma of the disc

o   Myopic crescent

o   Gliomas of the optic nerve

o   Avulsion of optic nerve

References

Kindler P: Morning glory syndrome: Unusual congenital optic disc anomaly. Am J Ophthalmol 69:376, 1970.

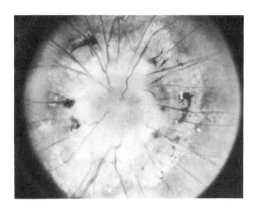

Fig. 3.24 This developmental anomaly of the optic disc has been called morning glory syndrome because of the deep central depression and the retinal vessels entering over the margins. Also shown in color section.

Fig. 3.25 Avulsion of the optic nerve after injury with a stick (a, left) and four years later (b, right). From Spizziri LJ: Avulsion of optic nerve. **Am J Ophthalmol** 58:1056, 1964. Used with permission.

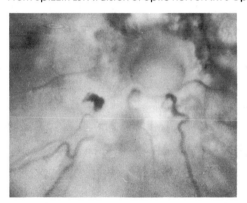 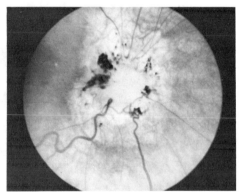

F. AVULSION OF DISC (Fig. 3.25)

Tearing of optic nerve from the eye is a severe orbital and ocular trauma disease.

Ophthalmoscopic findings

o In the acute stage, intravitreal hemorrhage may be extensive and obscure view, or may be limited to posterior eye around optic disc site and worsen later.

o Pallor of choroid and exposure of sclera.

o Disc tissue absent.

o Funnel depression at disc site.

o Retinal blood vessels disappear at disc site; blood column stagnated.

Symptoms & signs

o   No light perception.

o   Proptosis and pain in acute stage due to injury.

o   Limited eye motion due to swelling of orbital tissue or to ocular muscle involvement.

o   Patient may be unconscious; many of these injuries are due to gunshot wounds.

Other confirming findings

o   History of severe orbital trauma.

o   Radiologic studies.

Main differential diagnosis

o   Fracture of sphenoid bone with involvement of the optic foramen

o   Morning glory syndrome

o   Ischemic optic neuropathy

References

Spizziri LJ: Avulsion of optic nerve. Am J Ophthalmol 58:1056, 1964.

IV. THE TILTED DISC (Fig. 3.26)

This seemingly insignificant developmental anomaly is considered separately because it may take on great importance. It causes bitemporal field loss and must be differentiated from serious central nervous system disease. The term dysversion of the optic disc, sometimes seen in the literature, is synonymous with tilted disc.

Ophthalmoscopic findings

o   Tilting involves the inferior disc.

o   Crescent at margin of disc exposes the choroid and/or sclera.

o   Anomalies of central vessels, such as situs inversus and cilioretinal vessels, are common.

Symptoms & signs

o Visual acuity is normal with glasses or decreased in one eye by amblyopia from early childhood.

o Patient is usually unaware of field loss.

Other confirming findings

o Field loss crosses vertical meridian (Fig. 3.26b), unlike hemianopic defects due to central nervous system disease.

o Field loss nonprogressive.

o Field loss can be correlated well with defective area of disc.

o Radiologic studies for chiasmatic disease are negative.

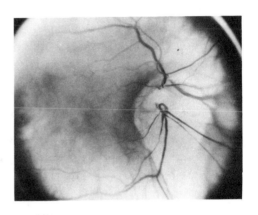

Fig. 3.26 In bilateral maldevelopment of the inferior disc (a, right), the patient may have normal vision but a superior bitemporal field defect that is confused with chiasmal compression. The bitemporal field defect in the tilted disc syndrome crosses the vertical meridian (b, below), whereas hemianopic field loss from chiasmal compression does not.

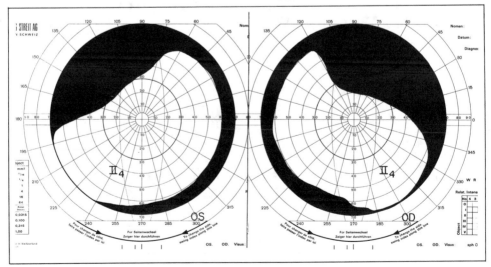

Main differential diagnosis

o   Bitemporal hemianopsia due to pituitary tumor or other disease at the chiasm

References

Walsh FB, Hoyt WF: Clinical Neuro-Ophthalmology, vol 1. Baltimore: Williams & Wilkins, 1969, p 660.

Young S, Walsh FB, Knox DL: The tilted disc syndrome. Am J Ophthalmol 82:16, 1976.

V. THE HIDDEN DISC

Some abnormalities partially or completely obscure the disc from view. The discussion is confined to conditions in which the view of the posterior eye is generally good, and the disc is the site of concern. Most abnormalities of the blood vessels on the disc are generally considered separately.

A. PROLIFERATIVE DIABETIC RETINOPATHY ON THE DISC
(see Chapter 4: VII A)

B. NEUROSENSORY RETINAL ELEVATION OVERHANGING THE DISC (see Chapter 5: III)

C. BERGMEISTER'S PAPILLA, PERSISTENT HYALOID ARTERY, AND PREPAPILLARY CYSTS (Fig. 3.27)

Remnants of the embryonic hyaloid vascular tree are common on the disc.

Ophthalmoscopic findings

o   Variations from a faint gray veil to a yellow-white strand ascending toward you from the central disc, ending in a white dot (Mittendorf's dot) on the back of the lens.

o   Prepapillary cyst may be present along the course of a persistent hyaloid artery.

o   Blood column may be present in the persistent vessel.

o   Hemorrhage rarely occurs, but may obscure the disc.

Fig. 3.27 Spontaneous hemorrhage over the disc in a 20-year-old male with bilateral persistent hyaloid artery remnants (a, left). Three weeks later, the blood on the disc had hemolyzed (b, right).

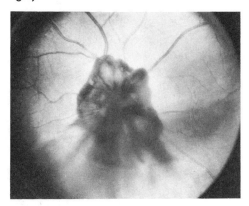 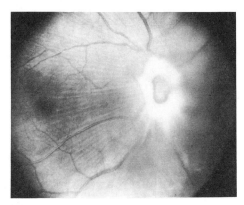

Symptoms & signs

o   Usually asymptomatic and found on routine examination.

o   Visual acuity is good, unless other developmental anomalies are associated.

o   Visual loss may occur from hemorrhage over the disc. This is rare.

o   There may be such other developmental anomalies as coloboma and falciform fold of the retina.

Other confirming findings

o   No hereditary pattern.

o   Occasionally bilateral.

o   Mittendorf's dot on lens.

o   Nonprogressive.

o   Fluorescein angiography confirms persistent hyaloid vessels.

Main differential diagnosis

o   Inflammatory cells in the vitreous over the disc

o   Proliferative diabetic retinopathy and other causes of disc neovascularization

o   Asteroid hyalosis

o   Cysticercosis in the vitreous

o   Endophthalmitis

o   Optic disc pit

References

Duke-Elder S: System of Ophthalmology, vol 3. St. Louis: Mosby, 1964.

Mann IC: Developmental Abnormalities of the Eye. Philadelphia: Lippincott, 1957.

D. POSTERIOR PERSISTENT HYPERPLASTIC PRIMARY VITREOUS
(Fig. 3.28; see 3.28a also in color section)

The embryonic vitreous is replaced in the developing eye by the clear adult gel. Replacement failure results in anterior vitreous opacities, a white pupil (leukocoria), and no view of the interior of the eye. Failure of posterior vitreous development does not always involve opacities that prevent ophthalmoscopy. Persistent primary vitreous is often accompanied by the remnants of the hyaloid artery system (see Fig. 8.3).

Ophthalmoscopic findings

o   White irregular membrane over disc.

o   Remnants of hyaloid artery or falciform retinal fold.

o   Sometimes associated with circumpapillary pigment disturbance resembling morning glory syndrome.

o   White membrane may be attached to and distort adjacent retinal vessels.

o   Stress lines may be present in the retina.

Symptoms & signs

o   Poor vision from birth, but sometimes unrecognized until child reaches school age. May be associated with strabismus.

o   Vision varies from 6/6 to light perception, depending on severity and structures involved.

o   Sudden visual loss may occur due to intravitreal hemorrhage or retinal detachment.

o   Acute glaucoma may occur in severe anterior and posterior maldevelopment associated with anterior chamber angle abnormality and swelling of the lens. It is accompanied by pain.

o   In one out of two cases, the affected eye has microcornea (small cornea).

Fig. 3.28 Posterior persistent hyperplastic primary vitreous in a 29-year-old man (a, left) with visual acuity limited to counting fingers and in a six-year-old (b, right) with a visual acuity of 6/18 (20/60). Fig. 3.28a also shown in color section.

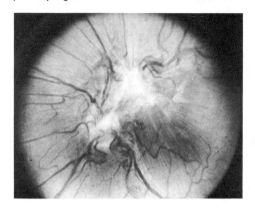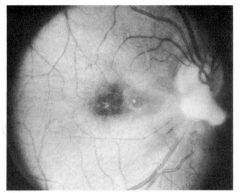

o   Hyaloid artery system remnants, such as Mittendorf's dot, tunica vasculosa lentis, may be seen on the lens.

o   Cataract may be present or developing.

o   Lens may subluxate when falciform retinal fold is present.

o   Vitreous membranes extend forward from disc to the equator and ora serrata.

o   Intravitreal hemorrhage and retinal detachment may occur in severe forms.

Other confirming findings

o   Generally no family history of disease.

o   Unilateral in most cases.

o   No history of postnatal oxygen therapy.

o   Full-term gestation.

o   Ultrasonography, electroretinogram, and computerized axial tomography aid diagnosis.

Main differential diagnosis

o   Peripheral uveitis of the young (pars planitis)

o   Parasitic disease, such as larval stage of Ascaris

o   Intraocular foreign bodies

o   Hamartomas of retinal pigment and retina

o   Retrolental fibroplasia

o   Retinal dysplasia

References

Hamada S, Ellsworth RM: Congenital retinal detachment and the optic disc anomaly. Am J Ophthalmol 71:460, 1971.

Joseph N, Ivry M, Oliver M: Persistent hyperplastic primary vitreous at the optic nerve head. Am J Ophthalmol 73:580, 1972.

Nankin SJ, Scott WE: Persistent hyperplastic primary vitreous. Arch Ophthalmol 95:240, 1977.

Pruett RC, Schepens CL: Posterior hyperplastic primary vitreous. Am J Ophthalmol 69:534, 1970.

E. PARASITIC DISEASE (Fig. 3.29)

Toxocara canis and cati (ascarid, dog and cat) and Taenia solium larva (cestode, pork tapeworm) are the organisms responsible for most of the intraocular parasitic disease on the North American continent. Neither exclusively invades the optic disc. They can be the cause of an inflammatory mass in or on the disc.

Ophthalmoscopic findings

o   Acute phase: varies from mild reaction to live worm to a gray, irregular mass, with radiating white lines in hazy adjacent vitreous; there may be subretinal hemorrhages and focal areas of depigmentation near the disc or scattered in the posterior eye. In some patients, you may see motile larvae in the vitreous or subretinal spaces; you may be able to identify the parasite from its scolex and alimentary canal while it is intraocular. You can see the worm undulate or move under the light of the ophthalmoscope.

o   Quiescent phase: white-gray mass with vitreous bands extending from it; retina and blood vessels distorted and pulled toward the main mass; focal areas of scarring with black pigmentation at the mass or at a distance from it.

o   Cysticercus may form a large cyst in vitreous with the white scolex visible within it.

o   Retinal and choroidal vessels may anastomose in the scar left at the site of the inflammatory mass.

Fig. 3.29 Tuft of cellular material on the disc (arrow, a, left) associated with a large granulomatous mass in the superior retina (b, right) in a nine-year-old male with a Toxocara canis larva.

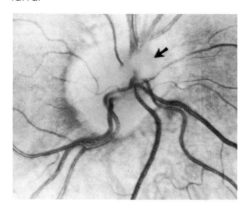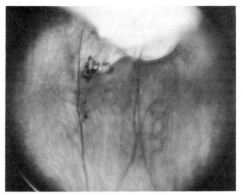

Symptoms & signs

o Poor vision may be discovered accidentally or during school examination; discovery of visual loss in children is often delayed.

o Strabismus or leukocoria (white pupil) may be the first sign.

o Red eye caused by associated iritis occasionally leads to detection.

o No pain unless iritis is present and then the most common symptom is photophobia.

o Adults may describe sensation of crawling movements of the larva.

Other confirming findings

o History of exposure to young dogs and cats, eating raw or undercooked meat, pica.

o No hereditary pattern.

o Usually unilateral.

o Occasionally elevated eosinophile count in acute phase.

o Calcification in liver, spleen, lungs, and occasionally in eye on radiologic study in longstanding disease.

o Hemagglutinin tests cross-react with other tests for Ascaris.

o Cross-reaction of blood type A agglutinins occurs but is nonspecific.

o Enzyme-linked immunoserum assay (ELISA) specific test for Toxocara is available.

Main differential diagnosis

o Retinoblastoma

o Peripheral uveitis of the young, pars planitis

o Posterior persistent hyperplastic primary vitreous

o Hamartoma of the retinal pigment and retina

o Intraocular foreign bodies

References

Barsante C: Cysticercus subretinalis. In Proceedings of International Symposium on Fluorescein Angiography (Shimizu K, ed). Tokyo: Igkau Shoin, 1974, pp 193-98.

Bird A, Smith J, Curtin V: Nematode optic neuritis. Am J Ophthalmol 69:72, 1970.

Santos R, Dalma A, Ortiz E, et al: Management of subretinal and vitreous cysticercosis:
Role of photocoagulation and surgery. Ophthalmology 86:1501, 1979.

F. TUMORS AT THE DISC

Neoplasms originating in optic disc tissue are rare. Some may be locally destructive, but the majority do not metastasize. Retinal and choroidal tumors arising near the disc are discussed in Chapters 5 and 7.

1. Melanocytoma (Fig. 3.30; see also in color section)

Ophthalmoscopic findings

o Black pigment overlying and obscuring part of the disc and retinal vessels.

o Usually flat; in superficial disc tissue.

o Generally there are no stress lines in the internal limiting membrane of the retina, and retinal vessel caliber and course are unaltered.

o Usually there is no distortion of central retinal vessels.

o Slight increases in size and pigmentation may occur.

Symptoms & signs

o Usually none; tumors are commonly discovered during routine examination of eyes with normal visual acuity.

o Mild vision loss may be present or occur.

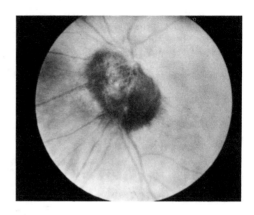

Fig. 3.30 Melanocytoma of the optic disc. This benign tumor requires observation only. Courtesy of Paul Torrisi, M.D., Syracuse, New York. Also shown in color section.

Other confirming findings

o   More common among black patients.

o   No hereditary tendencies.

o   Possible enlargement of the blind spot on visual field testing.

Main differential diagnosis

o   Juxtapapillary choroidal melanomas

o   Hamartomas of the retinal pigment epithelium

o   Gliomas and hemangiomas

o   Choroidal hemangiomas and retinal angiomas (angiomatosis retinae — von Hippel-Lindau disease)

References

Joffe L, Shields JA, Osher RH, et al: Clinical and follow-up studies of melanocytomas of the optic disc. Ophthalmology 86:1067, 1979.

Juarez CP, Tso MOM: An ultrastructural study of melanocytomas (magnocellular nevi) of the optic disc and uvea. Am J Ophthalmol 90:48, 1980.

Osher RH, Shields JA, Layman PR: Pupillary and visual field evaluation in patients with melanocytoma of the optic disc. Arch Ophthalmol 97:1096, 1979.

2. Choroidal melanoma (see Figs. 7.23-7.29; see 7.24-7.29 also in color section)

3. Gliomas of the optic nerve (Fig. 3.31)

Gliomas of the optic nerve cause optic atrophy and proptosis in children. The occasional presentation at the disc led to the original use of the term

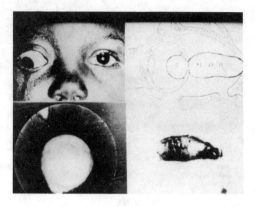

Fig. 3.31 Sketch and photographs of patient with a rare glioma involving the disc. Courtesy of Robert Ellsworth, M.D., Barrett Haik, M.D., and Algernon Reese, M.D., New York.

retinal glioma for retinoblastoma, a tumor indistinguishable from glioma on physical appearance.

Ophthalmoscopic findings

o Smooth, pale, elevated white mass that may partially or completely hide the disc from view.

o Unilateral.

o Venous congestion, disc edema, hemorrhage, and star-figure exudate may be present.

Symptoms & signs

o Poor vision in the affected eye; often only light perception or less.

o Proptosis with restriction of ocular rotation.

o Pupil reaction is poor or nonexistent.

o Pain from proptosis and corneal exposure may occur.

Other confirming findings

o Eighty-five percent of gliomas occur before age 20.

o Probably more common in patients with neurofibromatosis.

o Most arise in the intraorbital optic nerve, and the usual ophthalmoscopic presentation is optic atrophy.

o Ultrasonography.

o Computerized axial tomography.

o Biopsy.

Main differential diagnosis

o Retinoblastoma

o Astrocytoma

o Neurofibromatosis with astrocytoma

o Persistent hyperplastic primary vitreous

o Hamartoma of retinal pigment epithelium

o Toxocara canis

References

Hoyt WF, Baghdassarian SA: Optic glioma of childhood: Natural history and rationale for conservative management. Br J Ophthalmol 53:793, 1969.

Reese AB: Tumors of the Eye. New York: Hoeber, 1951, p 144.

Walsh FB, Hoyt WF: Clinical Neuro-Ophthalmology, vol 3. Baltimore: Williams & Wilkins, 1969, p 2083.

4. Astrocytic hamartoma (astrocytoma) and neurofibroma (Fig. 3.32; see also in color section; see Chapter 5: VIB, 2)

5. Meningioma (Fig. 3.33)

Meningiomas rarely present ophthalmoscopically. The patients seen have had a mass obscuring the disc, sometimes displacing retina and associated with splinter hemorrhages. Proptosis is common. More than 50 percent of patients are older than 30.

References

Reese AB: Tumors of the Eye. New York: Hoeber, 1951, p 169.

Fig. 3.32 Astrocytoma of the optic disc. Most astrocytomas occur in patients with tuberous sclerosis. Also shown in color section.

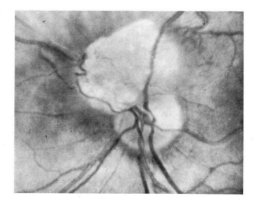

Fig. 3.33 Rendering of extension of a meningioma into the optic disc. Courtesy of Robert Ellsworth, M.D., Barrett Haik, M.D., and Algernon Reese, M.D., New York.

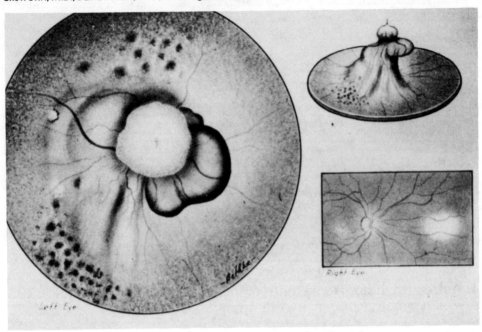

6. Hamartoma of the retinal pigment epithelium and retina
(Fig. 3.34)

Embryonal rests of retinal pigment epithelial cells on the disc or retina have an unusual appearance and occasionally diminish visual acuity.

Ophthalmoscopic findings

o   Slightly elevated tissue; vitreous is clear.

o   Charcoal-gray pigment with feathery edges and faint translucent membrane on surface.

o   Many small blood vessels in tumor, sometimes exudate nearby.

o   Stress lines in the surrounding retina.

o   May be on or near the disc, or in the adjacent periphery.

Symptoms & signs

o   Visual acuity often normal until stress lines develop into macula during adolescence. May cause strabismus in a child.

o   Field loss corresponding to the affected retina.

PHYSICIANS' GUIDE TO OCULOSYSTEMIC DISEASES

Other confirming findings

o Unilateral.

o Does not get larger.

o No history of prematurity or systemic disease.

o No hereditary pattern.

Main differential diagnosis

o Melanocytoma

o Juxtapapillary choroidal melanoma

o Posterior persistent hyperplastic primary vitreous

o Toxocara canis

References

Gass JDM: Differential Diagnosis of Intraocular Tumors. St. Louis: Mosby, 1974.

Vogel MH, Zimmerman LE, Gass JDM: Proliferation of the juxtapapillary retinal pigment epithelium simulating malignant melanoma. Doc Ophthalmol 26:461, 1969.

7. Hemangiomas of the optic disc (Fig. 3.35)

Ophthalmoscopic findings

o Elevated, circumscribed reddish-orange, round or oval lesions obscure part of the disc margin.

o Sometimes flatter (sessile), gray, ill-defined lesions.

Fig. 3.34 Hamartoma in a 49-year-old male. Visual acuity decreased to 6/12 (20/40) due to wrinkling of the macula.

Fig. 3.35 Angioma at the margin of the disc in a 30-year-old female with von Hippel-Lindau disease. The patient is paraplegic from a spinal cord angioma. Her father died of the disease.

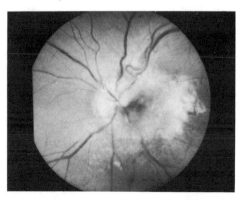

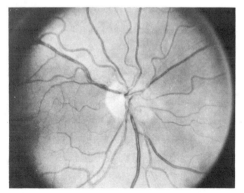

o Exudate may ring lesion, and subretinal hemorrhage may be present.

o Possible retinal elevation, macular edema, or retinal folds.

o Possible vitreous opacities or retinal folds.

o Possible extensive retinal detachment.

o Peripheral angiomas if von Hippel-Lindau disease is present.

Symptoms & signs

o Decreased visual acuity is the most common complaint. In some patients, a diagnosis of papilledema without symptoms has been given after routine examination.

o Distorted vision in the presence of macular edema.

o Pupil may be dilated and have a Marcus Gunn's sign if vision is poor.

o Field is impaired if retinal separation or nerve-fiber conduction is disrupted.

o Painful glaucoma may occur in late stages.

Other confirming findings

o Mean age 29 years at discovery.

o Males and females, right and left eyes, equally affected.

o Occasionally bilateral.

o Von Hippel-Lindau disease in 24 percent of patients.

o Hypertension, pheochromocytoma, cerebral tumors with convulsions may be associated.

Main differential diagnosis

o Papilledema

o Persistent posterior hyperplastic primary vitreous

o Drusen of disc

o Parasitic disease

o Sarcoidosis

o Metastatic tumor

o Retinoblastoma

o Choroidal melanoma

o Hamartoma of the retinal pigment epithelium

o Astrocytoma of disc

o   Melanocytoma

o   Disc neovascularization

References

Gass JDM, Braunstein R: Sessile and exophytic capillary angiomas of the juxtapapillary retina and optic nerve head. Arch Ophthalmol 98:1790, 1980.

Schindler RF, Sarin LK, MacDonald PR: Hemangiomas of the optic disc. Can J Ophthalmol 10:305, 1975.

8. Retinoblastoma (Fig. 3.36)

This tumor in children is discussed in Chapter 5: VIB, 1. Involvement of the optic disc is an ominous sign.

9. Metastatic tumor (Fig. 3.37; see also in color section)

While metastasis of breast, lung, kidney and neoplasms occur mostly to the very vascular choroid, nodules on the optic disc have been reported (see Chapter 7: VIC).

References

Kattah JC, Suski ET, Killen JY, et al: Optic neuritis and systemic lymphoma. Am J Ophthalmol 89:431, 1980.

Nicholls JV: Metastatic carcinoma of the optic nerve: Report of two cases. Trans Can Ophthalmol Soc 24:18, 1961.

Norton HJ Jr: Adenocarcinoma metastatic to the distal nerve and optic disc. Am J Ophthalmol 47:195, 1959.

Fig. 3.36 Retinoblastoma nasal to the disc has elevated the retina and invaded the disc tissue. Courtesy of Robert Ellsworth, M.D., and Barrett Haik, M.D., New York.

Fig. 3.37 Adenocarcinoma metastatic to the distal nerve and optic disc. Courtesy of Herman Norton, M.D., Rochester, New York. Also shown in color section.

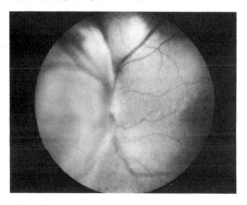
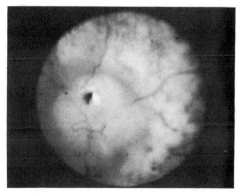

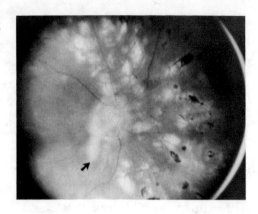

Fig. 3.38 Fibrovascular remnants on the disc (arrow) following vitrectomy and membrane resection for diabetic retinopathy.

VI. FOREIGN BODIES OR DISPLACED TISSUE

Accidents or surgical trauma may introduce foreign materials or intraocular tissue on the optic disc and obscure it from view. Various foreign materials have penetrated eyes (see Fig. 5.39).

Dislocation of the lens (see Fig. 8.17) may occur; the lens may remain clear or become opaque (cataractous). A rare phenomenon is total retinal detachment (traumatic or nontraumatic) resulting from a giant 360° tear, leaving the retina a small, shriveled gray mass over the disc (see Fig. 5.8). Fibrovascular remnants on the disc are common after vitrectomy (Fig. 3.38).

Because the history of trauma, surgery, and sudden visual loss are not specific for the optic disc area, they are discussed elsewhere.

It's unusual for foreign bodies smaller than 1-2 mm to have sufficient mass or velocity to penetrate the tough coats of the eye. This means that nearly every foreign body seen inside an eye is likely to be at least as large as the disc, or 1.5 mm.

References

Havener WH, Gloeckner SL: Atlas of Diagnostic Techniques and Treatment of Intraocular Foreign Bodies. St. Louis: Mosby, 1969.

VII. THE BULGING DISC

To distinguish the truly swollen disc, you must be familiar with the variations of normal anatomy that, at first glance, appear to be swelling. It's critically important to distinguish causes of disc swelling from papilledema, a term reserved for disc swelling due to increased intracranial pressure.

This section considers the bulging disc in a step-wise manner, as if it were an isolated physical finding.

A. FALSE APPEARANCE OF SWELLING (see Fig. 3.8)

In younger patients, it's not uncommon to see reflections around the disc. This reflection ring results from a slight flattening of the retina at the disc margin that mirrors the ophthalmoscope's light. It's not universally present in young people. The ring commonly disappears as the retina thins with aging. The reflection takes on significance only when it's absent in one eye. Unilateral absence may lead you to suspect the eye with the reflection of having a swollen disc when, in fact, just the opposite is correct. Swelling of the disc tilts the mirror-like surface at the disc margin and eliminates the reflection. This is a nonspecific finding, since it can occur with disc swelling from any cause.

In some patients, the central retinal vessels bifurcate deeply in the physiologic cup even before they can be seen. In others, this bifurcation may occur above the disc plane, and the vessels may curve back to the retinal level (see Fig. 3.9). This curve of the vessels may, at first glance, appear to be due to disc swelling. Such bifurcation patterns are usually bilateral, hereditary, and unrelated to symptoms or signs suggesting central nervous system disease.

The thicker nerve fiber layer of the retina on the nasal side of the disc obscures the view of the underlying retinal pigment margin. The nasal margin is naturally less distinct.

Even experienced examiners have been misled into thinking a disc is swollen when a corneal opacity, cataract, or cloudy vitreous partially obscures their view. Sometimes in such cases, the only way to see the disc is with the binocular indirect ophthalmoscope through a well-dilated pupil.

B. TRUE SWELLING

1. Disease next to the optic disc

a) INFLAMMATORY DISEASE (Figs. 3.39, 3.40)
Acute juxtapapillary choroiditis, or retinochoroiditis, is accompanied by some swelling of the adjacent disc (Fig. 3.41). Choroiditis and retinochoroiditis are discussed separately. Unless unusually severe, multifocal, or accompanied by hypotony, an inflammatory lesion causes disc swelling only on the affected margin.

Ophthalmoscopic findings

---

o   Hazy vitreous over the disc is common.

o   Gray or gray-white lesion with indistinct borders at the disc margin.

o   Localized hyperemia of the disc and possible displacement of vessels with ripples in the retinal pigment epithelium.

Fig. 3.39 Acute toxoplasmosis retinochoroiditis with swelling of the adjacent disc and hazy overlying vitreous.

Fig. 3.40 Sarcoidosis of the optic disc in a 29-year-old black patient. Visual acuity was 6/6 (20/20). The other eye was similar. From Jampol LM, Woodfin W, McLean EB: Optic nerve sarcoidosis. **Arch Ophthalmol** 87:355, 1972. Copyright © 1972, American Medical Association. Used with permission.

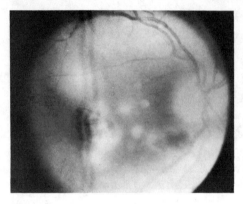

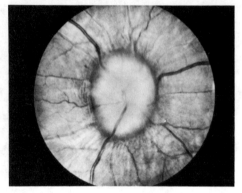

Fig. 3.41 Swelling of the disc and macula in severe peripheral uveitis (pars planitis). Note that no active lesions are present near the disc and macula, but inflammatory cells have accumulated.

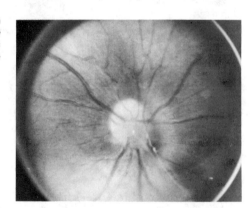

o Physiologic cup may be pushed in adjacent to lesion.

o Retinal vascular sheathing with "candle drippings" appearance or hard exudate sometimes as a partial star-figure on the disc side of the fovea.

Symptoms & signs

o Floaters, "cobwebs," dimness, loss of field are frequent complaints.

o Visual loss is determined by the location of the inflammatory site and the degree to which it affects the nerve fibers coming to the disc. If the papillomacular bundle is affected, loss of central vision may be profound. Visual loss from intravitreal inflammatory cells and protein is usually mild. Macular edema with visual loss can occur even in lesions remote from it.

o   No pain is present unless iritis occurs, in which case photophobia and ocular aching may also be present.

Other confirming findings

o   Past history of iritis or uveitis is common.

o   Physical or laboratory evidence of conditions such as toxoplasmosis, Toxocara canis, sarcoidosis, tuberculosis, syphilis (see Table 7.2).

Main differential diagnosis

o   Papilledema
o   Optic neuritis
ò   Toxoplasmosis
o   Sarcoidosis
o   Toxocara canis
o   Peripheral uveitis
o   Necrotic retinoblastoma
o   Histoplasmosis syndrome
o   Hypotony
o   Serpiginous choroiditis

References

Laties AM, Scheie HG: Evolution of multiple small tumors in sarcoid granuloma of the optic disc. Am J Ophthalmol 74:60, 1972.

Walsh FB, Hoyt WF: Clinical Neuro-Ophthalmology, vol 2. Baltimore: Williams & Wilkins, 1969, p 1503.

b) TUMORS (see VF, above)

c) VASCULAR DISEASE (see VIIB, 4, below)

2. Disease within the eye remote from the disc

a) PERIPHERAL UVEITIS, PARS PLANITIS (Fig. 3.41)

This disease of unknown etiology in young patients may be an immune complex disorder.

Ophthalmoscopic findings

o   Mild disc elevation (1 - 2 diopters).

o   Disc margins indistinct; adjacent retina slightly gray.

o   Veins engorged and slightly tortuous, and neovascularization may be present on the disc.

o   With some patients, there may be splinter hemorrhage near the disc or macula.

o   Macula may be edematous (use proximal illumination).

o   Yellow-white vitreous "puffballs," especially inferiorly.

o   Similar disease is invariably present in other eye but may be less pronounced.

o   Gray thickening of far peripheral retina inferiorly.

o   With indirect ophthalmoscope and scleral depression, you may see yellow "snowbanks" of exudate on the pars plana.

Symptoms & signs

o   Blurred vision in one eye is the usual complaint. Despite macular edema, patients rarely complain of distorted images. They are generally unaware that the second eye is also involved.

o   Floaters or "cobwebs" may be the chief complaint in the case of severe vitreous changes over the macula.

o   Photophobia and mild discomfort occur if iritis is also present.

Other confirming findings

o   Almost exclusively a disease of the first three decades of life; onset is usually before age 20.

o   No hereditary pattern.

o   Frequently afflicts children who have many pets.

o   No confirming laboratory findings to date.

o   If not bilateral, diagnosis in doubt.

Main differential diagnosis

o   Peripheral focal retinochoroiditis due to toxoplasmosis or unknown causes

o   Intravitreal hemorrhage (multiple causes)

o   Juvenile diabetes mellitus with retinopathy

o   Sarcoidosis

References

Hogan MJ, Kimura SJ: Cyclitis and peripheral chorioretinitis. Arch Ophthalmol 66:667, 1961.

Kimura SJ, Hogan MJ: Chronic cyclitis. Arch Ophthalmol 71:193, 1964.

Tasman W, ed: Retinal Diseases in Children. New York: Harper & Row, 1971.

b) HYPOTONY (Fig. 3.42)

Perforating injury, ocular surgery, uveitis, choroidal separation, and sudden decrease in aqueous production may lower intraocular pressure so much that the retina falls into folds.

Ophthalmoscopic findings

o   Media hazy due to corneal wrinkles (striae) and protein and cells in the aqueous and vitreous.

o   Mild disc elevation (1-2 diopters).

o   Disc margins indistinct and adjacent retina slightly gray and wrinkled.

o   Veins engorged and tortuous; occasional splinter hemorrhages.

o   Macula may be edematous.

o   Large, dark gray, highly elevated peripheral retina and choroid may approach the disc (see Chapter 7:VIE).

Fig. 3.42 Left disc in a young woman with acute bilateral hypotony following a drug reaction (a, left). Visual acuity was hand motion, both eyes. Six months later (b, right), vision had returned to 6/12 (20/40).

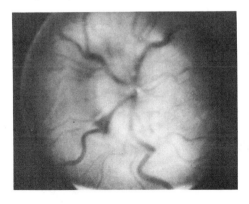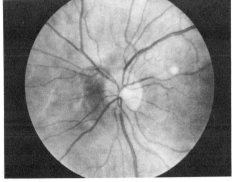

Symptoms & signs

o Visual acuity is poor — often 6/60 or less.

o Aching pain and photophobia are common.

o Pupil miotic and poorly reactive.

o Field generally constricted.

Other confirming findings

o History of trauma, ocular surgery (particularly cataract or glaucoma surgery), uveitis, or general patient collapse or debilitation, including diabetic acidosis. Severe reactions to medications must be considered.

o Intraocular pressure is diagnostic; usually gentle finger tension comparison between the two eyes confirms hypotony (this is to be avoided in obvious trauma).

o The disc swelling of hypotony is not characteristic and other causes for the swelling must be considered.

Main differential diagnosis

o Papilledema

o Optic neuritis

o Chorioretinitis

o Retinal detachment

o Chorioretinal folds

o Epiretinal membranes

o Retinoschisis

References

Fasanella RM: Complications in Eye Surgery. Philadelphia: Saunders, 1965, p 257.

Gass JDM: Stereoscopic Atlas of Macular Diseases. St. Louis: Mosby, 1977, p 148.

Kolker AE, Hetherington J Jr: Becker-Shaffer's Diagnosis and Therapy of the Glaucomas. St. Louis: Mosby, 1970, p 385.

3. Disease of retinal vessels

a) ACUTE VENOUS OCCLUSION (Fig. 3.43 a, b)

Occlusion of the central retinal vein or its branches results in mild disc elevation, blurring of the margins, venous distention, and other disorders. It is the subject of fuller discussion elsewhere (see Chapter 4:VIA).

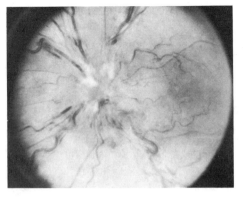
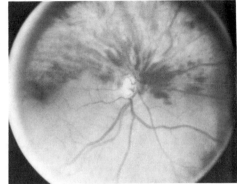

Fig. 3.43 Occlusion of the central retinal vein (a, above left). Note the disc swelling, obliteration of the physiologic depression, and marked venous congestion with hemorrhages. Occlusion of a branch of the central vein (b, above right). Note the swelling of the disc near the occluded vein. Embolus in the inferior temporal artery (c, right). Swelling of the infarcted retina obscures the disc margin.

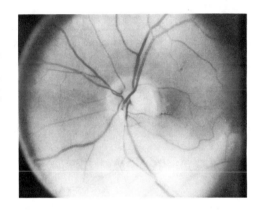

b) DIABETIC RETINOPATHY

Diabetic retinopathy is considered in detail in Chapter 4:VIC. Acute disc swelling may occur in both juvenile and adult-onset diabetics. It is usually bilateral and accompanied by symptoms of decreased vision that lead the patient to come for examination. Often the patient has had diabetes for several years and the disease has been out of control prior to onset of symptoms, perhaps due to an infection. Acute florid nonproliferative and proliferative diabetic retinopathy enter the differential diagnosis of the swollen disc.

c) ACUTE RETINAL ARTERIAL DISEASE (Fig. 3.43c)

Retinal arterial occlusion, particularly emboli lodging in a vessel on the disc, causes edema in addition to other findings (see Chapter 4:VB). Disc swelling in malignant hypertension must be included in the differential diagnosis of papilledema (see Chapter 4:VA).

Fig. 3.44 Ischemic optic neuritis in acute phase in a patient with giant cell (temporal) arteritis. The disc is swollen and pale. Note the marked narrowing of the retinal arterioles. Also shown in color section.

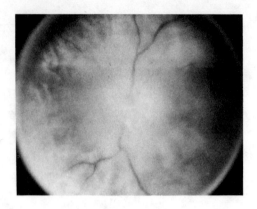

4. Acute disc and adjacent choroid vascular disease

a) GIANT CELL ARTERITIS (TEMPORAL ARTERITIS, CRANIAL ARTERITIS, POLYMYALGIA RHEUMATICA) (Fig. 3.44; see also in color section)

This systemic disease in older patients may have devastating ocular effects, producing bilateral blindness in a short time. Giant cell infiltrates more commonly involve the ophthalmic artery branches distal to the origin of the central retinal artery, but both may be affected.

Ophthalmoscopic findings

o Yellow-pink color gives way to white swelling of the disc; physiologic depression is filled in; disc is rarely elevated more than 2 diopters.

o The prepapillary capillaries are dilated with splinter hemorrhages on or near the disc. Arteriosclerosis is usually present.

o Cotton-wool infarcts often present near the disc.

o Deep subretinal, or intrapapillary blot hemorrhage may be present.

o Adjacent choroid is often pale.

o The narrowed blood column of the central retinal artery may close completely with boxcarring of the blood column when patient is upright. Retinal edema may follow.

o Optic atrophy, central retinal artery narrowing, and choroidal pallor are the end results.

Symptoms & signs

o Anorexia, low-grade fever, malaise, weight loss precede, by one to two weeks, head and body pains and loss of vision.

o Pain on one side of the head commonly associated with chewing or combing the hair often precedes the visual loss. The pain is often severe and may involve the pelvis or shoulder girdles (polymyalgia rheumatica). There may be hair loss and tenderness over a ropy temporal artery.

o Dimness of vision in the affected eye is a frequent complaint, and vision may improve measurably on lying down, only to dim on standing or sitting.

o Visual acuity varies from absence of light perception to normal. Patient may notice an altitudinal (upper or lower half) loss of field.

o Pupil will be fixed and dilated on the side of visual loss without giving a consensual response to the other eye (Marcus Gunn's sign). In altitudinal defects, light cast on the blind retina gives less response than from opposite direction.

o Corneal ulcers with pain may be a presenting complaint.

o Ptosis or diplopia due to muscle involvement can occur.

o Denial of poor vision may be part of the disease.

o Cerebrovascular disease, myocardial infarction, ruptured aortic aneurysm, and pneumonia result in a mortality of 20 percent.

o Rubeosis iridis and glaucoma may develop.

o Bilateral ocular disease occurs in giant cell arteritis, and one patient in two becomes blind in the second eye if it is left untreated.

Other confirming findings

o Mean age of patients 71 years (range 53 to 83).

o Equal sex distribution.

o Occipital and temporal arteries both involved often.

o Fifty percent of patients have normocytic anemia.

o White blood count may be 15,000 per cubic mm.

o Elevated sedimentation rate in 90 percent of patients.

o C-reactive protein elevated.

o Temporal artery biopsy usually positive (inflamed area can be missed by biopsy site selection).

o Electroretinogram may be abnormal with a large a-wave.

o Cerebral angiography may show vascular deficiency.

o Fluorescein angiography confirms disc and choroidal ischemia.

o Prompt response to steroids.

Main differential diagnosis

o Ischemic optic neuropathy or neuritis

o Optic neuritis

o Acute central retinal artery occlusion

o Papilledema

References

Eshaghian J, Goeken JA: C-reactive protein in giant cell (cranial, temporal) arteritis. Ophthalmology 87:1160, 1980.

Gerstle CC, Friedman AH: Marginal corneal ulceration (limbal guttering) as a presenting sign of temporal arteritis. Ophthalmology 87:1173, 1980.

Lessell S: Case records of the Massachusetts General Hospital. N Eng J Med 297:492, 1977.

Walsh FB, Hoyt WF: Clinical Neuro-Ophthalmology, vol 2. Baltimore: Williams & Wilkins, 1969, p 1878.

Fig. 3.45 Ischemic optic neuritis. This 58-year-old man had sudden loss of vision in the right eye (a, left). When he returned one year later with acute loss of vision in the left eye (b, right), the right disc was pale, but vision had returned to 6/7.5 (20/25). It had resembled the left eye in the acute phase. Giant cell arteritis has a similar appearance. Also shown in color section.

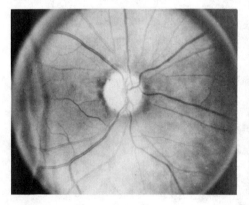 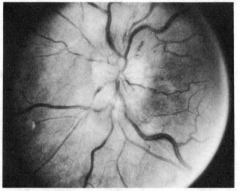

b) ISCHEMIC OPTIC NEUROPATHY (ISCHEMIC OPTIC NEURITIS)
(Fig. 3.45; see also in color section)

Localized closure of small vessels in the optic disc may cause severe irreversible visual loss without the systemic symptoms or findings of giant cell arteritis.

Ophthalmoscopic findings

o The findings are similar to those described for temporal arteritis.

o Arteriosclerotic, hypertensive, or embolic vascular disease are commonly present.

o Only a segment or half of disc may be most involved.

o Optic atrophy and attenuation of the central retinal artery are often the end result.

Symptoms & signs

o Visual loss in one eye is the presenting complaint. It may be preceded by hours or days of a vague discomfort, without tenderness, on the same side of the head as the affected eye.

o Dimness of vision is often described as a loss of the upper or lower half of the visual field (altitudinal hemianopsia).

o Pupil reaction on affected side varies with depth of visual loss; it may be fixed and dilated.

o In older, hypertensive, or diabetic patients, both eyes may be involved, but the interval may be weeks to years, and there is no association with systemic symptoms as in giant cell arteritis.

Other confirming findings

o Mean age of patients is 70 years (range 50-85).

o Equal sex distribution.

o Predisposing causes include preeclampsia, diabetes mellitus, hypertension, collagen disease, arteriosclerosis, cataract surgery, and carotid and/or aortic arch atherosclerosis.

o Blood count, sedimentation rate, C-reactive protein, temporal artery biopsy, and other such findings are normal.

o Fluorescein angiography is often characteristic.

o Carotid auscultation may confirm stenosis.

o Orbital plethysmography and cerebral angiography can aid diagnosis.

o No response to steroids.

Main differential diagnosis

o Giant cell arteritis

o Central retinal artery occlusion

o   Papilledema

o   Optic neuritis

References

Beck RW, Gamel JW, Willcourt RJ, et al: Acute ischemic optic neuropathy in severe pre-eclampsia. Am J Ophthalmol 90:342, 1980.

Hayreh SS: Anterior ischemic optic neuropathy: 4. Occurrence after cataract extraction. Arch Ophthalmol 98:1410, 1980.

Hollenhorst R: Symposium: Occlusive cerebrovascular disease. Carotid and vertebral-basilar arterial stenosis and occlusion: Neuro-ophthalmologic considerations. Trans Am Acad Ophthalmol & Otolaryngol 66:166, 1962.

Walsh FB, Hoyt WF: Clinical Neuro-Ophthalmology, vol 2. Baltimore: Williams & Wilkins, 1969.

5. Disease just behind the eye (Figs. 3.46 - 3.48)

Intraorbital pressure from mass lesions rarely creates swelling of the optic nerve, probably because of the gradual onset. Sudden changes in a growing mass may cause wrinkles and folds in the pigment epithelium (see Chapter 6:VIB). Acute tissue swelling from thyroid exophthalmos may cause optic disc edema, vascular congestion, and, sometimes, small superficial hemorrhages (Fig. 3.46). Trauma may increase orbital pressure enough to squeeze myelin out of the optic nerve (Fig. 3.48).

Ophthalmoscopic findings

o   Nonspecific disc swelling varies in degree.

o   Venous congestion and splinter hemorrhages.

o   Wrinkles in the pigment epithelium or stress lines in the retina may be present.

Symptoms & signs

o   Disc edema may diminish visual acuity to 6/120 (20/400) or worse, but usually the deficit is mild, unless the optic nerve is severed by trauma. Corneal exposure from proptosis causes epithelial irregularity and reduces vision.

o   Pain and photophobia from corneal exposure and orbital congestion.

o   Diplopia from restriction of ocular rotation usually is vertical and worse in up gaze. The patients may arrive with one eye covered to avoid double vision.

o   Nervousness from eye condition and thyrotoxicosis are common.

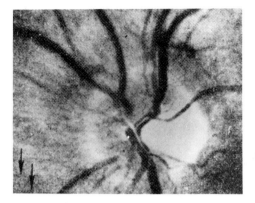

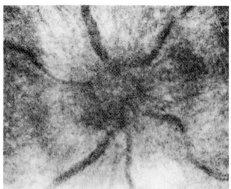

Fig. 3.46 Dysthyroid disc swelling. Mild edema, capillary dilatation, vein engorgement, and retinochoroidal striae (arrows, a, above left). Moderate and marked disc swelling (b, above right, and c, right, respectively) with superficial hemorrhages. From Trobe JD, Glaser JS, Laflamme P: Dysthyroid optic neuropathy. **Arch Ophthalmol** 96:1199, 1978. Copyright © 1978, American Medical Association. Used with permission.

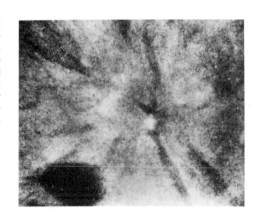

Fig. 3.47 Swollen disc and vascular tortuosity in a 49-year-old male found two years later to have lymphocytic lymphoma.

Fig. 3.48 Myelin squeezed into the retina by a gunshot wound of the orbit.

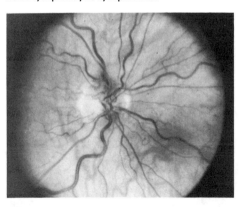

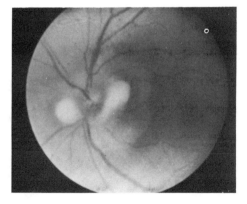

- Depending on the optic nerve damage from edema, visual field may be restricted or the blind spot may be enlarged.

- Exophthalmos, lid retraction, ocular muscle congestion, and restriction of eye movement may be unilateral or bilateral, especially in thyroid exophthalmos. Displacement of the globe and proptosis depend on the size and location of a space-taking lesion.

Other confirming findings

- History of medical or surgical treatment for thyroid disease or metastatic tumor. Acute orbital infectious disease may be preceded by an upper respiratory infection or by sinus disease. History of trauma to orbital tissues is easily elicited.

- Physical evidence of thyrotoxicosis: rapid pulse, cardiac arrhythmia, hot and dry skin, brittle hair.

- Radiologic and laboratory evidence of thyroid-pituitary and orbital disease. Computerized axial tomography aids tumor diagnosis.

Main differential diagnosis

- Papilledema
- Optic neuritis
- Drusen of the disc
- Orbital tumor, primary or metastatic

References

Trobe JD, Glaser JS, Laflamme P: Dysthyroid optic neuropathy. Arch Ophthalmol 96:1199, 1978.

Walsh FB, Hoyt WF: Clinical Neuro-Ophthalmology, vol 2. Baltimore: Williams & Wilkins, 1969, p 1084.

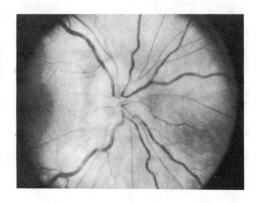

Fig. 3.49 Optic neuritis with acute loss of vision, centrocecal scotoma, and a swollen disc in a 22-year-old white female. Visual acuity improved from 6/120 (20/400) to 6/9 (20/30) in one and one-half weeks. The other eye was normal. Also shown in color section.

6. Intrapapillary disease

a) OPTIC NEURITIS AND OPTIC NEUROPATHY (Figs. 3.49-3.51; see 3.49 also in color section)

Inflammation in the neural tissue and supporting elements of the optic nerve arises from multiple infectious, toxic, demyelination, and possibly immune responses collectively called optic neuritis. In the inherited neuropathies, such as Leber's, the optic disc may initially be inflamed (Fig. 3.50). The effect on vision may be variable, depending on the amount, the reversibility of the damage, and whether the papillomacular fibers are compromised by swelling or the inflammation.

Ophthalmoscopic findings

o   Moderate elevation of the disc (1-2 diopters).

o   Filling in of the physiologic depression by swollen disc tissue (possibly segmental).

Fig. 3.50 Leber's optic neuropathy in the right (a, left) and left (b, right) eyes of a 19-year-old white male, two of whose cousins had a similar acute loss of vision in both eyes at age 19-20. Note the hyperemia of the discs and the dilated prepapillary capillaries (arrows). Optic atrophy followed.

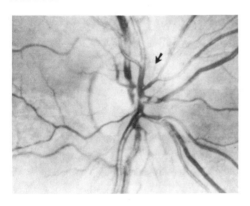 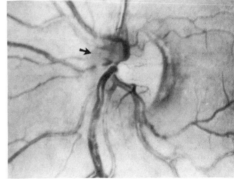

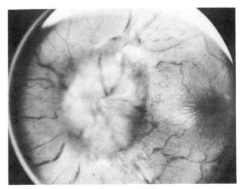

Fig. 3.51 Severe optic neuritis in a 25-year-old female. Visual acuity was 6/12 (20/40). Note the partial macular star-figure on the side toward the swollen disc.

o Sometimes yellowish discoloration of the disc and adjacent retina with dilated prepapillary capillaries.

o Splinter hemorrhages on disc and adjacent retina, but within 1-2 disc diameters of disc.

o Loss of usual light reflections; draping of vessels over disc margin.

o Cells in overlying vitreous may make the view of the disc hazy.

o Exudative star-figure in macula is more complete on disc side in optic neuritis (Fig. 3.51).

Symptoms & signs

o Visual acuity usually decreases suddenly — within 24 hours — and may fall to perceiving hand motion only. Recording the visual acuity in bright rather than dim light often gives a better result because of poor conduction in the optic nerve. After a period of poor sight visual acuity may improve nearly as rapidly as it was lost. This contrasts sharply with loss of vision associated with intracranial pathology.

Table 3.1

DISEASES AND CONDITIONS
ASSOCIATED WITH OPTIC NEURITIS, PARTIAL LIST

Actinomycosis	Neuromyelitis optica (Devic's disease)
Beriberi	Orbital inflammation
Carcinomatosis	Pellagra
Cryptococcosis	Pernicious anemia
Diabetes mellitus	Polyradiculoneuritis
Disseminated sclerosis	Postviral demyelinization
Encephalitis epidemica	Relapsing fever
Encephalitis periaxialis diffusa	Relapsing polychondritis
(Schilder's disease)	Rhodesian sleeping sickness
Epidemic Typhus	Sarcoidosis
Herpes zoster	Sinusitis
Hyperemesis gravidarum	Subacute bacterial endocarditis
Intraocular inflammation	Tropical vitamin deficiency
Leprosy	Tuberculosis
Malaria	Tularemia
Measles	Typhoid fever
Mumps	Varicella encephalitis
Myxedema	Viral hepatitis

o   Mild discomfort associated with ocular movements may be present, though this is more common with retrobulbar neuritis.

o   Scotoma may be an enlargement of the blind spot that includes fixation (centrocecal). Although this defect may be very large, it may also leave enough peripheral field for the patient to ambulate with the affected eye alone. Arcuate defects in the field may cause the patient to experience an upper or lower loss of vision.

o   Pupil may be dilated and fixed or respond weakly. Because of weak conduction in the affected optic nerve, the consensual response of the other eye is minimal or unsustained (Marcus Gunn's sign).

o   Color vision in the affected eye, especially blue-yellow, is often defective.

o   When asked about brightness of light, the patient is likely to describe it as 50 percent of illumination seen by the other eye.

Other confirming findings

o   History must cover inflammatory diseases or their preventive vaccinations; demyelinating diseases; metabolic disturbances such as pernicious anemia, hereditary optic neuropathy, exposure to toxins, and hypersensitivities. The treatment of any conditions must also be reviewed. Diseases and conditions associated with optic neuritis are listed in Table 3.1.

References

Hirst LW, Miller NR, Kumar AJ, et al: Medulloblastoma causing a corticosteroid-responsive optic neuropathy. Am J Ophthalmol 89:437, 1980.

Walsh FB, Hoyt WF: Clinical Neuro-Ophthalmology, vol 1. Baltimore: Williams & Wilkins, 1969, p 607.

b) DRUSEN (PSEUDOPAPILLEDEMA) (Fig. 3.52; see 3.52a and 3.52c also in color section)

Drusen may cause bulging of the optic disc. This condition, especially in children, results in considerable anxiety, expense, and risk in evaluating the possiblility of a brain tumor. Disc swelling found in an otherwise healthy patient is usually the original cause for concern. Distinguishing disc drusen from papilledema may be critical for the neurosurgical patient.

Ophthalmoscopic findings

o   Swollen disc is only mildly elevated (less than 1 mm).

o   Bilateral in many patients; discs often congenitally small.

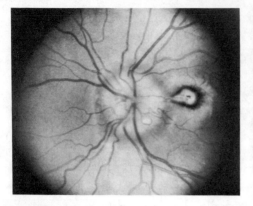
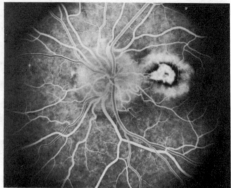
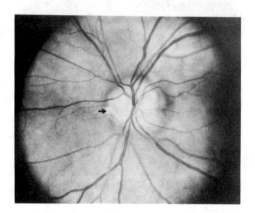

Fig. 3.52 Drusen buried in the disc of a child often cause concern that papilledema is present (a, above left). The absence of retinal vascular dilatation, hemorrhages, or edema and the presence of venous pulsation suggest the swelling is benign. Fluorescein angiography often helps confirm drusen (b, above right). In adults, the drusen (arrow) become exposed to view (c, right). Subretinal neovascularization and hemorrhage may occur (see a, to right of disc). Fig. 3.52a and 3.52c also shown in color section.

o No venous dilation, exudate, or edema.

o Vessel displacement, anomalous branching, or cilioretinal vessels are common; hemorrhages may occur as splinters on the disc surface or subretinally at the disc margin.

o In children, you often cannot see the drusen. In adults, drusen appear as single or multiple glistening, irregular yellow concretions visible in marginal disc substance.

o Drusen are seen best on proximal illumination.

o Drusen may make disc border irregular.

o In some patients, when associated with retinitis pigmentosa, they are seen in front or at the edge of disc.

Symptoms & signs

o Usually none.

o Visual acuity may decrease in hemorrhages, which are rare, or in swelling that disrupts nerve fibers.

o Scotomata are uncommon, but there may be peripheral field constriction characterized by a bizarre irregular pattern. Enlargement of the blind spot is possible.

Other confirming findings

o Family history of drusen of the optic disc; bilateral drusen are often dominantly inherited.

o Extremely rare among black and Oriental persons.

o Drusen may possibly be associated with tuberous sclerosis and retinitis pigmentosa.

o Drusen glow brightly on fluorescein angiography.

o If large, drusen may occasionally be seen on computerized axial tomography.

o If large, drusen will reflect ultrasound.

Main differential diagnosis

o Papilledema

o Optic neuritis

o Astrocytomas and hamartomas of retinal pigment epithelium

o Ischemic optic neuritis

o Giant cell arteritis

References

Frisen L, Scholdstrom G, Svendsen P: Drusen in the optic nerve head. Arch Ophthalmol 96:1611, 1978.

Sacks JG, O'Grady RB, Choromokos E, et al: The pathogenesis of optic nerve drusen. Arch Ophthalmol 95:425, 1977.

Spencer WH: Drusen of the optic disc and aberrant axoplasmic transport. Ophthalmology 85:21, 1978.

Walsh FB, Hoyt WF: Clinical Neuro-Ophthalmology, vol 1. Baltimore: Williams & Wilkins, 1969, p 673.

7. Papilledema due to increased intracranial pressure

Increased pressure in the cranial vault and spinal column has multiple causes. The optic disc, as a readily visible tissue at a bony opening of the cranial vault, is an important barometer of intracranial pressure. Acute papilledema can occur within 24 to 48 hours. If pressure is relieved, it may show signs of receding just as quickly. The magnitude of intracranial pressure is a factor in the rate of change. Spinal fluid pressure above 180-200 mm of H_2O is generally considered abnormal. Disruption of axoplasmic flow in the optic nerve tissue, rather than venous congestion, probably accounts for the swelling.

Papilledema is a nonspecific finding that by itself gives no clue to its cause. Hypertensive encephalopathy causing papilledema may be an exception, since, with this condition, hypertensive retinopathy is also present.

Papilledema may accompany spinal cord tumors; but in these cases its pathogenesis is not well understood.

a) ACUTE PAPILLEDEMA (Figs. 3.53 - 3.56; see 3.54a, 3.55, and 3.56 also in color section)

Ophthalmoscopic findings

---

o Red flush from hyperemia and dilation of capillaries; splinter hemorrhages may occur on disc or nearby retina. Subretinal and intravitreal hemorrhage may occur.

o No spontaneous venous pulsation; veins seem overfilled and tortuous. Light pressure on the globe does not initiate venous pulsation.

o Almost always bilateral (Kennedy's syndrome is rare); disc margins indistinct on all sides.

o Physiologic depression absent or partially obscured.

o Elevation of disc surface varies from mild to very high (3 diopters = 1 mm). There may be peaks of elevation in optic tract lesions (Fig. 3.56).

o Large retinal vessels hook over edge of disc down to retinal level.

o Usual ring of highlights is absent; adjacent retina may show ripples from displacement by swollen disc.

o White cotton-wool infarcts may be present on disc or nearby.

o In patients with hypertension, arteriolar spasm, narrowing, marked crossing changes, hemorrhages, and cotton-wool infarcts are seen in retina away from the disc.

Fig. 3.53 Bilateral papilledema in a 28-year-old white female with pseudotumor cerebri. Note the subretinal and splinter hemorrhage in the right eye (a, left) and the splinter hemorrhage in the left eye (b, right) away from the disc margin. The physiologic depression is absent and the circumpapillary light reflections are gone, despite the usual light reflections at the macula (b).

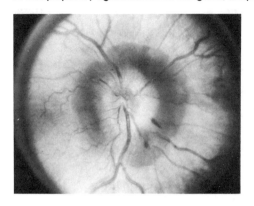 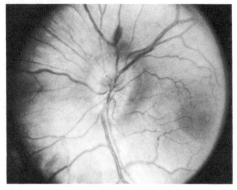

Fig. 3.54 Acute papilledema in a 28-year-old male with a diffuse frontal lobe glioma that confounded all diagnostic studies except biopsy. Right eye (a, left) and left eye (b, right). Fig. 3.54a also shown in color section.

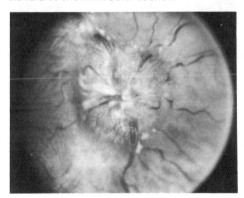 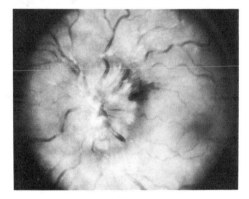

Symptoms & signs

o   Ocular symptoms are rarely the chief complaint. Symptoms are principally those of increased intracranial pressure, such as headache, unconsciousness, seizures, paralysis.

o   Some patients have transient (10-15 seconds) obscurations of vision in one or both eyes, especially on changing position. An occasional patient with intracranial disease causing hemianopsia may describe loss of peripheral vision.

o   Blurred vision may persist, but for the most part visual acuity is not markedly decreased.

Fig. 3.55 Bilateral papilledema in a slightly obese 19-year-old female (a, left). The patient complained of a paracentral scotoma. Peritoneal shunting for pseudotumor cerebri improved papilledema, leaving some optic atrophy (b, right). Also shown in color section.

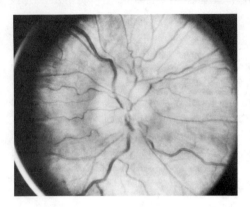 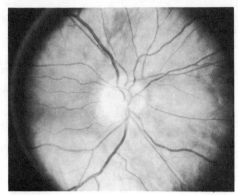

Fig. 3.56 Descending optic atrophy and papilledema. Optic tract lesions may cause horizontal band disc pallor on the same side and temporal half pallor in the opposite eye. The swelling of the disc tissue gives an appearance of "twin peaks" of papilledema. From Czarnecki JS, Weingeist TA, Burton TC, et al: 'Twin-peaks' papilledema. **Can J Ophthalmol 11:**279, 1976. Used with permission. Also shown in color section.

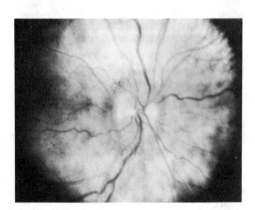

o   Patient may complain of dimness of light.

o   Diplopia due to sixth nerve paresis may occur; occasionally, third or fourth nerve may also be involved.

o   Pupil dilation may be present because of intracranial disease, but occasionally may be due to severe papilledema alone. In the latter case, the visual acuity is poor and the pupil reaction is not sustained on exposure to light (Marcus Gunn's sign).

o   Visual field changes may include enlargement of blind spots, general constriction of peripheral field, centrocecal scotoma (associated with decreased visual acuity), or a hemianopic defect from intracranial disease.

Other confirming findings

o History of obesity, drug and vitamin ingestion, head trauma, diseases with known intracranial pathology, unconsciousness, paralysis, or seizures. A general review of symptoms is essential.

o Physical evidence of disease with known intracranial or spinal cord manifestations, ranging from right-sided heart failure and extreme obesity to Schilder's disease. The full differential diagnosis of increased intracranial pressure is available in neuro-ophthalmologic texts.

o Radiologic evidence, including computerized axial tomography of brain swelling or displacement, bony erosion or displacement, or ventricular dilation or compression. Angiographic and pneumoencephalographic studies may be necessary to confirm the cause of increased intracranial pressure.

o Fluorescein angiography confirms optic disc hyperemia but cannot separate papilledema from optic neuritis. It helps define vascular disease, drusen, and some other causes of disc swelling.

o Cerebrospinal fluid pressure reading is the sine qua non for confirmation of increased intracranial pressure and papilledema. However, because of the risk of sudden death from brain impaction in the tentorial incisura or foramen magnum, it is done only with extreme caution under controlled circumstances.

Main differential diagnosis

o Drusen of the optic disc

o Optic neuritis

o Ischemic optic neuritis and giant cell arteritis

o Emboli to the optic disc

o Tumors, developmental anomalies, and inflammatory diseases near, over, or in the disc

References

Czarnecki JSC, Weingeist TA, Burton TC, et al: "Twin-peaks" papilledema. Can J Ophthalmol 11:279, 1976.

Hayreh MS, Hayreh SS: Optic disc edema in raised intracranial pressure. Arch Ophthalmol 95:1237, 1977.

Levin BE: The clinical significance of spontaneous pulsations of the retinal vein. Arch Neurol 35:37, 1978.

Walsh FB, Hoyt WF: Clinical Neuro-Ophthalmology, vol 1. Baltimore: Williams & Wilkins, 1969, pp 567, 585.

Fig. 3.57 Chronic papilledema in a 48-year-old male with pseudotumor cerebri. Note the opticociliary shunt (arrow, a, left) disappeared after a peritoneal shunt (b, right).

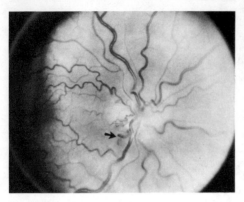 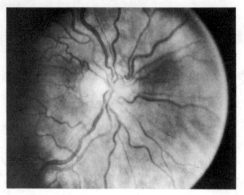

b) CHRONIC PAPILLEDEMA (Fig. 3.57)

Papilledema may go undiscovered for long periods of time in children or adults in whom the symptoms of increased intracranial pressure are mild or ignored. Reversal of papilledema in patients with pseudotumor cerebri and lead encephalopathy may also take many months.

Ophthalmoscopic findings

o   Dilated individual capillaries replace the general flush of acute papilledema.

o   Elevation of disc may decrease as atrophy follows prolonged swelling.

o   Opticociliary shunts often develop to improve venous return.

o   Disc and choroidal pallor are common with atrophy and clumping of circumpapillary pigment.

o   Hemorrhage and exudate along retinal veins may persist, but are scattered and mild, especially if opticociliary shunts have developed.

Symptoms & signs

o   Visual acuity may be mildly or severely affected. Children seem to withstand protracted papilledema better than adults.

o   Observant patients report dimness of light and decreased perception of color, particularly blue and yellow.

o   Some patients describe visual field loss. In contrast to the patient with acute papilledema, the chronic papilledema patient may have an altitudinal hemianopsia.

o   Afferent (Marcus Gunn's sign) pupil reaction is common.

Other confirming findings

o The confirming findings described for acutely elevated intracranial pressure apply for chronically elevated pressure.

o Fluorescein angiography is helpful in defining opticociliary shunts, drusen, optic disc ischemia, and the like.

Main differential diagnosis

o Drusen of the optic disc

o Ischemic optic neuritis and giant cell arteritis

o Retinal vein thrombosis

o Meningiomas and gliomas of the optic nerve

References

Walsh FB, Hoyt WF: Clinical Neuro-Ophthalmology, vol 1. Baltimore: Williams & Wilkins, 1969, p 580.

c) RESOLVING PAPILLEDEMA (Figs. 3.57, 3.58)

Resolution of papilledema after successful control of intracranial pressure is rarely complete in less than six to eight weeks. However, evidence of incipient resolution is often visible within one week. Recovery of visual loss depends upon damage to optic nerve blood supply, nerve fibers, and the intracranial pathology.

Ophthalmoscopic findings

o Elevation of the swollen disc tissue diminishes; the physiologic depression may reappear.

o Marks that resemble ripples in a pond may appear, indicating the effect of the swollen disc on the surrounding retina and retinal pigment epithelium.

o Hyperemia and venous congestion subside; spontaneous venous pulsations may reappear. Splinter hemorrhages may persist for a few weeks.

o Color of the disc changes from a hyperemic flush to yellow.

o Sharp disc margins may not appear for many weeks.

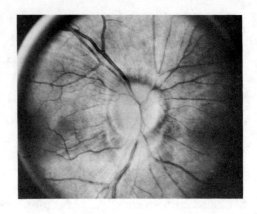

Fig. 3.58 Resolving papilledema. Note the demarcation line below the disc, indicating the limit of the previous swelling.

Symptoms & signs

o   If the cause of elevated intracranial pressure has been successfully resolved, optic nerve recovery follows. Visual acuity improves, depending on depth of injury.

o   Dimness of light diminishes; color perception improves.

o   Disappearance or diminution of visual field loss.

o   Pupil reactions may return to normal or near normal within 24 hours.

Other confirming findings

o   Clinical evidence of improvement; subsiding of such symptoms as paralysis and unconsciousness.

o   Lower cerebrospinal fluid pressure.

o   Fluorescein angiographic evidence of decreased optic disc hyperemia, shunting, and small vessel incontinence.

Main differential diagnosis

o   Optic neuritis

o   Peripheral uveitis and hypotonia

o   Vascular disease

o   Ischemic optic neuritis or giant cell arteritis

o   Drusen of the disc

References

Walsh FB, Hoyt WF: Clinical Neuro-Ophthalmology, vol 1. Baltimore: Williams & Wilkins, 1969, p 583.

VIII. THE PALE AND EXCAVATED DISC

It is sometimes difficult to determine pallor of the optic disc. Judgment is easier if the opposite disc is normal (Fig. 3.59; see also in color section). Disc pallor may be associated with extreme excavation (cupping) or may show minimal loss of disc substance. It may involve only a segment of the disc or all of it, and this may be different in each eye.

There are multiple causes of poor capillary perfusion, which is the cause of disc pallor. The loss of blood supply may result from direct or indirect vascular injury. Ganglion cell death in the retina, optic nerve, or brain may reduce vascular requirement, or there may be a combination of factors. Aside from central nervous system maldevelopment, optic disc atrophy is rarely caused primarily by disease posterior to the chiasm, but has been seen with optic tract and lateral geniculate body lesions.

It's often difficult to tell if the pallor that follows papilledema is from descending atrophy or secondary mechanical effects on optic nerve vasculature. When optic atrophy follows ascending (wallerian) degeneration due to ganglion cell damage in the retina, it is termed consecutive, because it follows the retinal injury. Primary optic atrophy denotes disease processes originating in the optic nerve tissue.

Disc pallor associated with excavation (cupping) is thought to be a function of optic disc ischemia combined with elevated intraocular pressure. When it occurs without elevated intraocular pressure, as in cavernous (Schnabel's) atrophy and high myopia, it is assumed that the disc is vulnerable to normal intraocular pressure or its diurnal variations.

The many causes of optic disc pallor mean that you have to sort through multiple overlapping presentations. General ophthalmoscopic findings described below emphasize specific findings to suggest the cause of the atrophy.

Fig. 3.59 Segmental optic atrophy of unknown cause in a 17-year-old male. Compare the right (a, left) and left (b, right) eyes. Also shown in color section.

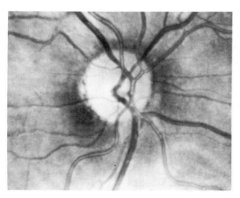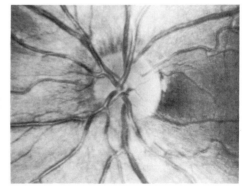

Fig. 3.60 Generalized consecutive optic disc pallor associated with extensive retinal damage from congenital syphilis. Note the attenuation of the retinal blood vessels and the circumpapillary chorioretinal pigment scarring. Also shown in color section.

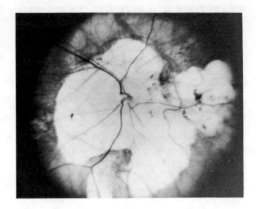

Fig. 3.61 Acute arterial occlusion (a, left) followed by segmental atrophy and pallor of the lower half of the optic disc (b, right). Also shown in color section.

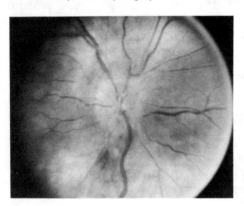 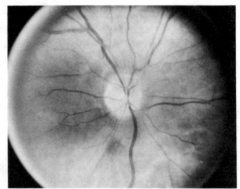

A. ASCENDING (CONSECUTIVE) OPTIC ATROPHY

(Figs. 3.60 - 3.62; see 3.60 and 3.61 also in color section)

Ophthalmoscopic findings

o   Narrowing of a branch or all of central retinal vessels suggests that the cause is in the eye (see Fig. 3.59). Emboli may be visible in arterioles.

o   Border of disc sharp, either all around (see Fig. 3.59) or only on the side of a destructive lesion (Fig. 3.61; see also in color section).

o   Retinal damage may be peripheral and not immediately visible, unless pupil is dilated.

o   To cause optic atrophy, retinal damage must be extensive, unless it is in the macula or close to the disc (see Fig. 3.59).

Fig. 3.62 Toxoplasmosis scar of the retina and choroid with consecutive pallor of the adjacent optic disc.

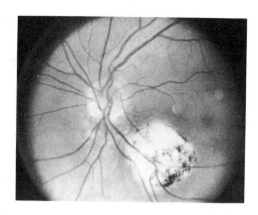

Symptoms & signs

---

o Visual acuity can be very poor if the macula is damaged, or it can be normal if the retinal destruction is peripheral. Absence of light perception is usual in most central retinal artery occlusions.

o Field loss is opposite the retinal damage.

o Nightblindness; patients who do not mention this should be directly asked about it.

o Possible partial color blindness.

o Flashing lights in the peripheral field are described by patients with retinal tears or detachment. Colored lights centrally may be described by some maculopathy patients.

o Pupil may show an afferent defect (Marcus Gunn's sign); it may be normal, or it may give a diminished response from the eye's blind side. Retinal destruction sufficient to cause optic atrophy also causes loss of pupil function.

o Visual field is invariably affected in some way, depending on the location of the retinal damage.

Other confirming findings

---

o History includes a review of systems for vascular, inflammatory, infectious, collagen disease, degenerations, neoplasms, toxicity, and trauma. The genetic history of such diseases as retinitis pigmentosa is essential.

o Physical examination includes all systems. Many congenital, hereditary, and acquired diseases have been associated with retinal disease.

o Fluorescein angiography, electro-oculography, and visually evoked potentials define the functional state of the retina, retinal pigment epithelium, and integrity of the visual pathway.

Main differential diagnosis

o Retinitis pigmentosa or other abiotrophy of the retina

o Toxoplasmosis

o Myopic degeneration

c Syphilitic retinitis

o Other severe traumatic, inflammatory, or infectious disease of the interior of the eye

References

Walsh FB, Hoyt WF: Clinical Neuro-ophthalmology, vol 1. Baltimore: Williams & Wilkins, 1969, p 583.

B. PRIMARY OPTIC ATROPHY (Fig. 3.63)

Ophthalmoscopic findings

o Initially, the central retinal vessels are of normal or near normal caliber; exceptions occur in cases of quinine intoxication and dominant Leber's optic atrophy.

o Retina and choroid are normal or insufficiently scarred to account for disc pallor.

o Usually the whole disc is pale in toxic and hereditary atrophy; segmental atrophy is more common in demyelinating disease.

o Bilateral, simultaneous pallor is common in toxic and hereditary disease; uncommon in demyelinating and vascular disease.

Symptoms & signs

o Visual acuity is usually 6/60 (20/200) or less, but depends on the stage of the disease.

o Field loss may be a general constriction or centrocecal scotoma or both. Vascular disease may give an altitudinal loss of field.

o The patient is likely to report dimness of light in the eye with poorer vision.

o Color vision may be defective.

PHYSICIANS' GUIDE TO OCULOSYSTEMIC DISEASES

- Pupil size and reactions vary considerably, depending on severity of the disease. Afferent pupil (Marcus Gunn's sign) is common.
- Esotropia or exotropia and/or nystagmus is common in congenital and hereditary optic atrophy.

Other confirming findings

- Family medical history must focus special attention upon genetics, gestation, drugs and chemical ingestion (see Table 3.2), previous subclinical episodes of visual loss, and developmental defects. Optic atrophy may be dominantly or recessively inherited.

Table 3.2

CHEMICALS KNOWN TO CAUSE OPTIC ATROPHY, PARTIAL LIST

Aminopyrine	Isoniazid
Aniline	Lead
Antimony	Mercury
Arsenicals	Methyl acetate
Aspidium (male fern, filix mas)	Methyl alcohol
Benzene	Methyl bromide
Carbon dioxide	Methyl chloride
Carbon monoxide	Methysergide maleate (Sansert)
Carbon tetrachloride	Naphthalene
Chloramphenicol (Chloromycetin)	Nialamide
Chlorodinitrobenzene	Nicotine
Chloroquine (Aralen)	Nitrites and nitrates
Chlorpropamide (Diabinese)	Nitroglycerin
Cortex granati (pomegranate bark)	Oil of chenopodium
Cyanides and hydrocyanic acid	Pamaquine
Dintrobenzene	Penicillamine
Disulfiram (Antabuse)	Picrotoxin
Emetine and ipecac	Primaquine
Ergotamine tartrate	Quinacrine (Atabrine)
Ethambutol (Myambutol)	Quinidine
Ethchlorvynol (Placidyl)	Quinine
Ethylbenzene	Thallium
Euprocin (Eucupin)	Tin
Fava beans	Trichloroethylene
Griseofulvin	Tricresyl phosphate
Hydrogen sulfide	Trinitrotoluene
Iodoform	Vinylbenzene (styrene)
Iodopyracet	

Fig. 3.63 Leber's optic atrophy in a 24-year-old white male with longstanding diabetes mellitus. The left eye was similar. The optic atrophy appears to have protected the patient from diabetic retinopathy, but best vision in each eye is 6/120 (20/400).

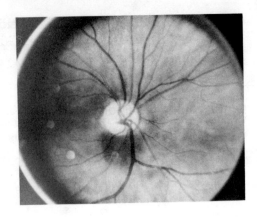

o Physical examination includes all systems.

o Radiologic study of the optic foramina must be carefully done; both sides must be compared.

o Electroretinogram, electro-oculogram, and visually evoked potentials as described above.

o Ultrasonography.

o Computerized axial tomography may demonstrate optic nerve atrophy behind the globe.

Main differential diagnosis

o Exposure to chemicals toxic to optic nerve

o Descending optic atrophy that is a result of central nervous system disease

o Glaucoma

References

Brinton GS, Norton EWD, Zahn JR, et al: Ocular quinine toxicity. Am J Ophthalmol 90:403, 1980.

Grant WM: Toxicology of the Eye. Springfield, Ill: Thomas, 1974.

Slamovits TL, Burde RM, Klingele TG: Bilateral optic atrophy caused by chronic oral ingestion and topical application of hexachlorophene. Am J Ophthalmol 89:676, 1980.

Walsh FB, Hoyt WF: Clinical Neuro-Ophthalmology, vol 1. Baltimore: Williams & Wilkins, 1969, p 909.

C. DESCENDING OPTIC ATROPHY (see Fig. 3.56)

Ophthalmoscopic findings

o   Central retinal vessels of normal or near normal caliber.

o   Pallor may occur in one eye, with papilledema in the other (Kennedy's syndrome).

o   In optic tract lesions, a "twin-peak" papilledema may occur with a horizontal band of pallor in the disc on the side with the pathology and pallor in the temporal half of the opposite disc (see Fig. 3.56).

Symptoms & signs

o   Visual acuity may be 6/6 (20/20) despite pallor, but may diminish considerably in dim light. Patients with optic tract lesions may complain bitterly about their poor vision, even though their field loss is peripheral and they can read the eye chart quite well. Patients with unilateral optic atrophy may have a visual acuity of no light perception in the affected eye and 6/6 (20/20) in the other.

o   Field loss due to optic nerve damage may be localized to the affected eye, but if the chiasm is injured, the crossing fiber from the nasal hemiretina causes a temporal field defect in the opposite eye.

o   Afferent pupil (Marcus Gunn's sign) is common; pupillary hemiakinesia (Wernicke's sign) may be found. If light is directed on the seeing hemiretina, there is a better response than when the blind hemiretina is illuminated.

o   Visual hallucinations from disease in the temporal lobe are specific, well-formed objects the patients can describe. Occipital lobe hallucinations are nonspecific lights and colors.

Other confirming findings

o   History includes a review of systems with inquiries about neurological symptoms, head trauma, and endocrinological problems. A partial list of central nervous system diseases associated with optic atrophy is given in Table 3.3.

o   Physical examination includes emphasis on neurological deficits.

o   Computerized axial tomography, arteriography, pneumoencephalography, electroencephalography, spinal fluid analysis are done as indicated after neurological or neurosurgical consultation.

Table 3.3

CENTRAL NERVOUS SYSTEM DISEASE
ASSOCIATED WITH OPTIC ATROPHY, PARTIAL LIST

Addison's disease	Laurence-Moon-Biedl syndrome
Arteriovenous aneurysm	Meningitis
Birth injury	Microcephaly
Carotid occlusion or aneurysm	Neurofibromatosis
Electric shock	Osteopetrosis
Fibrous dysplasia	Otitic hydrocephalus
Glucose 6-phosphate dehydrogenase deficiency	Paget's disease
	Pelizaeus-Merzbacher disease
Hand-Schüller-Christian disease	Schnabel's cavernous atrophy
Hereditary ataxias	Spastic diplegia and paraplegia
Hydrocephalus	Subdural hematoma
Idiopathic infantile hypercalcemia	Sydenham's chorea
Infantile neuroaxonal dystrophy	Syphilis
Krabbe's cerebral sclerosis	Syringomyelia

Main differential diagnosis

o Heredofamilial and degenerative central nervous system disease

o Optic neuritis

o Glaucoma

o Trauma of eye or central nervous system

o Heredofamilial and degenerative disease of the eyes

References

Czarnecki JSC, Weingeist TA, Burton TC, et al: "Twin-peaks" papilledema. Can J Ophthalmol 2:279, 1976.

Walsh FB, Hoyt WF: Clinical Neuro-Ophthalmology, vols 1, 2, 3. Baltimore: Williams & Wilkins, 1969.

IX. THE CUPPED DISC (Figs. 3.64-3.67; see 3.65 and 3.66 also in color section)

There are wide variations in the physiologic cupping of the optic disc. There's a striking similarity in the size and shape of physiologic cups in the two eyes of individual patients. Blood vessels passing through the rim tissue of the disc indicate that the cup is of developmental origin (Fig. 3.64).

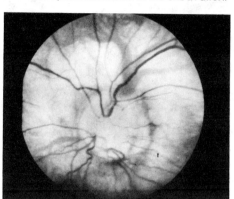

Fig. 3.64 Myopic eye with a large cup. The patient did not have glaucoma. Note how the vessels enter through the rim tissue confirming the developmental nature of the excavation.

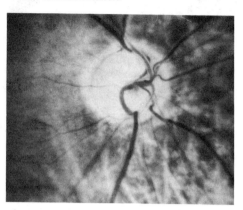

Fig. 3.65 Advanced cupping in a 79-year-old female with chronic glaucoma. There is no rim tissue, and the retinal vessels drape over the scleral rim. Note the atrophy of the retinal pigment and choroid around the disc. Also shown in color section.

Ophthalmoscopic findings

- Cupping with pallor involves the center of the disc and only extends to the disc rim in advanced glaucomatous atrophy (Fig. 3.65). The rim tissue may be involved earlier in optic disc infarction.

- Depth of cup is quite variable and can be measured with the lens wheel.

- Large central retinal vessels hook over the rim tissue and may disappear under a shelf. Splinter hemorrhages on the disc are a sign of progressive atrophy (Fig. 3.67).

- The lamina cribrosa, when exposed by cupping, has a sieve-like appearance with multiple gray openings (Fig. 3.65).

Symptoms & signs

- Slight aching in eyes or "steamy" vision is a rare complaint in chronic glaucoma. When it does occur, it is usually on awakening. These symptoms are more common with subacute attacks of angle-closure glaucoma. They may be relieved by the miosis of sleep or by pain medication. Acute glaucoma may cause cupping after a few months if pressure is not relieved or central artery occlusion occurs in the attack. Chronic glaucoma takes years to cause cupping.

- The extent of disease rarely is the same in both eyes; symptoms and signs are usually not similar bilaterally.

Fig. 3.66 Progressive cupping of the left disc in a 35-year-old male with an iron intraocular foreign body present undetected for two years. Extensive siderosis (darker pigmentation) has developed as well as cupping in the two-year interval between photographs a (left) and b (right). Also shown in color section.

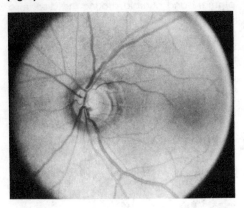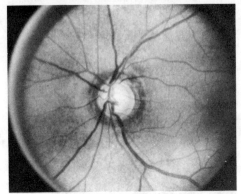

Fig. 3.67 Circumpapillary atrophy due to myopia and chronic glaucoma. Note the cupping of the disc and particularly the small splinter hemorrhage on the disc that indicates progressive disease.

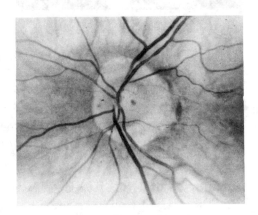

o   Visual acuity may be 6/6 (20/20) when only a tunnel of visual field remains. Further progression may destroy central vision, leaving only hand motion sight in the temporal field.

o   Limited field causes the patient to complain about walking or being afraid to drive.

o   Dark adaptation will be defective; it becomes exaggerated if the patient is on miotic eye drops.

o   Pupil reactions may be normal, even though only a small field of vision remains. However, if the patient takes miotic drops, pupils remain fixed and miotic.

Other confirming findings

o History includes a review of systems with emphasis on the family pattern of myopia, glaucoma, or other ocular disease, drug or chemical ingestion, of methanol, for example, previous visual loss, or central nervous system disease.

o Physical examination includes tonometry and visual fields. Carotid artery function should be evaluated by auscultation, ophthalmodynamometry, and other means.

o Fluorescein angiography helps define the optic nerve and choroidal vascular deficit.

Main differential diagnosis

o Coloboma of the optic nerve

o Myopic degeneration

o Drusen

o Central retinal artery occlusion

o Giant cell arteritis

o Ischemic optic neuropathy

References

Armaly MF: Genetic determination of cup/disc ratio of the optic nerve. Arch Ophthalmol 78:35, 1967.

Fishbein SL, Schwartz B: Optic disc in glaucoma. Arch Ophthalmol 95:1975, 1977.

Kolker AE, Hetherington J Jr: Becker-Shaffer's Diagnosis and Therapy of the Glaucomas. St. Louis: Mosby, 1970, p 132.

Lichter PR, Henderson JW: Optic nerve infarction. Am J Ophthalmol 85:302, 1978.

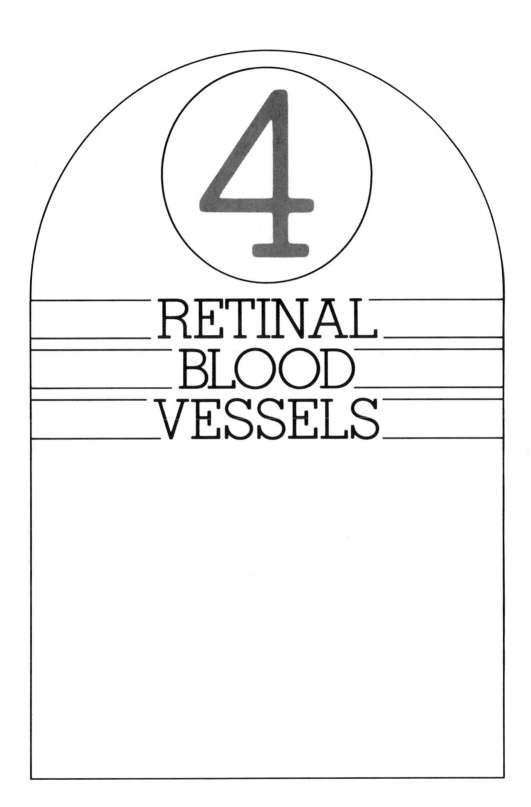

4

RETINAL BLOOD VESSELS

The ophthalmoscope provides a superb view of functioning blood vessels (Fig. 4.1; see also in color section). Under 15 times magnification, you can — without expensive equipment, special preparation, or patient risk and discomfort — see details of blood quality, flow, and vascular structure.

The central retinal artery arises from the ophthalmic artery in the orbit (see Fig. 3.6). After piercing the meninges, it enters the optic nerve approximately 10 mm behind the globe. It comes into view for the first time in the nasal disc tissue (Fig. 4.2a). It may divide before it reaches that point or, in some patients, above the disc surface, arching back to the retinal plane. Branching usually occurs at the disc, with major branches running to all the four quadrants in a uniform fashion. The central retinal artery is commonly aided by a separate artery from the vascular plexus of Zinn-Haller behind the globe. These cilioretinal arteries enter the retina through the marginal disc tissue (see Fig. 3.10). The blood vessels on and about the disc are described in Chapter 3.

Fig. 4.1 By permission from **Anatomy of the Eye and Orbit** by Eugene Wolff. London: H. K. Lewis & Co., Ltd. Also shown in color section.

Fig. 4.2 Developmental variations in the course of the central retinal vessels. The inferior temporal vein exits separately from the central retinal vein (a, immediately below), the superior temporal artery independent of the central artery (b, bottom page).

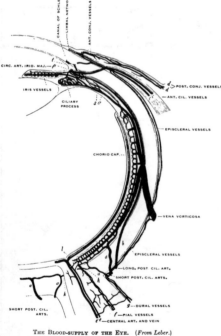

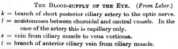

THE BLOOD-SUPPLY OF THE EYE. *(From Leber.)*
k = branch of short posterior ciliary artery to the optic nerve.
l = anastomoses between choroidal and central vessels. In the case of the artery this is capillary only.
s = vein from ciliary muscle to vena vorticosa.
t = branch of anterior ciliary vein from ciliary muscle.
o = recurrent artery.

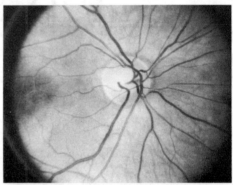

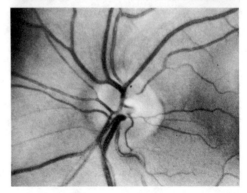

PHYSICIANS' GUIDE TO OCULOSYSTEMIC DISEASES

Venous drainage of the retina closely follows arterial perfusion, usually exiting from the eye just temporal to the artery in the disc. Occasionally in health, and frequently in disease, venous flow may leave the eye by entering the choroidal or ciliary circulation through the margins of the disc (Fig. 4.26; see also Fig. 3.57a).

Several vascular disease processes may be present at one time. For example, it is not uncommon to find arteriosclerotic, diabetic, and hypertensive vasculopathy all in the same patient. The retinal findings overlap, and only by experience can you appreciate their relative significance for that patient. Sometimes it's only with repeated observations as the disease processes are controlled, cured, or continue that you can reach conclusions about what has been affecting the patient.

I. OPHTHALMOSCOPIC ANATOMY

A. COLOR

In the healthy retina, there's a distinct difference in color between the arteries and veins (Fig. 4.3). The greater concentration of oxyhemoglobin in the arterial blood accounts for brighter red appearance when compared to the adjacent vein. The thicker arterial wall adds slightly to the difference. In the periphery, where the caliber of the vessels is smaller, the color difference is not so apparent. To determine if it is of arterial or venous origin, you may find it necessary to go back to the disc area and follow a vessel to the periphery (Fig. 4.4).

Fig. 4.3 The color, caliber, and width of the light reflection distinguish artery (A) and vein (V). Note the thickness of the artery and vein walls where they are seen on-end (arrow).

Fig. 4.4 Large retinal arteries (A) and veins (V) are easily distinguished, but in smaller peripheral vessels the difference is not so apparent. The caliber of the artery and of the vein and width of the light reflection from each should be noted.

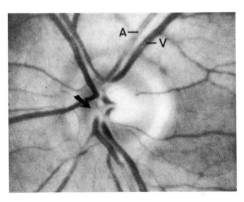

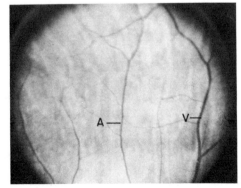

B. CALIBER

Near the disc the lumen (visible blood column) of the central retinal artery is about 100 μ and its wall about 15 μ thick. The adjacent vein has a lumen of 200 μ, and the wall is considerably thinner. In normal patients, the ratio of artery to vein — in diameter — appears clinically to be close to 3:5, and that approximate ratio is maintained throughout the retinal vascular tree. When a vessel is seen "on-end," the substance of its wall is more readily appreciated (Fig. 4.3). The difference between the thickness of the artery and vein walls should be noted carefully, since alterations of vessel caliber by disease are important. Light reflection and transparency of vessels are indirect indicators of vessel caliber.

C. LIGHT REFLECTIONS

The width of the light reflection from the surface of a vessel wall can indicate its thickness, a fact used in assessing blood vessel damage (Fig. 4.5). Though the artery has a smaller visible blood column, its overall diameter may equal a nearby vein. The artery, therefore, presents a flatter external surface to mirror light back to the observer.

D. VESSEL TRANSPARENCY

It's essential from the outset to keep in mind that only the blood column of the retinal arteries and veins is visible under ordinary circumstances. This transparency allows light transmission to the rods and cones under the blood vessels. If this were not the case, we would see a shadow of our own blood vessels all the time. You can see such a shadow or angioscotoma by placing a light to your closed eye in a darkened room.

Vessel transparency is especially important at arteriovenous crossings. The darker blood column of the vein is readily seen through the artery (Fig. 4.6a, b; see 4.6b also in color section). The reverse is also true but not as easily distinguished through the darker venous blood (Fig. 4.6c).

Fig. 4.5 Both tubes have the same internal diameter. Light reflection is wider from the tube with the greater external diameter.

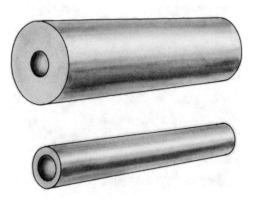

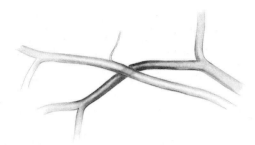

Fig. 4.6 Sketch demonstrates how the dark venous blood shows through the artery at crossings (a, right). The darker blood column of the vein can be seen through the artery (b, below left). Loss of this transparency at crossings is the first evidence of thickening of vessel walls. The arterial blood column is not seen as well through venous blood (c, below right). Fig. 4.6b also shown in color section.

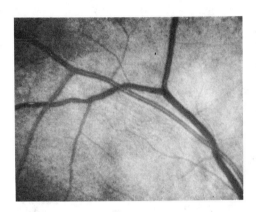

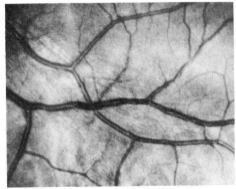

E. COURSE

The temporal retinal vessels arch above and below the fovea (Fig. 4.7a); retinal vessels in general obviously circumvent the foveola (Fig. 4.7b). Variations in vessel branching are common, and it's not unusual to see a major branch of a retinal artery or vein arise from an unexpected source. (Fig. 4.7c). A cilioretinal vessel (see Fig. 3.10) can serve as a major vessel for a retinal quadrant. There are no arteriovenous shunts in the retina. Large capillaries communicate near the ora serrata, but do not cross the ora to anastomose with the ciliary body blood supply.

F. CROSSINGS

Retinal arteries and veins commonly cross each other, but, in a normal eye retinal arteries never cross other retinal arteries, and the same applies to veins. Vessel crossings have been counted in very many patients and found to be more frequent in the superior temporal retinal quadrant, a fact sometimes used to explain pathology in these vessels (Fig. 4.8).

G. CAPILLARIES

The capillary bed is a two-layered meshwork throughout most of the retina. The tighter meshwork layer lies at the level of the inner nuclear layer of the

Fig. 4.7 Rendering from photographs. Note how the temporal vessels arch around the macula (a, right). Retinal vessels do not supply the fovea but course around it; foveal blood supply comes from the choroid (b, below left). Branch of superior temporal artery supplies inferior temporal quadrant in a normal variation (c, below right).

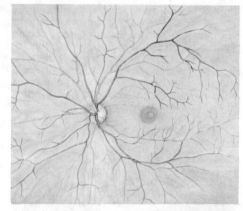

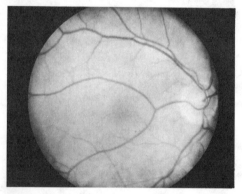

Fig. 4.8 Multiple artery-vein crossings along the superior temporal vessels. Note the difference from the inferior vessels. The patient has diabetic retinopathy.

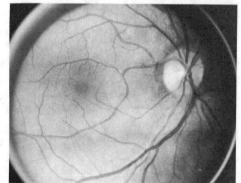

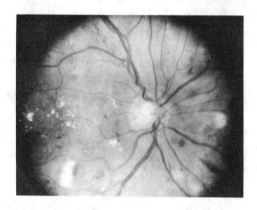

retina, while a slightly looser net is present in the nerve fiber and ganglion cell layer (Fig. 4.9a). A third capillary plexus in the peripapillary retina has a radial orientation in the superficial nerve fiber layer (Fig. 4.9b). These capillaries do not appear to have the intercommunications of the others, a fact considered important in some diseases. In retinal digest preparations, it's possible to see a broad capillary-free zone along retinal arterioles and a

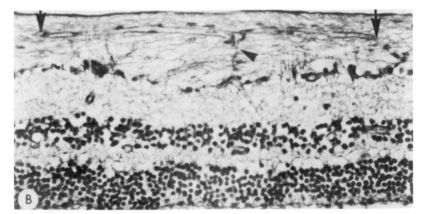

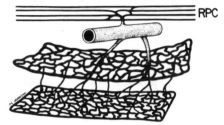

Fig. 4.9 The loose superficial retinal capillaries (arrows) communicate with the deeper capillaries (arrowhead) in the inner nuclear layer (a, above). From Henkind P: New observations on the radial peripapillary capillaries. **Invest Ophthalmol** 6:103, 1967. Used with permission. A third capillary layer, the radial peripapillary capillaries, is present near the disc (b, right). From Henkind P: Microcirculation of the peripapillary retina. **Trans Amer Acad Ophthal Otolaryng** 73:890, 1969. Used with permission.

Fig. 4.10 The capillary bed thins out and stops short of the foveola, leaving a capillary-free zone seen here on fluorescein angiography.

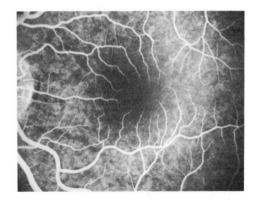

narrow one along the veins. Near the foveola, the two capillary beds described above become one and thin out, leaving a capillary-free zone (Fig. 4.10). The retinal capillaries vary in diameter from 15 to 130μ, putting only the larger ones in the visible range of the ophthalmoscope.

H. AGING

Even histologists don't agree on the differences in retinal vascular changes brought on by aging from those caused by diseases. Ophthalmoscopically, the vessels of older patients may appear no different from those of a much

Fig. 4.11 One of these photographs is of a 75-year-old, the other a 15-year-old. It is difficult to tell them apart, indicating that arteriosclerosis is not due to aging.

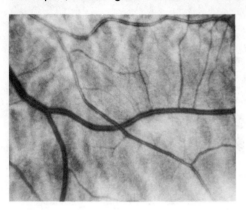 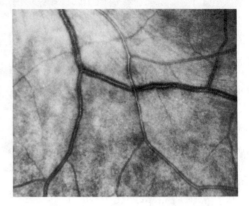

younger person (Fig. 4.11). Collagen in the vascular walls appears to increase with age, and this is accompanied by replacement of smooth muscle by fibrous tissue. The vessels increase in diameter, but there is not always an associated decrease in caliber of the blood column. An increase in width of the light reflex is attributed to the increased diameter. Whether there is lengthening and more vessel curvature with age remains to be proven. Thinning of the neurosensory retina is a result of aging that brings the retinal vessels closer to the retinal pigment epithelium. While often difficult to appreciate — and even more difficult to photograph — the shadow casting of the retinal vessels seen in young patients is less obvious in the elderly.

II. HEMORRHAGE

Escape of blood from its normal intravascular location may be massive or minute. Most hemorrhages come from small vessels; even in severe trauma it's unusual to see disruption of a major branch of the central retinal artery or vein. Hemorrhage is an accident and therefore related to any number of pathologic conditions. In some systemic diseases, retinal hemorrhages are a major diagnostic clue. On the other hand, not all red spots are hemorrhages.

A. CHOROIDAL HEMORRHAGE (see Chapter 7:VF)

B. HEMORRHAGE UNDER THE RETINAL PIGMENT EPITHELIUM
(see Chapter 6:IIID,4)

C. HEMORRHAGE UNDER THE NEUROSENSORY RETINA

(Fig. 4.12; see also in color section)

The source of bleeding may be vessels of retinal or choroidal origin. Subretinal blood is red, in contrast with hemorrhage beneath the retinal pigment epithelium or in the choroid.

Ophthalmoscopic findings

o   Blood is red but may be darker red in areas of greater thickness; where hemolyzed, it is gray-yellow.

o   Retinal blood vessels are visible over the blood and may be elevated over a large hemorrhage; occasionally a retinochoroidal anastomosis is present.

o   Margins of the hemorrhage are smooth.

o   Blood does not move with changes of the patient's position.

o   Neurosensory retina may be elevated, thickened, or cystic over a clot.

o   Blood appears black with red-free light of the ophthalmoscope or on proximal or transillumination.

Symptoms & signs

o   Loss of vision is usually localized to the affected area. It may vary from very poor (hand motion only) if the fovea is involved, to normal if fovea is not involved.

o   Subretinal hemorrhage away from the macula diminishes sensitivity of the overlying retina and gives a scotoma on visual field testing. The patient with a displaced retina experiences distorted images.

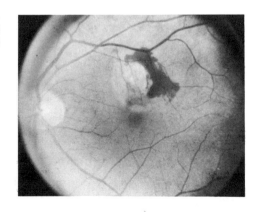

Fig. 4.12 Hemorrhage from neovascularization under the retina. Note that retinal vessels can be seen over the blood. Also shown in color section.

o   Pain and, in some patients, acute glaucoma may occur with a large hemorrhage.

o   Greenish discoloration of the iris, sclera, and vitreous occurs from hemosiderosis in longstanding hemorrhage. Loss of both dark adaptation and color vision accompanies permanent damage to the rods and cones from iron toxicity.

Other confirming findings

o   History and physical evidence of ocular, chest, neck, or abdominal trauma, macular degeneration, hypertension, diabetes mellitus, primary or metastatic choroidal malignancy or inflammation, etc.

o   Physical and laboratory evidence of a disease or treatment with hemorrhagic consequences, such as leukemia and anticoagulation.

o   Fluorescein angiography assists in defining the source and level of the hemorrhage.

o   Ultrasonography defines retinal elevation by large (3 mm) subretinal hemorrhages and helps distinguish blood from tumor or swollen tissue.

Main differential diagnosis

o   Senile macular degeneration

o   Primary or metastatic choroidal malignancy

o   Ocular trauma, including surgery

o   Ocular or orbital inflammation, such as scleritis, histoplasmosis syndrome, toxoplasmosis

o   Myopic degeneration

o   Optic nerve drusen

o   Papilledema

o   Coats's disease

o   Angioid streaks and pseudoxanthoma elasticum

o   Purtscher's disease from crush injuries to the chest, neck, or abdomen

o   Severe Valsalva's maneuver

References

Freeman HM, ed: Ocular Trauma. New York: Appleton-Century-Crofts, 1979, pp 59-60.

Pandolfi M: Intraocular hemorrhages: A hemostatic therapeutic approach. Surv Ophthalmol 22:322, 1978.

Wise GN, Dollery CT, Henkind P: The Retinal Circulation. New York: Harper & Row, 1971, pp 167, 495.

D. HEMORRHAGE IN THE RETINA (Figs. 4.13 - 4.16)

Ophthalmoscopic findings

o   Deep retinal hemorrhages are circular, and superficial ones are linear.

o   Blood vessels may be visible over a deep hemorrhage, but are obscured by a superficial hemorrhage on the nerve fiber layer; the retinal pigment epithelium and choroid are hidden by both.

o   Blood does not move with position changes of the patient or eye.

o   Hemolysis may cause some hazy yellow spots, but most intraretinal blood stays red until its disappearance.

o   Red-free light makes blood look black.

Fig. 4.13 Multiple round hemorrhages in a young diabetic patient.

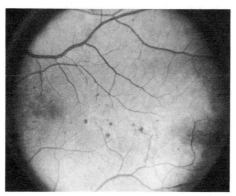

Fig. 4.14 Deep retinal hemorrhage .in the fovea has spread along Henle's layer. Superficial hemorrhage is present near the disc.

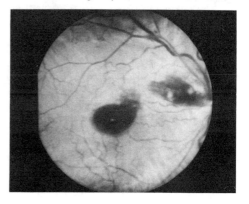

Fig. 4.15 Superficial retinal hemorrhage follows the nerve fiber layer.

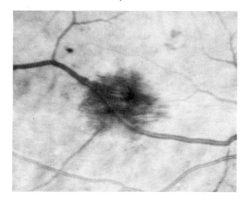

Fig. 4.16 Multiple superficial hemorrhages following the distribution of the nerve fibers.

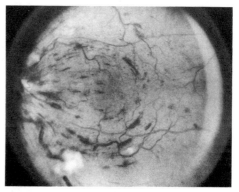

Symptoms & signs

o   Loss of vision may be severe with hemorrhage in the fovea. Hemorrhage is a sign of vascular disease, and the effect on visual acuity is more often related to vascular insufficiency than to hemorrhage alone.

o   Field loss may be localized to the area of hemorrhage, to concomitant vascular disease, or nerve fiber damage.

o   Intraretinal hemorrhage does **not** cause pain and it infrequently displaces the retina, except microscopically.

Other confirming findings

o   History and physical evidence of hematologic, endocrine, vascular, infectious, autoimmune, collagen, and neoplastic disease. Trauma, including birth trauma, carbon monoxide poisoning, decompression, crush injury, and gravitational "red out" must be considered.

o   Family history of retinal vascular disease.

o   Laboratory, radiologic, and other evidence to support a specific diagnosis.

o   Fluorescein angiography assists in defining the source and level of the hemorrhage.

o   Ultrasonography to help analyze large hemorrhages.

Main differential diagnosis

o   Diabetes mellitus

o   Hypertension

o   Retinal vein occlusion

o   Papilledema

o   Embolic disease: arteriosclerotic, infectious, and from injection

o   Trauma

o   Other retinal vascular disorders

o   Retinal tears, posterior vitreous detachment

o   Leukemia

o   Malaria

o   Rickettsial disease (Rocky Mountain spotted fever)

o   Sickle cell disease

o   Juvenile retinoschisis

References

Wise GN, Dollery CT, Henkind P: The Retinal Circulation. New York: Harper & Row, 1971, p 131.

E. HEMORRHAGE NEAR OR ON THE SURFACE OF THE RETINA (Fig. 4.17)

Ophthalmoscopic findings

o Blood may be trapped under the delicate internal limiting membrane of the retina or between the posterior hyaloid (vitreous) face and the retina. In both locations, it often has a fluid level consistent with the patient's position.

o Blood under the internal limiting membrane usually does not move quickly with changes in patient's position, but preretinal blood usually does, if the vitreous is separated from the retina. Blood in this location does not clot.

o Hemolysis gives a smudged, gray-yellow color to the blood, and the hemolyzed blood, too, has a fluid level.

o The overlying vitreous may develop an orange or ocher appearance.

o All retinal and choroidal details are obscured by the blood.

o Retina and disc are obscured by blood on transillumination ophthalmoscopy.

Fig. 4.17 Blood trapped between the vitreous and retina has formed a fluid level and started to hemolyze (arrow).

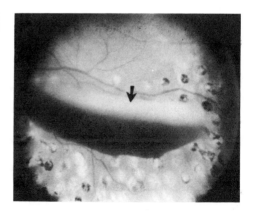

Symptoms & signs

o   Vision is poor if blood covers the macular area. The patient may describe poor vision after lying down that improves on assuming an upright position. The obscuration of vision is black to the patient, not red. If the vitreous is liquid, patient activity may disperse the blood and decrease vision.

o   Shifting scotomata can be found on visual field testing.

o   Hemosiderosis (see IIC, above) may occur.

Other confirming findings

o   History and physical evidence of hematologic, endocrine, vascular, infectious, autoimmune, collagen, and neoplastic disease. Trauma, including birth trauma, carbon monoxide poisoning, decompression, crush injury, and gravitational "red out" must be considered.

o   Family history of retinal vascular disease.

o   Laboratory, radiologic, and other evidence to support a specific diagnosis.

o   Fluorescein angiography assists in defining the source and level of the hemorrhage.

o   Ultrasonography to help localize large hemorrhages.

Main differential diagnosis

o   Diabetes mellitus

o   Hypertension

o   Retinal vein occlusion

o   Papilledema

o   Embolic, arteriosclerotic, and septicemic disease

o   Trauma

o   Other retinal vascular disorders

o   Retinal tears, posterior vitreous detachment

o   Leukemia

o   Malaria

o   Rickettsial disease (Rocky Mountain spotted fever)

o   Sickle cell disease

o   Juvenile retinoschisis

References

Duke-Elder S: System of Ophthalmology, vol 14. St. Louis: Mosby, 1972, p 717.

Walsh FB, Hoyt WF: Clinical Neuro-Ophthalmology, vol 2. Baltimore: Williams & Wilkins, 1969.

Wise GN, Dollery CT, Henkind P: The Retinal Circulation. New York: Harper & Row, 1971.

III. EXUDATE

Lipid and protein deposits under or within the retina, like hemorrhage, may be minute or massive. True exudates need to be distinguished from focal accumulations of leukocytes, retinal infarctions (cotton-wool spots), excrescences at the retinal pigment epithelial level that are dystrophic or degenerative, and hemolyzing blood. True exudate represents vascular decompensation, allowing extravasation and delayed absorption of lipid and protein. Its presence is a nonspecific finding characteristically associated with vascular insufficiency, retinal edema, and tissue death, sometimes remote from the site of exudate deposition.

A. TRUE (HARD) EXUDATES (Figs. 4.18 - 4.20)

Exudates usually deposit along decompensated vessels or surround small areas of capillary insufficiency. The exception is the macular retina. It often accumulates exudate from even remote pathology.

Fig. 4.18 Exudate forms a circle (circinate figure) around an area of retinal ischemia in a diabetic patient (a, left). Two years later, the exudate was gone, leaving the retina atrophic and the vision poor (b, right).

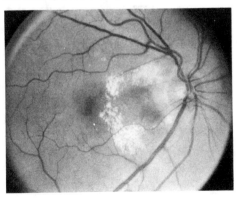
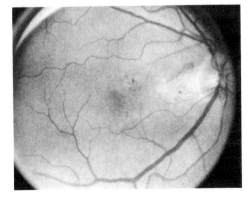

Ophthalmoscopic findings

o Most exudates are deep to the retinal vessels.

o Exudates often surround diseased retina in a circinate (circular) or semicircular pattern.

o In the macula, exudate follows Henle's layer and forms a star-figure (Fig. 4.19).

o Evidence in the retina of arteriosclerosis, diabetes mellitus, hypertension, or other vascular diseases.

o As exudate clears, the margins become blunt and less distinct. In the macula, a white fibrous scar with some pigment hyperplasia often remains. Elsewhere in the retina, there may be no sign of the previous exudate.

o Longstanding subretinal or intraretinal glistening crystals are common. Some may be iridescent and move with eye movement. They are cholesterol crystals and suggest hemorrhage was part of a disease process.

Symptoms & signs

o Central vision is poor if exudate has been deposited in the fovea. The vessel closure or leakage may be remote from the fovea. With foveal exudate, vision is rarely better than 6/12 (20/40).

o Peripheral field loss is associated with vascular occlusion. In Coats's disease, this loss may be in the extreme periphery.

Fig. 4.19 Exudate along a temporarily occluded retinal artery. A star-figure is present in the macula remote from the injured artery (arrow).

Fig. 4.20 Subretinal exudate nasal to the disc in a 59-year-old male with macular degeneration. The brighter central exudate has become crystalline and glistening.

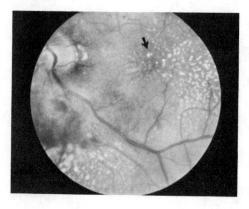
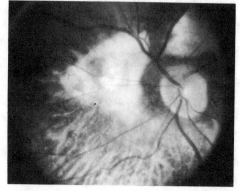

o   Pupil reactions are often abnormal in those patients suffering from longstanding diabetes mellitus and in those patients with exudative maculopathy.

o   Exudation rarely is associated with pain, except in end-stage disease when retinal detachment, secondary glaucoma, and phthisis bulbi ensue.

Other confirming findings

o   History and physical evidence of diabetes mellitus, arteriosclerosis, hypertension, or other vascular disease. The family history of vascular disease should not be overlooked.

o   Laboratory, angiographic, or radionuclear confirming evidence of the above diseases.

o   Fluorescein angiography of the retinal vasculature helps define the decompensated or occluded vessels.

Main differential diagnosis

o   Diabetes mellitus

o   Arteriosclerosis with retinal vascular occlusion or insufficiency

o   Hypertension with retinal vascular occlusion or insufficiency

o   Von Hippel-Lindau disease

o   Leber's miliary aneurysms

o   Macroaneurysms of retina

o   Coats's disease

o   Familial exudative retinopathy

o   Other causes of retinal vascular decompensation, such as sickle cell disease

o   False exudates

References

Leinfelder PJ: Ophthalmoscopy: An investigative challenge. Am J Ophthalmol 61:1211, 1966.

Little HL, Sacks A, Vassiliadis A, et al: Current concepts on pathogenesis of diabetic retinopathy: A dysproteinemia. Trans Am Ophthalmol Soc 75:397, 1977.

Wise GN, Dollery CT, Henkind P: The Retinal Circulation. New York: Harper & Row, 1971, p 131.

B. FALSE EXUDATES (Figs. 4.21 - 4.26; see 4.25 also in color section)

Everything white or yellow seen with the ophthalmoscope is not extravasated lipoprotein, even though it may be associated with vascular decompensation.

Ophthalmoscopic findings

o Cotton-wool (soft exudate) infarcts result in swelling of the ganglion cells and opacification of the retina. Arterioles or arteriolar capillaries are invariably closed or show segmentation. These infarcts are most common in the superficial peripapillary plexus because they do not anastomose as do deeper capillaries.

o Accumulations of leukocytes around the disc often cannot be distinguished from cotton-wool infarcts. When they are peripheral or associated with old scars or vascular disturbances, the distinction may be possible.

o Hemolyzed blood may resemble true exudate. When it is seen without an accompanying hemorrhage, the distinction is impossible.

o Multiple white or yellow-white defects or deposits in the retinal pigment epithelium do not form the typical star-figure pattern of exudates in the macula. Their deep location is unassociated with retinal vascular disturbance early in the disease.

o Superficial myelinated nerve fibers away from the disc have a characteristic striation and feathery distal border.

Fig. 4.21 A cotton-wool (soft exudate), or retinal, infarction in a young man with hypertension. Note the location in the superficial prepapillary capillaries and the indistinct margins.

Fig. 4.22 An old retinal and choroidal scar that exposes the sclera should not be confused with exudate. The patient had toxoplasmosis.

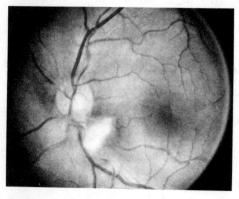

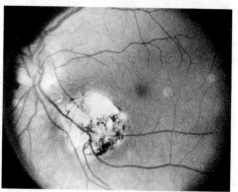

Symptoms & signs

o Cotton-wool infarcts do not involve the fovea, since it is a capillary-free zone. Scotomata associated with capillary occlusions usually are in the peripapillary plexus.

o Septic emboli may lodge anywhere. When the macular arcades, papillomacular bundle, or disc are involved, visual loss is often severe.

o Blood in the macula causes severe visual loss.

o Multiple drusen or other retinal pigment epithelial defects may or may not disrupt function of the overlying neurosensory retina. Vision varies with adequacy of retinal nutrition.

Fig. 4.23 Septic embolus in a patient with bacteremia. Note the vascular tortuosity and the small yellow true exudates also present.

Fig. 4.24 Blood under the retinal pigment epithelium (small arrows) and the neurosensory retina (large arrow). The subretinal blood has started to hemolyze (white area).

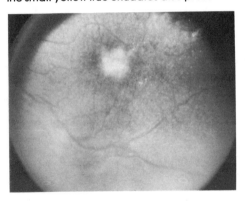

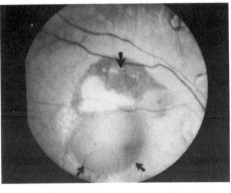

Fig. 4.25 Drusen in the retinal pigment epithelium do not take the star-figure configuration of exudate in Henle's layer. Also shown in color section.

Fig. 4.26 The fine striations of myelin along the nerve fibers, even away from the disc, make them distinct from exudate. No other abnormality is present to suggest disease.

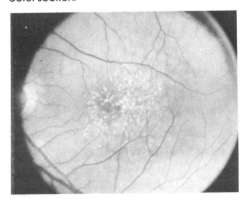

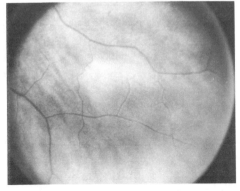

o   A scotoma may be plotted on visual field testing when myelinated fibers are present, but it's relative and often absent altogether. Field defects are present with retinal infarcts, vascular occlusions, septic emboli, or hemorrhage. The patient may describe a blind spot or distortion.

o   If the macula has been damaged, the pupil may be dilated and give a poor consensual response to the other eye.

Other confirming findings

o   History and physical evidence of diabetes mellitus, arteriosclerosis, hypertension, or other vascular disease, including sepsis, leukemia, or rickettsial infection.

o   Laboratory, radiologic, radionuclear, and biopsy evidence to support the above diagnoses.

o   Fluorescein angiography of the retina.

Main differential diagnosis

o   Diabetes mellitus

o   Hypertension

o   Arteriosclerosis and embolism

o   True exudates, as described above

o   Trauma

o   Retinochoroiditis

o   Solar, photocoagulation, or diathermy burns

o   Other vascular disease, such as periarteritis

References

Jampol LM, Goldberg MF, Busse B: Peripheral retinal microaneurysms in chronic leukemia. Am J Ophthalmol 80:242, 1975.

Klien BA: Comments on the cotton-wool lesion of the retina. Am J Ophthalmol 59:17, 1965.

Wise GN, Dollery CT, Henkind P: The Retinal Circulation. New York: Harper & Row, 1971.

IV. BLOOD VESSEL WALLS

We base many of our judgments about blood vessel walls on alterations in the appearance of the visible blood column. The vessel walls themselves are nearly invisible (see Fig. 4.3). Hemorrhage and exudation, described above, are manifestations of poor perfusion of the vascular bed; they are rarely isolated findings. Similarly, the vascular wall diseases rarely occur alone. They are isolated here solely for clarity.

A. LOSS OF VESSEL TRANSPARENCY (THICKENING, SHEATHING, AND EDEMA)

Decreased light transmission through vessel walls usually, but not always, is related to an increase in thickness. You can judge that there is opacification of vessel walls if adjacent tissues or the vessel blood column are hidden from view. Some information may be derived from increased light reflection from the vessel surface. Increased thickness of the wall of a tube does not necessarily mean the internal diameter is decreased, but this is often the case in diseases affecting retinal vessels. This effect may be both focal and generalized. Years of observation by many observers indicate the condition of retinal vessel walls to be a good clinical estimate of vessels of similar caliber in other organs.

1. Arteriosclerosis

Ophthalmoscopic findings

o Hiding of venous blood by a crossing artery (Fig. 4.27a; see also in color section; compare with Fig. 4.6b).

o Nicking occurs at arteriovenous crossings where thickening of the artery wall hides the blood column of the vein (Fig. 4.28). Where artery and vein run side by side, the vein is often masked (Fig. 4.27b; see also in color section).

o Burnishing (polishing) of the arteries, as the thicker walls reflect more light.

o Arterial walls may become opaque, hiding the blood column completely and resembling silver wires in the retina (see Fig. 4.68).

Fig. 4.27 Earliest sign of arteriolar wall thickening is a loss of transparency hiding the venous blood column at crossings (arrow, a, left). When an artery and vein run side by side (see just below the disc) the same hiding occurs (b, right). Also shown in color section.

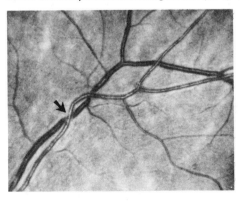
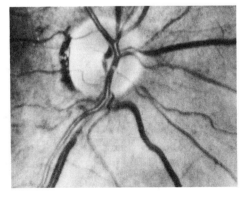

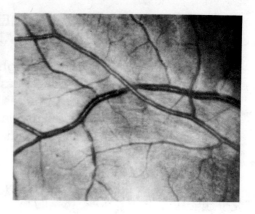

Fig. 4.28 The arterial light reflection is widened and the underlying vein is hidden on either side of the crossing artery (nicking) and cannot be seen through the arterial blood column.

o All the above findings may be seen in the same patient in advanced disease. See Table 4.1 for a clinical grading system for arteriosclerosis.

o Ophthalmoscopic findings need to be related to the patient's age.

o Sheathing (cuffing) of vessels, often localized, frequently in the peripheral retina, may be associated with angulation of vessels and usually does not affect the blood column (Figs. 4.29 - 4.31; see 4.31 also in color section). By definition it consists of a visible coating on the vessels rather than a change in the wall. It's more commonly seen on veins and in the inferior retina.

o Edema of vessel walls hides and often narrows the blood columns, giving the vessel a segmented appearance. The appearance may resemble multiple emboli, but in most embolic diseases, more than one or two emboli in the same vessel is rare (Fig. 4.32).

Symptoms & signs

o Visual loss associated with vessel wall changes occurs only with interruption of blood flow. This interruption may be permanent or temporary. The retina, being of neural origin, is vulnerable to even transient ischemia. Vascular occlusions are considered in VB, below. Probably chronic retinal ischemia is a significant factor in some maculopathies (see Chapter 5:IVB, 3b).

o Visual loss from vascular occlusion may be total — no light perception — or a localized scotoma (see VB, below).

o Pupil reactions to light are normal, unless there are large areas of retinal or optic nerve infarction. The pupil response to light directed into a seeing area may differ from the response to light directed into a nonseeing area.

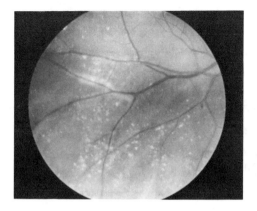

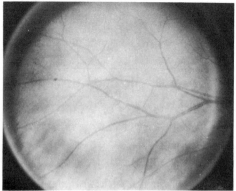

Fig. 4.29 Sheathing of peripheral retinal vessels and exudate (a, above left) in a 39-year-old white female cleared in six months (b, above right). A small A/V shunt (arrow) was present peripherally (c, right).

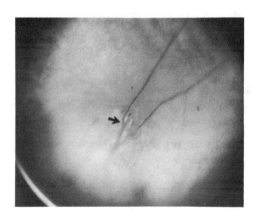

Fig. 4.30 Venous sheathing in a patient with longstanding diabetes mellitus (arrow). Note that the blood column is not narrowed.

Fig. 4.31 Venous sheathing in a patient with possible sarcoidosis. Appearance is sometimes described as candle-wax drippings. Also shown in color section.

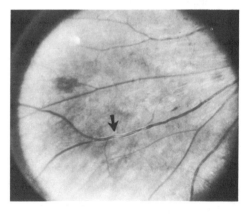

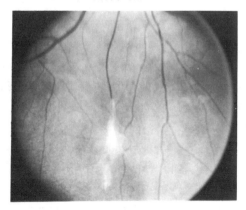

o Sheathing is often associated with acute inflammatory responses in the vitreous. The patient may have photophobia, ocular pain, floaters, miosis, ciliary flush, and glaucoma.

Other confirming findings

o History and/or physical evidence of arteriosclerotic heart, carotid, aortic, or peripheral vascular disease, including acute abdominal pain. The presence of hypertension, diabetes, collagen, and other vascular diseases contributing to vessel wall thickening needs to be considered.

o Other ocular evidence to be correlated include xanthelasma and arcus senilis.

o Physical examination for carotid, aortic, cardiac, cerebral, and other areas of poor vascular function are necessary. Collagen disease study, including lupus erythematosus preparations, antinuclear antibody, VDRL titers, cholesterol levels, and muscle biopsy may be of value.

o Vitreous or uveal biopsy in severe ocular inflammatory disease with vascular cuffing has yet to be found of proven value.

Main differential diagnosis

o Arteriosclerosis, including carotid artery occlusion

o Hypertension of all types

o Diabetes mellitus

Table 4.1

CLINICAL CLASSIFICATION
OF ARTERIOSCLEROTIC RETINOPATHY

Grade I	Hiding of blood column at arteriovenous crossings or side by side overlapping; wide light reflection
Grade II	Hiding plus nicking, banking, and masking of adjacent vessels and tissues; wide light reflection
Grade III	All of above plus nearly complete hiding of arterial blood column by light reflection — copper-wire effect
Grade IV	All of above plus complete hiding of blood column — silver-wire effect

PHYSICIANS' GUIDE TO OCULOSYSTEMIC DISEASES

Fig. 4.32 Acute necrotizing vasculitis in left eye of a 54-year-old white female with collagen disease, uveitis, arthritis, cataracts, heart disease, and hypertension. Photograph for Fig. 4.32a (left) was taken on routine examination five weeks before photograph for Fig. 4.32b (right). The opacities are in the walls of arterioles. They disappeared in one month on steroids. Compare with Fig. 4.47.

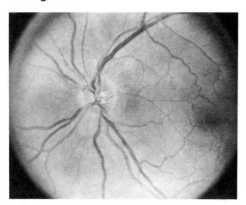 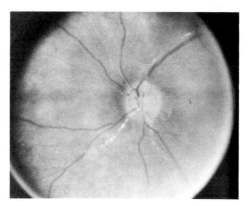

o Embolic disease — infectious, traumatic, and arteriosclerotic

o Coats's disease

o Collagen disease, periarteritis, necrotizing angiitis

o Sarcoidosis

o Macroaneurysms of retinal arteries

o Behcet's syndrome

o Leber's miliary aneurysms

o Arteriovenous shunts of unknown cause

o Von Hippel-Lindau disease

o Juvenile retinoschisis

o Leukemia

References

Michelson EL, Morganroth J, Nichols CW, et al: Retinal arteriolar changes as an indicator of coronary artery disease. Arch Intern Med 139:1139, 1979.

Wise GN, Dollery CT, Henkind P: The Retinal Circulation. New York: Harper & Row, 1971.

2. Hypertension (see VA, below)

3. Necrotizing angiitis (collagen disease) (see VA, below)

B. LOCALIZED INCREASES IN VESSEL SIZE

Important changes may be in the large rather than the narrow vessels. Vessel narrowing is considered in VA, below. Local retinal vessel dilatation is described here.

1. Angiomatosis retinae (von Hippel-Lindau disease)
(Figs. 4.33 - 4.35)

Ophthalmoscopic findings

o Characteristic finding is a dilated artery and vein from the vessels at or near the disc to a peripheral red or white, slightly elevated lesion. Vessels join only at an angioma.

o The tumors may be multiple in the same or both eyes.

o Tumors may be different sizes and often are subtle.

o Both eyes are affected in 50 percent of patients when first seen, and eventually both eyes are affected in nearly all patients.

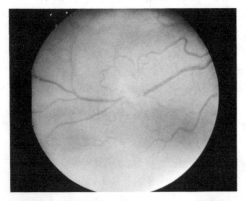
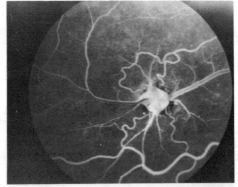
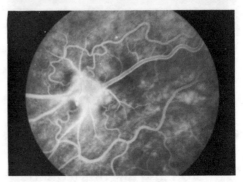

Fig. 4.33 Subtle retinal angioma in a 20-year-old female with angiomatosis retinae (a, above left). Intravenous fluorescein confirms the rapid arteriovenous shunting through the tumor (b, above right) and its "leaky" nature (c, right).

o Exudates, retinal edema, and hemorrhage may surround the tumors and reach the macula.

o Retina may be detached in late stages, and eye may have a dense cataract blocking a view.

o Tumors at the disc may obscure the short, deep, large vessels. You may see vessels resembling neovascularization on the disc (see Fig. 3.35).

o Following treatment with photocoagulation or cryotherapy and occasionally after spontaneous closure, the large vessels atrophy and exudation stops.

o Papilledema may occur in acute central nervous system tumor growth or hemorrhage.

Symptoms & signs

o Loss of vision is variable. Among its causes, the most frequent are exudates or edema in the macula. It's caused less frequently by retinal detachment and only occasionally by hemorrhage. In longstanding disease, cataract may be present, accompanied by retinal detachment and even phthisis bulbi.

o Dilated pupil associated with loss of vision and loss of visual field from retinal detachment, exudation, or hemorrhage.

o Ocular pain is rare, except in late stages of disease with beginning phthisis bulbi.

o Presenting symptoms may be due to ocular or central nervous system disease (Lindau's description). Angiomas involve the cerebellum, medulla, or spinal cord and may run the whole gamut from ataxia to paralysis and collapse. Headache, nausea, and vomiting are common in the acute central nervous system disease.

Other confirming findings

o Dominantly inherited disease without sex prediction; 50 percent have both eyes affected when first seen.

o Onset is usually before age 30, but rarely before age 10.

o Cysts or tumors of the pancreas, kidney, adrenals, or epididymis may occur. No skin lesions.

o Radiographic evidence, including angiographic findings of central nervous system tumors.

o Fluorescein angiographic confirmation of the retinal disease.

Fig. 4.34 Another peripheral angioma in the same patient seen in Fig. 4.33 before (a, left) and after (b, right) cryotherapy. The characteristic large artery and vein are markedly reduced after treatment.

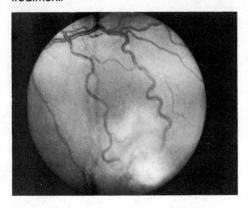 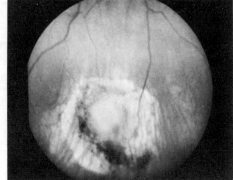

Fig. 4.35 Angiomatosis retinae at the edge of the disc has very short dilated arteries and veins hidden from view by the tumor.

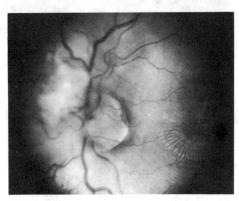

Main differential diagnosis

o Retinoblastoma

o Coats's disease

o Leber's miliary aneurysms

o Cirsoid arteriovenous malformation

o Retinal macroaneurysm

o Toxocara canis

o Cavernous hemangioma of retina

o Sickle cell retinopathy

o Choroidal hemangioma

o Poikiloderma

References

Walsh FB, Hoyt WF: Clinical Neuro-Ophthalmology, vol 2. Baltimore: Williams & Wilkins, 1969.

Wise GN, Dollery CT, Henkind P: The Retinal Circulation. New York: Harper & Row, 1971.

2. Coats's disease (Leber's miliary aneurysms)
(Fig. 4.36; see 4.36a and 4.36b also in color section)

This sporadic retinal vascular disease in children and young adults is thought to be due to an embryonal rest activated by growth hormone.

Ophthalmoscopic findings

o Massive exudation involving the macula is common.

o Almost always involves one eye only, with perhaps a slight predilection for the left.

o Tortuous, knobby vessels with arteriovenous shunts mostly in the retinal periphery. Vessels are often sausage-like and involve one quadrant more than others, although often the whole peripheral vasculature has some abnormality.

o Edema around the abnormal vessels may extend to the macula, and localized intraretinal hemorrhage may be seen.

o Knobby retinal elevation, with mounds of yellow and sometimes crystalline exudate that float in the subretinal space.

o Vitreous may have a hazy greenish discoloration.

Symptoms & signs

o Painless loss of vision detected on routine vision examination may vary from 6/60 (20/200) to counting fingers.

o Pupil dilatation or a white pupil reflex is an occasional complaint.

o Ocular pain, greenish discoloration of the iris, and hemorrhagic glaucoma in end-stage disease may be associated with a cataract that blocks a view of the retina.

Other confirming findings

o Four times more common in males than females.

o Four times more often unilateral than bilateral.

o Discovery may be at birth, but usually between ages four and 16 years.

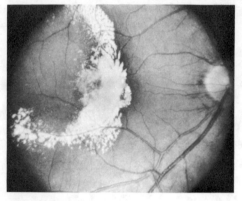

Fig. 4.36a

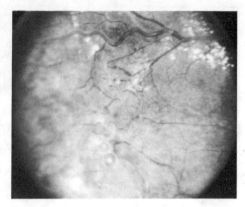

Fig. 4.36b

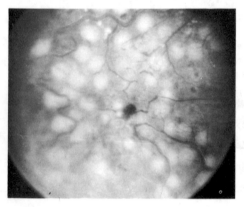

Fig. 4.36c

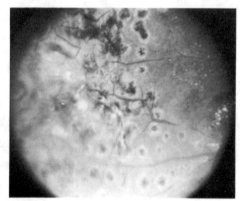

Fig. 4.36d

Fig. 4.36 Coats's disease in a 20-year-old male (a). Visual acuity was reduced to counting fingers at 1 meter. The peripheral aneurysms (b) were treated with photocoagulation (c, immediately after treatment) and disappeared six months later (d). Macular exudate gradually disappeared (e), but vision returned only to 6/60 (20/200). Fig. 4.36a and 4.36b also shown in color section.

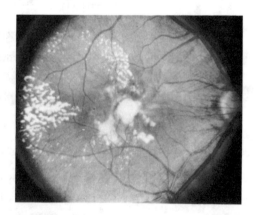

Fig. 4.36e

o Family history is rarely positive for similar disease, but there occasionally is family history of muscular dystrophy.

o Fluorescein angiography defines the abnormal vasculature.

o Ultrasonography is helpful if no view of retina is possible.

Main differential diagnosis

o Sickle cell disease

o Retinoblastoma

o Angiomatosis retinae (von Hippel-Lindau disease)

o Toxocara canis and other parasites

o Diabetic retinopathy

o Choroidal rupture (trauma)

o Persistent hyperplastic posterior vitreous

o Retinal artery and/or vein occlusion

o Cavernous hemangioma of the retina

o Poikiloderma

References

Coats G: Forms of retinal disease with massive exudation. Ophthalmol Hosp Rep 17:440, 1908.

Wise GN, Dollery CT, Henkind P: The Retinal Circulation. New York: Harper & Row, 1971.

Wise GN, Horava A: Coats's disease. Am J Ophthalmol 56(1):17, 1963.

3. Retinal macroaneurysms (Fig. 4.37)

Ophthalmoscopic findings

o Macroaneurysms are usually single and may be saccular or fusiform. The arteriolar and venous abnormalities seem to be confined to one pair of vessels in a localized spot.

o The abnormality comes to attention when it's in the posterior part of the eye; aneurysms may occur more peripherally.

o Exudation around aneurysms has a circinate (circular) pattern; separate exudate may involve the macula.

o Small intraretinal hemorrhages may be present, and in some patients, severe intravitreal hemorrhage obscures all details.

Fig. 4.37 Isolated macroaneurysm of the retina (arrow) in a 52-year-old white female with previously normal vision (a, left). With intravenous fluorescein, the aneurysmal nature of lesion is better defined and demonstrates the sluggish blood flow in the aneurysm (b, right).

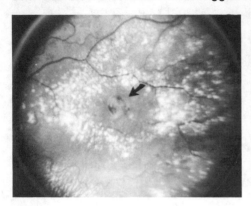 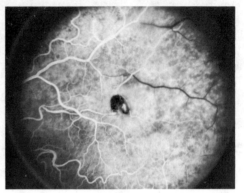

o   Hypertensive and arteriosclerotic retinopathy are often present.

o   Severe subretinal hemorrhage may cause a smooth, dark retinal detachment.

Symptoms & signs

o   Visual loss may be mild to severe and is related to the degree of exudation and proximity of the aneurysms to the macula.

o   Pupil dilatation and scotomata are related to degree of visual loss.

o   Pain is a rare complaint, except in end-stage disease associated with severe hemorrhage or in rare subretinal pigment epithelial hemorrhage of sudden onset. This pain is transient and usually due to elevated intraocular pressure. The anterior chamber may be flat.

Other confirming findings

o   Retinal macroaneurysms occur most often in middle- to older-age hypertensive females.

o   They are usually unilateral.

o   No hereditary pattern has been established.

Main differential diagnosis

o   Coats's disease

o   Diabetic retinopathy

o   Retinal artery and/or vein occlusion

o   Angiomatosis retinae (von Hippel-Lindau disease)

o   Cavernous hemangioma of the retina

o   Sickle cell retinopathy

o   Poikiloderma

References

Cleary PE, Kohner EM, Hamilton AM, et al: Retinal macroaneurysms. Br J Ophthalmol 59:355, 1975.

Gold DH, LaPiana FG, Zimmerman LE: Isolated retinal arterial aneurysms. Am J Ophthalmol 82:848, 1976.

Lewis RA, Norton EWD, Gass JDM: Acquired arterial macroaneurysms of the retina. Br J Ophthalmol 60:21, 1976.

Wise GN, Dollery CT, Henkind P: The Retinal Circulation. New York: Harper & Row, 1971.

4. Diabetic retinopathy (see VIIA, below)

5. Cirsoid (racemose) arteriovenous malformation (Wyburn-Mason disease) (Fig. 4.38)

This dominantly inherited disease has serious central nervous system and cardiovascular complications.

Ophthalmoscopic findings

o   Large, dilated, tortuous retinal vessels, usually arising from or consisting of major retinal vessels.

o   Rarely involves the macula.

o   May be difficult to tell the artery from the vein.

Fig. 4.38 Cirsoid (racemose) arteriovenous anastomosis unchanged for years and without symptoms.

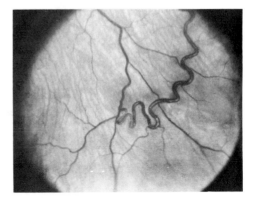

o Vessels may be of irregular caliber.

o Normal vessels seem to branch from the dilated, abnormal vessels.

o Vessels may involve one or more quadrants and the optic disc.

o No exudate or hemorrhage, and condition remains unchanged for years.

Symptoms & signs

o Usually no ocular symptoms; often the disease is discovered as an incidental finding. Double vision and ptosis occur if oculomotor palsy is part of the disease.

o Rarely is the vision reduced, even when the vessels are close to the macula.

o Central nervous system symptoms include oculomotor palsy, hemiplegia, seizures, and ataxia.

Other confirming findings

o Almost always unilateral.

o Family history of similar findings is usually present.

o Fluorescein angiography confirms the arteriovenous anastomosis.

o Arteriography and computerized tomography demonstrate vascular malformation in the orbit, sylvian fissure, or midbrain in 75 percent of patients.

Main differential diagnosis

o Angiomatosis retinae (von Hippel-Lindau disease)

o Retinoblastoma

o Arteriovenous retinal anastomosis (trauma)

o Chorioretinal anastomosis (trauma)

o Opticociliary shunts

References

Geeraets WJ: Ocular Syndromes. Philadelphia: Lea & Febiger, 1976.

Rosen E: Vascular malformations in the human retina. Am J Ophthalmol 67:501, 1969.

Walsh FB, Hoyt WF: Clinical Neuro-Ophthalmology, vol 3. Baltimore: Williams & Wilkins, 1969.

Wise GN, Dollery CT, Henkind P: The Retinal Circulation. New York: Harper & Row, 1971.

6. Cavernous hemangioma of retina (Fig. 4.39)

This subtle vascular abnormality is easily overlooked.

Ophthalmoscopic findings

o Red, blotchy cluster of flat saccular red vessels, sometimes with fluid levels between red cells and plasma that seem to be independent of adjacent vessels.

o Vessels remain unchanged for years.

o Vessels rarely leak plasma and even more rarely bleed.

Symptoms & signs

o Plasma or hemorrhage into the vitreous or on the retinal surface affects vision. This usually clears spontaneously within one to two weeks.

o Cavernous hemangiomas of the prerolandic cerebral cortex may occasionally cause neurologic symptoms and seizures.

Other confirming findings

o Rare hereditary history.

o Skin hemangiomas may be present.

o Fluorescein angiography has a characteristic appearance.

o Angiography is necessary to confirm central nervous system lesions (may not be indicated without symptoms).

Fig. 4.39 Cavernous hemangioma of the retina (arrow, a, left). Intravenous fluorescein indicates blood flow is very poor in the hemangioma. Transudation may interfere with vision (b, right).

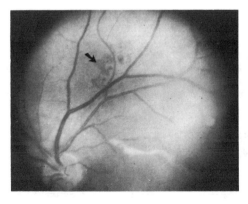 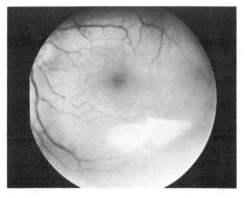

Main differential diagnosis

o Leber's miliary aneurysms, retinal macroaneurysms, and Coats's disease

o Von Hippel-Lindau disease

o Cirsoid (racemose) malformation

o Chorioretinal anastomosis (trauma)

References

Gass JDM: Stereoscopic Atlas of Macular Diseases. St. Louis: Mosby, 1977.

Rosen E: Vascular malformation in the human retina. Am J Ophthalmol 67:501, 1969.

Wise GN, Dollery CT, Henkind P: The Retinal Circulation. New York: Harper & Row, 1971.

7. Poikiloderma (Rothmund-Thomson syndrome) (see Fig. 4.36)

This rare skin disease starts between the third and sixth month of life. Skin telangiectasis, pigmentation, and hypopigmentation are inherited in 70 percent of patients. Females are more commonly affected. Cataracts occur in 52 percent of patients. There have been reports of dilated peripheral retinal vessels resembling those seen in Coats's disease.

References

Silver HK: Rothmund-Thomson syndrome: An oculocutaneous disorder. Am J Dis Child 3:182, 1966.

Tasman W: Retinal changes in congenital poikiloderma. Am J Ophthalmol 72:979, 1971.

Table 4.2

CLINICAL CLASSIFICATION OF HYPERTENSIVE RETINOPATHY

Grade I	Mild arteriovenous crossing, overlap, and light reflection changes unexpected for the patient's age
Grade II	More advanced arteriovenous crossing, overlap, and light reflection changes unexpected for patient's age
Grade III	Above, plus local and generalized arteriolar narrowing, splinter hemorrhages, cotton-wool infarcts
Grade IV	Above, plus disc edema

V. TOO LITTLE BLOOD

Attention is directed here to diseases from the aortic arch, carotid, and the retinal vessels. Failure to adequately perfuse the retina may accompany central nervous system ischemia with its attendant symptoms. None of the ophthalmoscopic findings stand alone. They are isolated here for clarity.

A. VESSEL NARROWING (HYPERTENSION)
(Figs. 4.40 - 4.47; see 4.42 - 4.45 and 4.47 also in color section)

Retinal vessel narrowing follows decreased vascular demand in retinitis pigmentosa or following panretinal photocoagulation for diabetic reti-nopathy (see Fig. 4.78). Here we are concerned with intrinsic blood and vascular disease associated with narrowing of the blood column.

Ophthalmoscopic findings

o   Mild generalized artery narrowing is subtle. Comparison with the other eye or known normal eyes is essential. Poor arterial perfusion means less venous return, so veins are narrow, too, and the usual artery-vein comparison is not helpful.

o   Focal narrowing is often present at the same time.

o   Artery-vein crossing changes are more advanced than expected for the patient's age.

o   Splinter hemorrhages, cotton-wool infarcts, and retinal edema hiding or smudging the view of the retinal pigment may be present.

o   The findings may be unilateral in aortic arch, carotid, or central retinal artery insufficiency, but are bilateral in hypertension. A useful clinical grading system for hypertension is given in Table 4.2.

o   Ophthalmodynamometry requires comparison between two eyes. The differences of 30-50 percent in diastolic and 20-40 percent in systolic are considered evidence of decreased flow.

Symptoms & signs

o   Visual acuity may be normal. Transient loss of vision in one eye may follow getting up from a lying or sitting position in optic nerve ischemia, and in carotid and aortic arch disease. Episodes usually last 10-15 seconds.

o   Transient visual loss may be altitudinal or central and occasionally hemianopic in vertebral-basilar artery insufficiency.

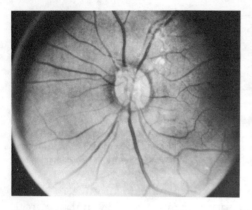

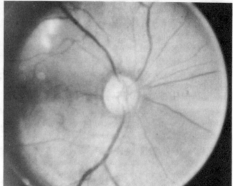

Fig. 4.40 Generalized arterial narrowing in both eyes in a patient with progressive carotid artery stenosis. Vessels of the left eye (a, above left) were less affected than the right (b, above right), which went on to extreme narrowing and poor vision in five months (c, right). The hazy photograph was due to protein transudate in the aqueous. Note the absence of hemorrhage, edema, exudate. Both veins and arteries are narrowed.

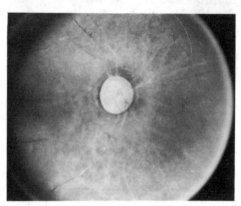

Fig. 4.42 Advanced hypertensive retinopathy (Grade IV) with focal and generalized arteriolar narrowing, exudates, hemorrhages, and retinal and disc edema in a 65-year-old male. Blood pressure was 210/150 mm Hg. Also shown in color section.

Fig. 4.41 Early hypertensive retinopathy with generalized and focal (arrow) arteriolar narrowing.

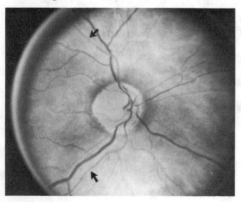

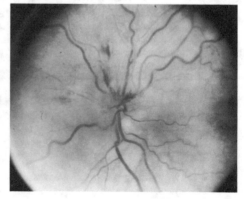

- Patients may describe visual defect as only a shading of their vision rather than loss. In some patients the defect may be the total inability to see light.

- Pupil reactions are usually normal, unless severe visual loss or rubeosis iridis occurs.

- Scotomata may be present if local retinal (cotton-wool) infarctions are present.

- Iris atrophy, rubeosis of the iris with poor pupil reaction to light, hyphema, glaucoma, and cataract may accompany carotid occlusion.

Other confirming findings

- Historical, familial, and physical evidence of aortic, carotid, vertebral-basilar, hypertensive, collagen, and other vascular disease.

- Malignant hypertensive retinopathy is usually associated with a diastolic blood pressure of 125 mm Hg or more.

- Carotid insufficiency is sometimes accompanied by symptoms of mental confusion and transient unconsciousness. Carotid bruit frequently means 50 percent stenosis. There may be absence of preauricular pulse, coolness of skin, and even hair loss on the affected side. The patient may experience lightheadedness on getting up from a lying or sitting position or on turning his head suddenly. Vertebral-basilar artery insufficiency may be accompanied by severe vertigo. Angiography, Doppler ultrasonography, and radioactive scanning are diagnostic aids.

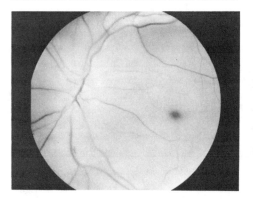

Fig. 4.43 Central retinal artery occlusion with retinal edema. The choroidal blood supply to the fovea is intact. Also shown in color section.

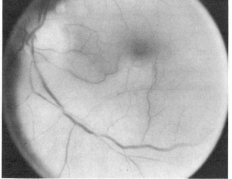

Fig. 4.44 Occlusion of a branch of the central retinal artery. Note that only the lower half of the macula is infarcted. Visual acuity was counting fingers in the lower field. Also shown in color section.

Fig. 4.45 Occlusion of the central retinal artery that did not result in total blindness because a cilioretinal artery spared the macula, while the rest of the retina lost transparency. Visual acuity was 6/15 (20/50). Also shown in color section.

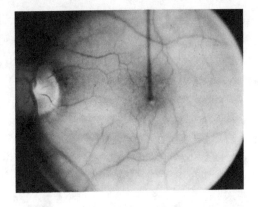

Fig. 4.47 Even in arterial occlusion, red blood cells still can be seen in the vessel lumen. The blood column may be segmented and move to and fro with the pulse. Visual acuity was hand motion temporally. Also shown in color section.

Fig. 4.46 Occlusion of a double cilioretinal artery nasal to the disc in a 30-year-old white male with hypertension. Visual acuity was 6/6 (20/20).

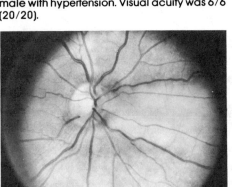

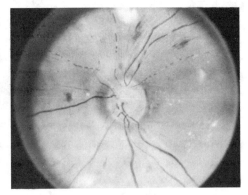

o   High sedimentation rate and positive temporal artery biopsy in giant cell arteritis. Other laboratory evidence of vascular, hematologic, and collagen disease.

o   Fluorescein angiography for confirmation of retinal and choroidal blood-flow patterns.

o   Electroretinogram and visually evoked potentials.

Main differential diagnosis

o   Hypertension (all causes)

o   Giant cell (temporal) arteritis

o   Chorioretinal scarring, optic nerve disease that decreases blood-flow requirements in part or all of an eye, such as retinitis pigmentosa, optic atrophy, glaucoma, toxoplasmosis scarring, trauma, photocoagulation

o   Carotid and/or vertebral-basilar artery insufficiency

o   Embolic disease (all causes)

o   Collagen diseases, necrotizing angiitis

o   Pulseless disease (Takayasu's disease, syphilitic aortitis)

o   Behcet's disease

References

Harnish A, Pearce ML: Evolution of hypertensive retinal vascular disease: Correlation between clinical and postmortem observations. Medicine 52:483, 1973.

Wise GN, Dollery CT, Henkind P: The Retinal Circulation. New York: Harper & Row, 1971.

B. ARTERIAL OCCLUSION (Figs. 4.48 - 4.51; see 4.48 and 4.49 also in color section)

Occlusion of major retinal arteries may be transient or permanent. Often the occlusion is transient (a passing embolus), but its effects are permanent. The effects of vascular occlusion and the recovery from it are easily observed in the eye.

Ophthalmoscopic findings

o   The retina in the distribution of the occluded artery is gray-white, opaque, and readily visible. This may be the whole central retinal artery or a branch. In some cases, a cilioretinal artery supplies the macula, but this artery, too, may be occluded. The gray retinal color is less noticeable peripherally. The foveola retains its normal color, because its blood supply is choroidal.

o   Small hemorrhages, usually superficial (splinter) may be present, but are sparse. There may be cotton-wool infarcts near the disc.

o   The occluded artery may have reopened by the time you see the patient, but you'll probably recognize a thread-like quality to it in comparison to similar branches in the same or other eye. If it remains closed there is segmentation (boxcarring) of the blood column and there may be to and fro movement of the blood with the pulse.

o   Emboli may be visible in the lumen. They are usually lodged at vessel bifurcations. The embolus is often distal to the point of occlusion, having moved on after the initial spasm. The emboli may be crystalline or

Fig. 4.48 Embolism to the superior temporal artery (arrow, a, left). Fluorescein injected intravenously has started to fill the proximal branches of the vein before the artery distal to the embolus receives any flow (b, right). Fig. 4.48a also shown in color section.

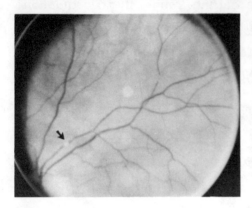
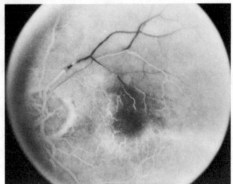

Fig. 4.49 Saddle embolus in a 65-year-old male with diabetes mellitus, hypertension, and loud carotid murmurs. Visual acuity was 6/60 (20/200). Also shown in color section.

Fig. 4.50 Emboli in peripheral branches of the inferior temporal artery (arrows). Macular edema reduced visual acuity to 6/12 (20/40).

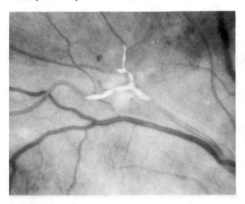
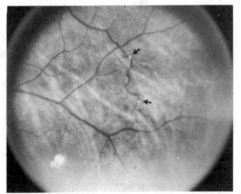

Fig. 4.51 Talc emboli in a 38-year-old drug addict. From Kresca LJ, Goldberg MF, Jampol LM: Talc emboli and retinal neovascularization in a drug abuser. **Am J Ophthalmol** 87:334, 1979. Used with permission.

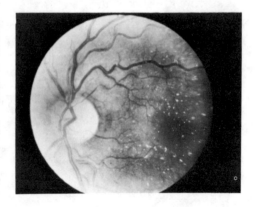

amorphous (the former are said to arise in the aorta or carotid artery, the latter from the atrium). They may be multiple, particularly in drug abusers (Fig. 4.51).

o   Old arterial occlusions may be difficult to detect, and only a generalized narrowing, loss of the nerve fiber layer (red-free light), thinning of the retina (decreased shadow casting), and gliotic sheathing of the vessel give clues to the previous events. When the blood column is thread-like and tortuous within a nearly all-white vessel, recanalization has occurred. Neovascularization and intravitreal bleeding may occur three months to several years after occlusion.

Symptoms & signs

o   Instantaneous, painless loss of vision must be considered as due to arterial occlusion until proven otherwise.

o   Transient loss of vision lasting 10-15 seconds may precede the final loss or occur repeatedly as small emboli pass. In temporal (giant cell) arteritis, vision may be better lying down than when sitting or standing. The patient may report scintillations.

o   Visual loss is total in the affected field: There is total blackness if the whole central retinal artery is occluded and there is no cilioretinal artery supplying some part of the retina (Fig. 4.45). Occlusion of the superior or inferior branches results in an altitudinal field loss.

o   If central nervous system vessels are also affected, the patient may have a headache on the same side.

o   If the whole central retinal artery is closed, the pupil is dilated and fixed, and there is no consensual response to light in the other eye (Marcus Gunn's sign). In branch occlusions, a small light directed at the functional retina may cause a pupil response, but less response if it's directed on infarcted retina (it's difficult to keep the light from scattering).

o   Iris atrophy, rubeosis of the iris, poor pupil reactions, hyphema, glaucoma, and cataract give evidence of more generalized ischemia from carotid or aortic arch disease.

Other confirming findings

o   History of previous vascular disease in patient and family.

o   Physical evidence of vascular insufficiency, including ophthalmodynamometry.

o   Radiologic, ultrasonic, plethysmographic, Doppler, radionuclear, and fluorescein angiographic evidence of blood-flow deficiency.

Table 4.3

CAUSES OF RETINAL ARTERIAL OCCLUSION, PARTIAL LIST	
Most common causes under age 30	**Most common causes over age 30**
Amniotic fluid embolus	Arteriosclerotic retinal artery disease
Chorioretinal inflammation	Cardiac or aortic arch emboli
Coagulation disease	(including mitral valve prolapse,
Intravenous drug abuse	artificial valve emboli)
Malaria	Carotid stenosis or emboli
Migraine	Coagulation disease
Oral contraceptives	Hypertensive retinal artery disease
Rheumatic heart and collagen disease	Injections in region of the eye, nose, and teeth
Rubeola retinopathy	Septic emboli
Sickle cell trait and disease	Sickle cell disease
Trauma: orbit, eye, or crush injury	Surgery of carotid, aorta, and heart
	Surgery of eye and orbit

o   Appropriate laboratory studies for blood oxygen content, sedimentation rate, syphilis, and other variables.

o   Electroretinogram.

Main differential diagnosis

o   See Table 4.3.

References

Caltrider ND, Irvine AR, Kline HJ, et al: Retinal emboli in patients with mitral valve prolapse. Am J Ophthalmol 90:534, 1980.

Duke-Elder S: System of Ophthalmology, vol 14. St. Louis: Mosby, 1972.

Fischbein FI: Ischemic retinopathy following amniotic fluid embolization. Am J Ophthalmol 67:351, 1969.

Kresca LJ, Goldberg MF, Jampol LM: Talc emboli and retinal neovascularization in a drug abuser. Am J Ophthalmol 87:334, 1979.

Rush JA, Kearns TP, Danielson GK: Cloth-particle retinal emboli from artificial cardiac valves. Am J Ophthalmol 89:845, 1980.

Sorr EM, Goldberg RE: Traumatic central retinal artery occlusion with sickle cell trait. Am J Ophthalmol 80:648, 1975.

Tse DT, Ober RR: Talc retinopathy. Am J Ophthalmol 90:624, 1980.

Whiteman DW, Rosen DA, Pinkerton RMH: Retinal and choroidal microvascular embolism after intranasal corticosteroid injection. Am J Ophthalmol 89:851, 1980.

Wise GN, Dollery CT, Henkind P: The Retinal Circulation. New York: Harper & Row, 1971.

C. DIABETIC RETINOPATHY (see VIIA, below)

D. BEHCET'S DISEASE (Fig. 4.52)

This systemic disease that affects mucus membranes of the mouth and genitals may also have devastating ocular and central nervous system manifestations. It's now believed to be a vaso-occlusive immune complex disease.

Ophthalmoscopic findings

o   Hazy view due to cells and protein in the anterior chamber and vitreous.

o   Edema of retina or retinal detachment may be present in acute phase.

o   Disc may be swollen from optic neuritis or central nervous system disease (papilledema).

o   Exudate deep in retina or on retinal pigment epithelium.

o   Perivascular sheathing is common, and venous or arterial occlusions occur.

o   Retinal pigment epithelial atrophy and pigment clumping are late manifestations.

o   Vessel obliteration and optic atrophy are often the final outcome.

o   Both eyes are affected.

Symptoms & signs

o   Blurred vision, often decreased to hand motion in severe cases. Both eyes may be affected. Blindness or severe visual loss common.

o   Photophobia and aching pain secondary to iritis are common. Hypopyon may be present (see Fig. 2.21).

Fig. **4.52** Recurrent anterior and posterior uveitis associated with intraretinal hemorrhages and vascular occlusive disease in a 19-year-old white male with Behcet's disease. Visual acuity was 6/18 (20/60) OD, 6/60 (20/200) OS.

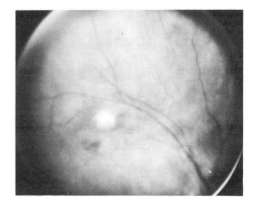

o Pupil reactions vary with severity of retinal injury and the iritis.

o Loss of visual field corresponding to vascular occlusion or retinal detachment.

Other confirming findings

o Reported more commonly in males in some studies.

o Mean age of onset 33 years.

o Protracted course and diagnosis often delayed (6.3 years, according to one study).

o Oral and genital ulcers, synovitis, cutaneous vasculitis, meningoencephalitis, and retinal vasculitis are principal manifestations of the disease.

o Principal eye findings other than those seen ophthalmoscopically are iritis, hypopyon, skin lesions on eyelids.

o Neurological disease reported: increased intracranial pressure, cranial nerve palsies (III, IV, V, VI, and VII), and hemianopic field loss.

o Skin biopsy, cerebrospinal fluid analysis, radiologic study, urine sediment analysis, bowel biopsy, HL-A B_{27} elevated.

o Fluorescein angiography.

Main differential diagnosis

o Herpes simplex infection

o Cytomegalovirus infection

o Moniliasis

o Reiter's disease

o Inflammatory bowel disease

o Vogt-Koyanagi-Harada disease

o Sympathetic ophthalmia

References

Colvard DM, Robertson DM, O'Duffy JD: The ocular manifestations of Behcet's disease. Arch Ophthalmol 95:1813, 1977.

Elliot AJ: Thirty-year observation of patients with Eales's disease. Am J Ophthalmol 80:404, 1975.

Shimizu T: Clinical and immunological studies on Behcet's syndrome. Folia Ophthalmol Jap 22:801, 1971.

VI. TOO MUCH BLOOD

Although hemorrhage may be part of the picture, overfilling of the vessels is significant in itself.

A. VENOUS OCCLUSION (Figs. 4.53 - 4.60;
see 4.53 and 4.54c also in color section)

Many retinal vascular problems are attributed to local ocular disease, although in fact systemic disease is an important factor. Often venous and arterial diseases coexist and this causes some confusion about the symptoms, signs, and results of treatment. For example, many central retinal vein occlusions in elderly patients are accompanied by arteriolar insufficiency, though it may be only transient. This provides the appearance of a central retinal vein occlusion, but with a more profound visual loss than would be expected. Most central retinal vein occlusions appear to be at the lamina cribrosa. Branch vein occlusions are at arteriovenous crossings, and artery occlusions are most often at the branch origin.

In poor arterial perfusion, the deprived retina is pale. On the other hand, venous occlusion suffuses the retina with blood unable to return to the heart. The term venous stasis retinopathy has been used for cases in which the disease seems confined to the veins alone. When arterial insufficiency accompanies the venous disease, the term hemorrhagic retinopathy has been used.

As elsewhere in the body, retinal veins vary considerably in their exact course, even though in general they take the same route in all of us. The course accounts for some of the differences in the appearance of venous occlusions. For example, the superior and inferior retinal veins may join to form a common central retinal vein while still visible on the disc. In the other eye of the same patient, the two may join out of view, deep in the optic nerve.

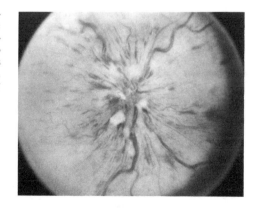

Fig. 4.53 Central retinal vein occlusion (hemorrhagic retinopathy). Blurred nasal disc margins, tortuous engorged veins, cotton-wool infarcts around the disc, and both deep and superficial hemorrhages. Hemorrhages could be seen all the way to the ora serrata. The physiologic depression is still just barely visible. Also shown in color section.

Fig. 4.54 Occlusion of the inferior temporal retinal vein at an arteriovenous crossing. Note the edema in the fovea (a) and the star-figure as the edema subsides (b). Two weeks later, the exudate of the star-figure is less discrete (c). Visual acuity was 6/21 (20/70) when first seen, and 6/7.5 (20/25) two years later without treatment (d). Star-figure usually means improvement has started. Fig. 4.54c also shown in color section.

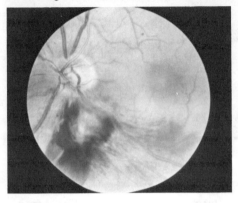

Fig. 4.54a

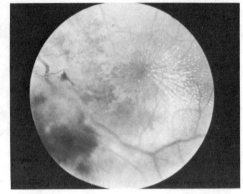

Fig. 4.54b

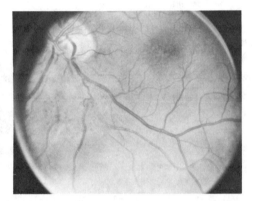

Fig. 4.54c

Fig. 4.54d

Fig. 4.55 Occlusion of the venous drainage of the lower half of the retina. It may happen that the upper and lower retinal venous drainage do not join to form a single central retinal vein, and either may become occluded.

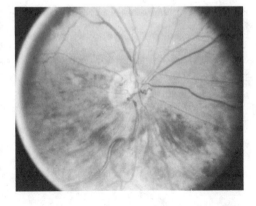

The occlusion of one venous branch, while the other remains patent, determines the distribution of hemorrhages and whether, and how, collateral circulation develops. The location of the occlusion, the efficiency of the collateral circulation, and retinal infarction (arterial insufficiency) also determine the immediate visual loss. Secondary effects, such as macular edema and neovascularization, are discussed later.

Ophthalmoscopic findings

o   Venous occlusion is rarely bilateral and even more rarely simultaneously bilateral.

o   Acute venous occlusion — deep and superficial hemorrhages all the way to the ora serrata in the distribution of the blocked retinal vein branch or all branches of the central retinal vein (a point that helps distinguish venous occlusion from diabetic retinopathy). The exception is occlusion of a small vein that drains the macula only.

o   Cotton-wool infarcts (soft exudates) are only around the disc.

o   Disc margins are indistinct because of retinal and optic nerve swelling. This involves the whole disc in central retinal vein occlusion or only the affected segment in branch retinal vein occlusion. Rarely does the swelling equal that of papilledema as measured with the ophthalmoscope, and often the temporal disc margin remains sharp and the physiologic depression visible.

o   Occasionally, preretinal or intravitreal hemorrhage occur. Most intravitreal hemorrhages occur later — after two years on the average — when retinal neovascularization follows hemorrhagic retinopathy.

Fig. 4.56 Central retinal vein occlusion (a, left) cleared completely in one year (b, right). Visual acuity was 6/60 (20/200) when photograph for Fig. 4.56a was taken and improved to 6/12 (20/40) three years later.

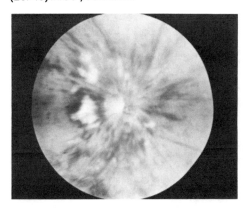 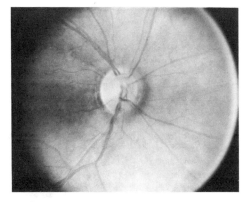

Fig. 4.57 Superior temporal branch vein occlusion in a 40-year-old male (a, left). Visual acuity was 6/9 (20/30) due to macular edema. In the fluorescein angiogram, note the sluggish perfusion and dilatation of the venous capillaries, the shunting through the macular capillaries to the inferior temporal vein, and how the blood blocks choroidal fluorescence (b, right).

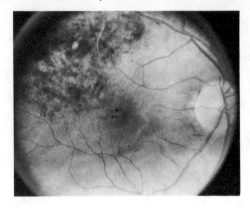

Fig. 4.58 Opticociliary shunts on the disc following central retinal vein occlusion in a 74-year-old female.

Fig. 4.59 Venous stasis retinopathy in a 25-year-old asymptomatic male. Note the absence of cotton-wool infarcts and the corkscrew, dilated veins. Visual acuity was 6/7.5 (20/25). The other eye was similar.

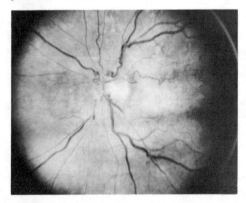

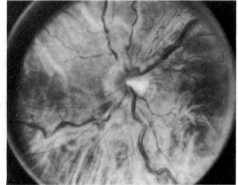

Fig. 4.60 Occlusion of a small branch of the superior temporal vein with an effect on central vision because it drains the foveal area. Visual acuity of 6/9 (20/30) never improved.

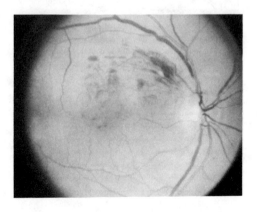

o Hemorrhages following branch or central vein occlusion may be present for many months before clearing.

o For a further classification of ophthalmoscopic findings, see Table 4.4.

Symptoms & signs

o Painless loss of vision may be undetected by the patient until the other eye is inadvertently covered. In venous stasis retinopathy in young patients, there may be vague visual symptoms and no visual loss. In hemorrhagic retinopathy in older, arteriosclerotic patients, visual loss may be severe (hand motion only) and is frequently discovered on awakening in the morning.

o Field loss is an altitudinal defect in branch vein occlusion, central scotoma in hemorrhagic retinopathy associated with extensive peripheral field loss, and mild relative central scotoma in venous stasis retinopathy. Partial retinal detachment may be present and alter the expected scotoma.

o Pupil reactions vary with the extent of retinal damage. Longstanding vein occlusions are occasionally associated with rubeosis iridis, irregular pupil, and glaucoma.

o In late disease, patient may describe dimness of light, partial loss of color perception, and distortions. Intravitreal hemorrhage and retinal detachment may reduce vision severely. Hemorrhagic glaucoma and rubeosis iridis occur in about three months in less than one percent of branch vein occlusions and 15-20 percent of central retinal vein occlusions.

Other confirming findings

o Venous stasis retinopathy occurs more commonly in young adults (usually 15-30 years old). Hemorrhagic retinopathy is most frequent in arteriosclerotic adults.

o Historical and physical evidence of arteriosclerosis, hypertensive disease, or hyperviscosity syndromes.

o Fluorescein angiography confirms blood-flow deficiency, collateral circulation, and neovascularization.

Main differential diagnosis

o Diabetes mellitus with retinopathy

o Papilledema

Table 4.4

OPHTHALMOSCOPIC FINDINGS IN VENOUS OCCLUSION

	Venous stasis retinopathy	Hemorrhagic retinopathy
Early cases		
Retinal veins	Markedly engorged, turgid, and tortuous	Markedly engorged, turgid, and tortuous
Retinal hemorrhages	Vary from few flame-shaped and punctate to very many centrally and punctate peripherally	Central gross hemorrhage, progressive early, less peripherally
Cotton-wool	Rare	Common
Disc	Hyperemic and maybe edematous	Usually covered with hemorrhage and swollen
Macula	Normal, occasionally edematous	Hemorrhages and edema common
Retinal arterioles	Normal, occasionally sclerotic	Usually sclerotic and narrow
Late cases		
Retinal veins	Mild to moderate engorgement, sometimes sheathed	Mild to moderate engorgement, often sheathed
Retinal hemorrhage	May be none or a few, mainly peripherally	May be none or only a few
Retina	Normal	Microaneurysms, dilated capillaries, neovascularization, preretinal or intravitreal hemorrhage
Disc	Normal or slightly hyperemic with retinociliary shunts	May be pale with retinociliary shunts
Macula	Normal or pale cystoid degeneration	Macular degeneration, pigmentary disturbance, preretinal fibrosis

Adapted from Hayreh SS: Central retinal vein occlusion: Differential diagnosis and management. Trans Am Acad Ophthalmol Otolaryngol 83:381, 1977. Used with permission.

PHYSICIANS' GUIDE TO OCULOSYSTEMIC DISEASES

- o Hyperviscosity states, such as leukemia, macroglobulinemia, polycythemia vera

- o Decompression disease

- o Crush injury to neck, chest, or abdomen

- o Carbon monoxide poisoning

- o Congenital heart disease

- o Dehydration

- o Von Hippel-Lindau disease

- o Rocky Mountain spotted fever

- o Fabry's disease

References

Chan CC, Little HL: Infrequency of retinal neovascularization following central retinal vein occlusion. Ophthalmology 86:256, 1979.

Hayreh SS: Hemorrhages after central retinal vein occlusion. Arch ophthalmol 96:1921, 1978.

Hayreh SS: So-called "central retinal vein occlusion." Ophthalmologica 172:1, 1976.

Hayreh SS, van Heuven WAJ, Hayreh MS: Experimental retinal vascular occlusion: 1. Pathogenesis of central retinal vein occlusion. Arch Ophthalmol 96:311, 1978.

Priluck IA, Robertson DM, Hollenhorst RW: Long-term follow-up of occlusion of the central retinal vein in young adults. Am J Ophthalmol 90:190, 1980.

Savir H, Wender T, Creter D, et al: Bilateral retinal vasculitis associated with clotting disorders. Am J Ophthalmol 84:542, 1977.

Sinclair SH, Gragoudas ES: Prognosis for rubeosis iridis following central retinal vein occlusion. Br J Ophthalmol 63:735, 1979.

Wise GN, Dollery CT, Henkind P: The Retinal Circulation. New York: Harper & Row, 1971, p 349.

B. HYPERVISCOSITY STATES (Figs. 4.61, 4.62)

Unusual sludging of blood flow has been reported in leukemia, dysproteinemia (multiple myeloma, Waldenström's macroglobulinemia, cryoglobulinemia), polycythemia, rickettsial disease, severe respiratory distress, and chronic cystic fibrosis. Blood viscosity increases rapidly with the hematocrit above 50, but increased amounts of large molecular globulins in the plasma are even more critical to flow in small vessels. White blood cells apparently are the cause of the reduced blood flow in leukemia. Intravascular clotting may occasionally be a factor. The result of poor blood rheology (flow) is inefficient oxygen delivery.

Ophthalmoscopic findings

o Marked venous engorgement, beading, and crossing changes are the most striking findings; one eye may have more involvement than the other.

o Intraretinal deep and superficial hemorrhages are present, often with microaneurysms and exudates.

o Cotton-wool infarcts may be present.

o Both disc and retina may be swollen, so that disc margins and the choroidal vessels are indistinct. Papilledema due to central nervous system disease may also be present.

o In leukemia, white patches surrounded by hemorrhage resemble large Roth spots.

o Large gray-white scalloped areas of edema may hide retinal vessels, and the arteries and veins may be thread-like in severe involvement; this may be related to cytomegalovirus, and similar findings can be seen in Rocky Mountain spotted fever and herpes simplex retinitis.

Symptoms & signs

o Vision varies from normal to light perception, depending on the degree and extent of retinal and optic nerve disease. Ophthalmologists may be the first to see patients because of blurred vision or field loss.

o Pupil reactions vary with the degree of retinal and optic nerve damage.

o Altitudinal, centrocecal, or central field defects may be present.

Other confirming findings

o History of fatigue, repeated infections, shortness of breath, Raynaud's phenomenon, respiratory distress, bone pain, rash, fever, and the like.

o Physical evidence of poor peripheral circulation, hepatosplenomegaly, enlarged nodes; skin, nail bed, lip, or conjunctival discoloration.

o Laboratory evaluation for abnormal blood count and proteins as well as radiologic and radioactive bone scanning may be needed. Bone biopsy may also be required.

Main differential diagnosis

o Central retinal vein occlusion

o Venous stasis retinopathy

o Dehydration

Fig. 4.61 Intraretinal hemorrhages in left (a, left) and right (b, right) eyes of a patient with acute myelogenous leukemia. The eye findings were the first evidence of the disease. Note some hemorrhages have white centers and resemble Roth's spots.

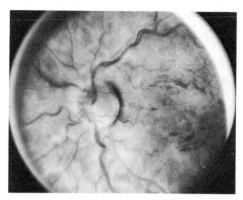 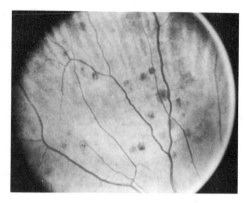

Fig. 4.62 The single microaneurysm in the fovea (a, left) and small blot hemorrhages in the peripheral retina (b, right) of both eyes led to a diagnosis of macroglobulinemia.

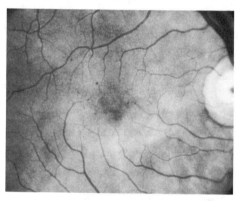 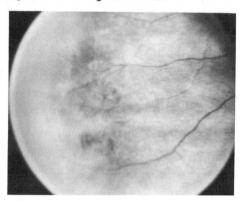

o Congenital heart disease with cyanosis

o Diabetic retinopathy

o Sturge-Weber syndrome with "tomato catsup" fundus

References

Carr RE, Henkind P: Retinal findings associated with serum hyperviscosity. Am J Ophthalmol 56:23, 1963.

Culler AM: Fundus changes in leukemia. Trans Am Ophthalmol Soc 49:445, 1951.

Delaney WV Jr, Liaricos SV: Chorioretinal destruction in multiple myeloma. Am J Ophthalmol 66:52, 1968.

Luxenberg MN, Mausolf FA: Retinal circulation in the hyperviscosity syndrome. Am J Ophthalmol 70:588, 1970.

Wise GN, Dollery CT, Henkind P: The Retinal Circulation. New York: Harper & Row, 1971, p 392.

C. DIABETIC RETINOPATHY (NONPROLIFERATIVE, BACKGROUND DIABETIC RETINOPATHY)

The facts concerning the etiology of diabetic retinopathy are slowly emerging. The severity of diabetes, as gauged by insulin dependence, seems less a factor in the etiology than the duration of poor control, age of onset, and unknown susceptibility factors of the individual patient. The following hypothesis illustrates many of the known facts:

o   Insulin deficiency with hyperglycemia stimulates increased plasma levels of growth hormone.

o   Concentrations of growth hormone and of insulin critically influence hepatic cell synthesis of plasma protein components, probably accounting for increased synthesis of fibrinogen and alpha-2 globulin and decreased albumin.

o   Increased concentrations of plasma (macroglobulins) lead to red cell aggregation and platelet clumping.

o   Alpha-2 globulin inhibits leukocyte proteases and results in increased thickening of capillary basement membranes.

o   Clumped red cells in presence of thickened capillary basement membrane causes impaired capillary perfusion and consequent retinal ischemia.

o   Finally, the sequelae of retinal ischemia and hypoxia are vasodilatation, capillary leakage, microaneurysms, and retinal neovascularization.

Diabetic retinopathy is an ischemic disease, even though it may at first appear there is too much blood because of venous congestion, vessel segmentation, hemorrhage, and vascular shunting.

Detailed photographic classification of diabetic retinopathy rose out of the Arlie House symposium on the disease and has been expanded in the collaborative study by the Diabetic Retinopathy Research Group (see references below). Practicality in the management of diabetic patients has resulted in the separation of nonproliferative (background) from proliferative (new vessel growth) diabetic retinopathy. Patients with background retinopathy may be visually handicapped, while those with proliferative disease may become incapacitated. This separation is not fixed. A patient with nonproliferative retinopathy is not protected from developing proliferative disease. The first sign of true neovascularization, no matter how minor, is considered as a change to proliferative disease. The importance lies in the visual prognosis.

1. Chronic nonproliferative diabetic retinopathy (Figs. 4.63 - 4.70; see 4.64, 4.65, and 4.68 also in color section)

Ophthalmoscopic findings

o The appearance of diabetic retinopathy is most severe posterior to the equator of the eye. Because small vessels are involved, the standard ophthalmoscope is invaluable in early detection. The disease is nearly always bilateral when first discovered. It may vary from a single aneurysm to extensive hemorrhage, exudate, edema, venous dilatation, and capillary shunts in all four quadrants.

o Microaneurysms are small, round, red spots, usually not much larger in diameter than the smallest visible vessel. Larger ones may be present, and some with a white rim are thought to be fibrosed. They may disappear, and new ones appear in the course of the disease. The number may vary from one to thousands.

o Small intraretinal hemorrhages deep in the retina are round; because of vertical orientation of the Müller's fibers they may be difficult to distinguish from microaneurysms. Superficial hemorrhages are flame-shaped.

o Exudates often make a circinate (circular) pattern around a cluster of aneurysms and edematous retina.

o Cotton-wool retinal infarcts are rarely more than 6 disc diameters from the disc, and tortuous small vessels may course through or near them, suggesting a shunt in the capillary bed. Venous beading is usually present nearby.

Fig. 4.63 Cluster of fine microaneurysms and exudate near the fovea in a 50-year-old male with diabetes for five years. Visual acuity 6/9 (20/30).

Fig. 4.64 Circinate pattern of exudates around a microaneurysm and an edematous and poorly perfused retina in a 62-year-old treated with insulin for 30 years. Also shown in color section.

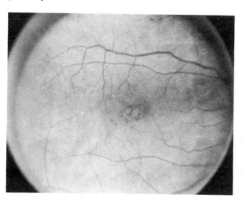
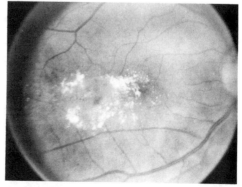

Fig. 4.65 Dilated and tortuous capillary bed (intraretinal microvascular abnormalities), retinal edema, hemorrhages, and cotton-wool exudates in a 49-year-old man with diabetes and hypertension for five years. The retinopathy became proliferative in three months. Also shown in color section.

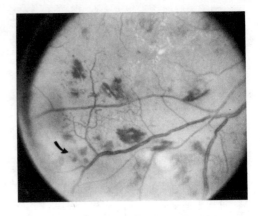

Fig. 4.66 Nonproliferative retinopathy in a 63-year-old male with diabetes 15 years (a, left). On fluorescein angiography, multiple areas of poor capillary perfusion can be seen temporal to the fovea as black areas surrounded by dilated capillaries and microaneurysms (b, right). Some black areas correspond to hemorrhage hiding the dye.

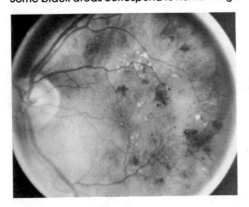
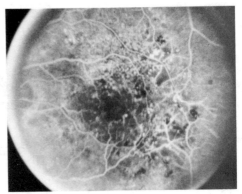

Fig. 4.67 Compare the two photographs. Venous loops are common in diabetic retinopathy (a, left). They do not bleed, but are often in eyes with neovascularization that does bleed. Arterial loops are rare in diabetic retinopathy (b, right). They do not bleed and may be seen in mild retinopathy.

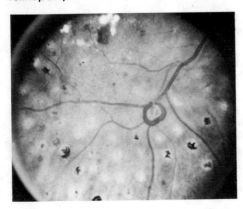
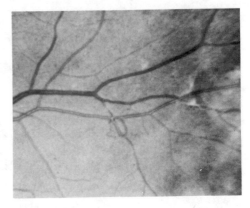

o Macular edema associated with aneurysms and circinate exudates may be seen in progressive disease and as an isolated finding in advanced disease with capillary closure. The neurosensory retina may contain multiple small cysts or occasionally larger cysts or even a macular hole. A silvery glial membrane on the retinal surface associated with silver-wire arterioles, increased tortuosity of small retinal vessels, and converging lines in the retina can be seen in advanced maculopathy.

o Venous loops are common and may remain unchanged for years. Arterial loops are seen less frequently.

o Acute onset of retinal edema, disc swelling, venous congestion associated with multiple hemorrhages, cotton-wool (soft exudate) infarcts, and capillary dilatation in juvenile onset diabetes out of control may be confused with florid proliferative retinopathy. The disc swelling may be confused with papilledema.

o The choroidal and retinal vessels may be filled with pale blood in the acidotic diabetic with lipemia retinalis.

o Hypertensive, arteriosclerotic, embolic, and vascular occlusive disease are often superimposed on diabetic retinopathy, and those findings should be reviewed.

o Laser photocoagulation results in pigmented scars in the retina and pigment epithelium. Immediately after treatment, the photocoagulation lesions may resemble spaced cotton-wool infarcts (see VIIA, below).

Symptoms & signs

o Patients are unaware of nonproliferative retinopathy, unless the macula is involved and visual acuity decreases. The visual loss in one eye may go unnoticed for a long time. The loss is gradual. In many patients, the first symptom is inability to read. The patient who is a good observer reports for examination when the first eye loses vision; the poor observer comes when the second eye becomes defective. Patients with macular edema may describe distortions of vision.

o Dimness, "fog," or light reflections around lights may accompany cataracts, and these may occasionally develop within a week. Some patients may note inability to see well when their blood sugar is high and they are spilling sugar in their urine. This induced myopia from lens swelling is useful to some patients in their diabetes regulation. Glasses prescribed for this myopia will be of no value to the patient when control is established.

o Field loss, when present, consists of a central scotoma or smaller paracentral scotomata corresponding to areas of poorly nourished retina or optic nerve.

Fig. 4.68 Diabetic, hypertensive, and arteriosclerotic retinopathy in a 41-year-old man with a 20-year history of diabetes and heart disease. Also shown in color section.

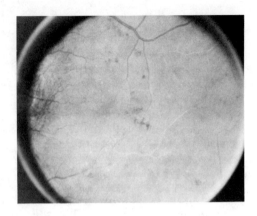

Fig. 4.69 Background diabetic retinopathy before (a, left) and after (b, right) laser coagulation. Photocoagulation improved circinate figure. Visual acuity improved from 6/7.5 (20/25) to 6/4.5 (20/15) in the three years after treatment (compare with Fig. 4.70).

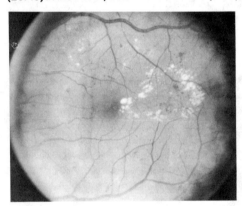 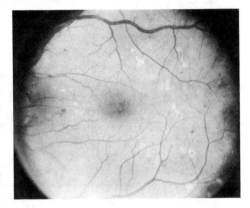

Fig. 4.70 Left eye of a 45-year-old diabetic male 15 years after the onset of the disease (a, left). Two years later a marked clearing of the retinopathy had occurred (b, right). No photocoagulation treatment was given.

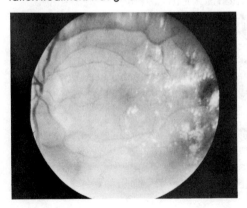 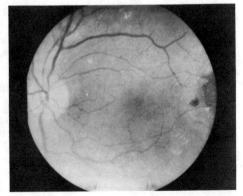

- Pupil reactions to light may be decreased when the patient's vision is severely affected. In longstanding diabetes, pupil responses may also be abnormal due to peripheral neuropathy, direct diabetic atrophy of the iris pigment, or rubeosis iridis. Corneal hypesthesia may be present.
- Loss of color vision is a rare complaint.

Other confirming findings

- Retinopathy is rarely seen in juvenile onset diabetes before three to five years of the disease. This may be accelerated in poorly controlled disease and is definitely accelerated in adult (after age 30 years) onset diabetics. In adults, the initial diagnosis of diabetes may be by ophthalmoscopic examination. The insulin-deficient adult diabetic probably has an earlier onset of retinopathy than the juvenile. This is often difficult to confirm, because there is less likely to be an acidotic crisis to pinpoint the diagnosis.

- There is some evidence that polycythemia, scleroderma, severe respiratory disease such as mucoviscidosis, sickle cell disease, carotid or aortic arch disease, hypertension, retinal vein occlusions, and ocular hypotony may accelerate the onset and contribute to the severity of diabetic retinopathy.

- The prognosis for life in patients with only microaneurysms is similar to that of a normal population. Spontaneous improvement may occur, and five years after discovery 36 percent of patients with only aneurysms have no visible lesions. Fifty percent will have hemorrhages and exudates. Sixty-three percent of the latter group survive five more years. Eleven to 12 percent of the blind population owe their sightlessness to diabetes.

- The historical, general physical, laboratory, and radiologic evidence for the diagnosis of diabetes mellitus are well described elsewhere.

- Note that intraretinal hemorrhages, aneurysms, and other disorders are often concentrated in the posterior retina and do not follow the distribution of a particular vessel — a point of some importance in distinguishing diabetic retinopathy from a vein occlusion.

- Pigment dispersion in the aqueous either spontaneously or particularly after pupil dilatation is best seen by split lamp microscopy. Cystic degeneration of the iris pigment epithelium may allow spotty iris transillumination.

- Fluorescein angiography defines the extent and nature of vessel disease characteristic of diabetic retinopathy.

Main differential diagnosis

o Retinal vascular occlusion

o Arteriosclerotic retinopathy

o Hypertensive retinopathy

o Coats's disease or Leber's miliary aneurysms

o Von Hippel-Lindau disease

o Collagen disease

o Sickle cell disease

o Macroaneurysm of retina

o Polycythemia and leukemia

o Chronic uveitis

o Subacute bacterial endocarditis

o Anemia

o Leukemia

References

Bresnick GH, Davis MD, Myers FL, et al: Clinicopathologic correlations in diabetic retino-pathy: 2. Clinical and histologic appearances of retinal capillary microaneurysms. Arch Ophthalmol 95:1215, 1977.

Caird FI, Pirie A, Ramsell TG: Diabetes and the Eye. Oxford: Blackwell, 1969.

The Diabetic Retinopathy Research Group: Preliminary report on effects of photocoagulation therapy. Am J Ophthalmol 81:383, 1976.

Goldberg MF, Fine SL, eds: Treatment of Diabetic Retinopathy. Arlie House, 1968.

Knowler WC, Bennett PH, Ballintine EJ: Increased incidence of retinopathy in diabetics with elevated blood pressure: A six-year follow-up study in Pima Indians. N Engl J Med 302:645, 1980.

Little HL, Sacks A, Vassiliadis A, et al: Current concepts on pathogenesis of diabetic retino-pathy: A dysproteinemia. Trans Am Ophthalmol Soc 75:397, 1977.

Wise GN, Dollery CT, Henkind P: The Retinal Circulation. New York: Harper & Row, 1971.

2. Acute florid nonproliferative diabetic retinopathy
(Fig. 4.71; see also in color section)

The ophthalmoscopic findings described in chronic disease occur in a period of a few weeks or months. In juvenile diabetics, the acute change may be from no retinopathy to the full presentation of background diabetic retinopathy after a few weeks of poor control. Usually they have had dia-betes for eight to 10 years or more. Adult onset diabetics may present with a

Fig. 4.71 Edema, aneurysms, and intraretinal hemorrhage of acute onset in a 15-year-old diabetic associated with a febrile illness and poor control (a, left). Both eyes were similar. Note the disc edema resembles papilledema. Same eye seven months later after good control (b, right). Also shown in color section.

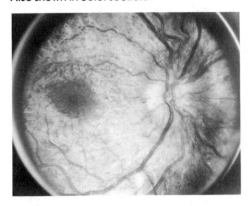 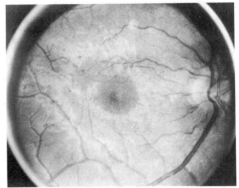

similar picture, unaware they have diabetes and seeking help for their failing vision. Both eyes are simultaneously involved.

It's sometimes difficult to distinguish acute nonproliferative from acute proliferative retinopathy. Marked prepapillary capillary vessel dilatation resembles fine neovascularization; it may take fluorescein angiography to demonstrate the difference. The acute process is sometimes reversible over a few months (Fig. 4.71b) with good diabetes control.

VII. NEOVASCULARIZATION

Inflammation, trauma, tumors, hypoxia, and probably other stimuli initiate new growth from retinal vessels. Whether there's a common, identifiable angiogenesis factor remains to be determined.

Retrolental fibroplasia in the premature — and occasionally the full-term — newborn has been demonstrated as an exaggerated growth response of retinal blood vessels. Somewhere between this abnormal response of immature vessels and neovascularization by mature, previously normal vessels, as in diabetic retinopathy, lies a group of diseases that includes hereditary retinal neovascularization, Eales's disease, Coats's disease, and others in which some abnormality may have been present from birth.

Certainly hypoxia is a major factor in new vessel proliferation from mature retinal vessels. The causes of hypoxia are multiple. In some circumstances, we understand the pathogenesis well, while in others it remains obscure. There's some clinical evidence that destroying hypoxic retina can reverse vessel proliferation, as with photocoagulation in diabetic retinopathy. Obviously, destruction of retina to prevent neovascularization and its complications is a compromise, not a solution.

A. PROLIFERATIVE, NEOVASCULAR DIABETIC RETINOPATHY
(Figs. 4.72 - 4.81; see 4.73a, 4.74, and 4.78 also in color section)

The pathogenesis of diabetic retinopathy has been described in VIC, above.

1. Chronic proliferative retinopathy
Fifty to 60 percent of all eyes with early proliferative diabetic retinopathy are legally blind — 6/60 (20/200) — in five years if untreated. Eyes with neovascularization on the disc do worse than eyes with neovascularization elsewhere. Fifty percent of eyes with neovascularization on the disc will be blind in two years if untreated.

Ophthalmoscopic findings

o   Diabetic retinopathy is most severe posterior to the equator. Because small vessels are involved, the hand-held monocular ophthalmoscope is invaluable in early detection. The disease is nearly always bilateral, but often more advanced in one eye.

o   Neovascularization is usually superimposed on nonproliferative retinopathy, but may occur where only minimal nonproliferative disease is visible.

o   Prior examination, carefully noted or photographed, confirms the presence of new vessels. New vessels are usually fine and naked in early disease, but may exceed normal retinal vessels in caliber in advanced disease. New vessels may appear within a few weeks, especially in juveniles, and regular observation is essential.

o   Early in development, new vessels lie on the retinal or disc surface and partly obscure the normal retinal vessels. Later, they may be lifted up by

Fig. 4.72 Fine neovascularization on the disc barely visible with the ophthalmoscope (a, left) may be confirmed by fluorescein angiography (b, right). New vessels leak fluorescein.

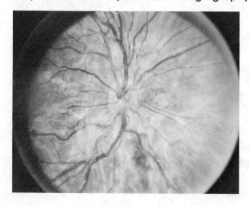
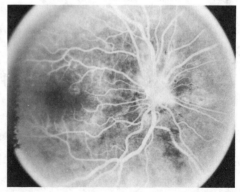

vitreous attachment and come into focus several diopters above the retinal plane. They may sway with eye movement.

o New vessels form a rete, or net, with scalloped distal edges. These distal edges are deep red and form grape-like clusters.

o It's difficult to define the feeding artery and draining vein in neovascular fronds, because there's no color difference. If you can identify them, you may see arterial feeders cross retinal arteries and veins cross veins — something that never occurs with normal vessels.

o Gray veils of supporting tissue follow vessel proliferation. After photocoagulation or spontaneous improvement, they persist, sometimes with fine vessel remnants.

o New vessel growth may originate more distally in late diabetes associated with severe arteriosclerosis and hypertensive disease. Abrupt loss of a visible arterial blood column may be associated with proliferating fronds. Usually, all four quadrants are affected.

o Preretinal or intravitreal blood may obscure part or all of the retina or disc. Intraocular blood does not clot and may flow back and forth with changes of position.

o Fibrovascular attachment of the vitreous exerts traction, tenting up the retina, causing stress lines in it and even holes and retinal detachment. This requires focusing at several levels, and the choroidal details will not be seen well. In some patients, vitreous traction may tear a plug out of the retina, which can then settle back on the pigment epithelium, occasionally with visual improvement.

o Spontaneous regression of neovascularization may occur, especially if the vitreous separates from the retina.

Fig. 4.73 Proliferative retinopathy at the disc in a 21-year-old female who developed diabetes at age 10 (a, left). Similar disease away from the disc in a 19-year-old diabetic (b, right). Fig. 4.73a also shown in color section.

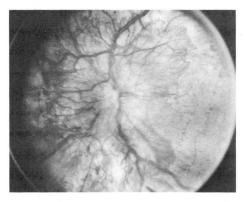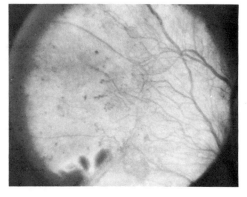

Fig. 4.74 Fibrous stage of severe proliferative diabetic retinopathy in a 42-year-old man. The other eye was similar. No change has occurred over a five-year period. Visual acuity was 6/18 (20/60) OD, finger counting at 1 meter OS. Also shown in color section.

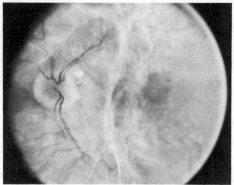

Fig. 4.75 White arteriole in the peripheral retina of a 34-year-old patient with diabetes 30 years. Neovascularization has developed at the point of apparent occlusion of the arterial blood column. This is a late form of neovascularization in patients with superimposed hypertensive and arteriosclerotic disease.

Fig. 4.76 Fibrovascular growth along the superior temporal vessels in a 19-year-old female with diabetes since age five. Note the retinal elevation and stress lines through the fovea. Visual acuity was 6/15 (20/50).

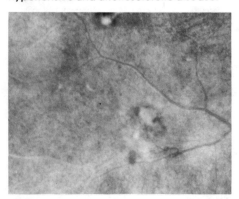

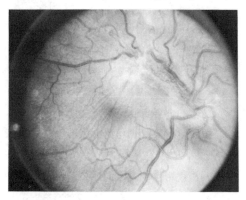

Fig. 4.77 Right eye of a 34-year-old male diabetic for 26 years who was advised to have photocoagulation for retinopathy (a, left). A sudden, unexplained decrease in his insulin requirements was accompanied by improvement (b, right). Three years later, retinopathy was worse again.

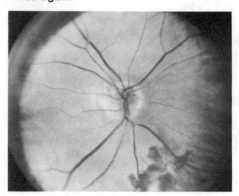

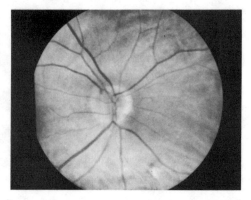

o Photocoagulation may cause regression of neovascularization, and multiple pigmented scars may dot the interior of the eye away from the macula. The scars vary in size from ⅓ to 1 disc diameter.

o Dense fibrous avascular bands remain after the active, proliferating, and often hemorrhagic stage of the disease. You can sometimes see these bands after vitrectomy.

Symptoms & signs

o The symptoms and signs of nonproliferative retinopathy (see VIC, above) often occur in the patient with proliferative disease.

o Pupil reactions to light and accommodation are often sluggish, minimal, or nonexistent. There may be a relative corneal hypesthesia.

o Intravitreal hemorrhage varies from that responsible for transient clouds of fine black specks before the patient's vision to a massive hemorrhage that nearly obscures light perception. It's common for patients to describe multiple small episodes of black floaters ("showers") before a massive hemorrhage that brings them for examination. These episodes may be related to lifting, straining, or stress.

o Thin layers of preretinal blood may act as a filter, and the patient may describe a red discoloration and obscuration of vision in the affected eye. This unilateral symptom needs to be distinguished from yellow or green bilateral dicoloration of vision in digitalis intoxication or the erythropsia described by aphakic patients after exposure to ultraviolet light.

o Aching ocular pain, sometimes referred to the head above the affected eye, occurs in hemorrhagic glaucoma from vessel proliferation on the iris and trabecular meshwork. Vision may be described as "steamy" or "foggy." Hazy cornea, nonreactive pupils, dilated blood vessels on the iris, hyphema, and elevated intraocular pressure confirm this diagnosis.

o Cicatricial or rhegmatogenous (rip or tear) retinal detachment gives the patient a shadow that obscures part of field of vision. The patient may describe flashes of light associated with entering a dark room or on head movement. The flashes are usually in the temporal field.

o Of patients with proliferative diabetic retinopathy and intravitreal hemorrhage, 55 percent survive five years, less than 40 percent survive 10 years.

o After the first intravitreal hemorrhage, about one-third are legally blind 6/60 (20/200) in both eyes in one year. One-third are economically blind 6/18 (20/60) in one year in their better eye. One-third have 6/12 (20/40) or better vision in their better eye in one year.

Fig. 4.78 Advanced proliferative retinopathy in the right eye of a 55-year-old patient who developed the disease at age 35 (a, left). Photocoagulation (black scars) away from the actual neovascularization (b, right) resulted in remission and improvement of vision from 6/120 (20/400) to 6/12 (20/40). Also shown in color section.

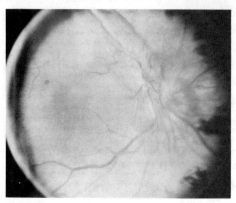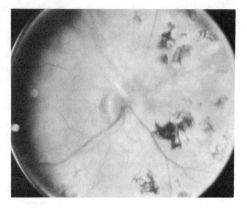

Fig. 4.79 Ochre vitreous in a 29-year-old male diabetic 17 years and blind in both eyes for two years (a, left). Dense fibrous bands surround the fovea (arrow) after vitrectomy (b, right). Visual acuity 6/6 (20/20).

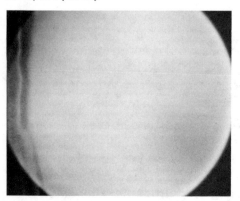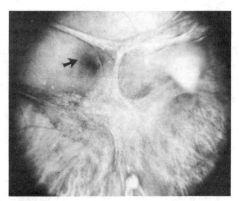

Fig. 4.80 Proliferative retinopathy in a 16-year-old female with diabetes since age six. She also has scleroderma. Response to photocoagulation is poor (arrow) and may be due to the relationship of the two diseases.

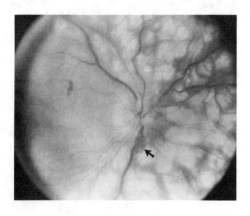

Other confirming findings

o The confirming findings described in VIC, above, apply in proliferative diabetic retinopathy as well.

o Slit lamp biomicroscopic evidence of depigmentation and vascularization of the iris and cataracts is essential.

o Fluorescein angiography demonstrates retinal and iris neovascular disease.

o Kidney function needs to be assessed in all proliferative diabetic retinopathy patients. Proliferative diabetic retinopathy and Kimmelstiel-Wilson syndrome often go together.

o Hypertensive, cardiovascular, and peripheral vascular disease are common in proliferative diabetic retinopathy patients.

Main differential diagnosis

o Retinal vascular occlusion associated with arteriosclerosis, embolization, or hypertension

o Carotid or aortic arch disease

o Retinal tear or detachment

o Sickle cell disease

o Coats's or Eales's disease

o Sarcoidosis

o Leukemia and anemia

o Macroglobulinemia and hyperviscosity states

o Ocular trauma

Fig. 4.81 Proliferative retinopathy in a 25-year-old male diabetic 20 years. The response to photocoagulation is poor (arrow). He has had respiratory disease due to cystic fibrosis throughout life.

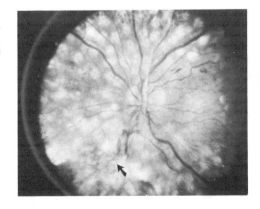

o Collagen disease

o Familial neovascularization of the retina

o Juvenile retinoschisis

o Subdural hematoma or subarachnoid hemorrhage

o Retinal vascular occlusive disease of unknown type

o Persistent hyaloid artery

o Von Hippel-Lindau disease

o Rocky Mountain spotted fever

References

The Diabetic Retinopathy Research Group: Photocoagulation treatment of proliferative diabetic retinopathy. Ophthalmology 85:82, 1978.

The Diabetic Retinopathy Research Group: Preliminary report on effects of photocoagulation therapy. Am J Ophthalmol 81:383, 1976.

Goldberg MF, Fine SL, eds: Treatment of Diabetic Retinopathy. Arlie House, 1968.

Merin S, Ber I, Ivry M: Retinal ischemia (capillary nonperfusion) and retinal neovascularization in patients with diabetic retinopathy. Ophthalmologica 177:140, 1978.

Wise GN, Dollery CT, Henkind P: The Retinal Circulation. New York: Harper & Row, 1971, p 421.

2. Acute florid proliferative retinopathy (Fig. 4.82)

Change from mild or moderate background diabetic retinopathy to neovascularization (proliferative diabetic retinopathy) may occur in a period of a few weeks in some juvenile onset diabetes patients. Diabetic control usually has been stable, unlike with patients with acute nonproliferative retino-

Fig. 4.82 Right eye of a 27-year-old female diabetic for 24 years. In one month, the appearance changed from mild nonproliferative retinopathy (a, left) to neovascularization on the disc (b, right).

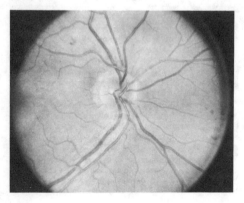 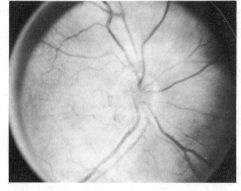

pathy. Both eyes are usually affected simultaneously, but to different degrees. Similar rapid vessel proliferation in adult onset diabetics may occur; in adults, however, the course is more protracted.

B. OCULAR VASCULAR ACCIDENT (OCULAR STROKE) AND NEW BLOOD VESSELS (Fig. 4.83)

Hypoxia rather than anoxia seems critical in stimulating new vessel growth. Neovascularization of the optic disc or retina is rare after the anoxia of total and permanent central retinal artery occlusion. Hypoxia may originate from disease in the eye, carotid arteries, or aorta. Some time passes before neovascularization develops. For example, hemorrhagic glaucoma due to rubeosis iridis has been named "90-day glaucoma" because of the interval following retinal vessel occlusion. Neovascularization on the retina often takes a similar interval to develop.

It's important to distinguish true neovascularization from shunt vessels, sometimes extensive, that bypass an obstruction (see opticociliary shunts).

The sequelae of neovascularization are hemorrhage, hemosiderosis, fibrous proliferation, vitreous opacification, and retinal detachment. Hemorrhage occurs from spontaneous rupture of the abnormal vessels or traction by the vitreous.

Ophthalmoscopic findings

---

o   The appearance of retinal arteriolar and venous occlusive disease has been described in VB and VIA, above.

o   Neovascular growth may be on the disc or the peripheral retina; it may be flat or elevated, but is confined to the distribution of the occluded vessel, starting just proximal to the point of occlusion, or arises from adjacent unoccluded vessels.

Fig. 4.83 Neovascularization on the disc in a 62-year-old arteriosclerotic female who suffered a branch venous occlusion. Note the white superior temporal vein. Recurrent intravitreal hemorrhage brought the patient in for examination.

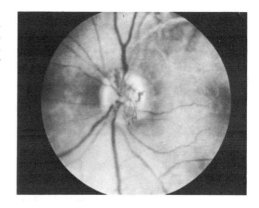

o The fronds often have grape-like, dark red clusters at the distal margin. The neovascularization is indistinguishable from that seen in diabetic retinopathy.

o White vessels, emboli, vessel narrowing, etc. may be present.

o There may be preretinal or intravitreal blood.

o Large shunts are likely after venous occlusion.

Symptoms & signs

o The symptoms and signs of the acute vascular occlusive process should be reviewed (see VB and VIA, above).

o Optic disc and retinal neovascularization is asymptomatic, unless preretinal or intravitreal hemorrhage occurs (see Chapter 8:IVA), retinal tear or detachment results from vitreous traction, or hemorrhagic glaucoma develops.

o The usual history given is a brief episode of decreased vision, perhaps altitudinal field loss followed by recovery. An asymptomatic interval, often two to three years, is followed by showers of black specks or even severe intravitreal hemorrhage that obscures vision.

o The possibility that intravitreal bleeding is due to something other than the neovascularization, for example, a retinal tear, should not be overlooked.

Other confirming findings

o History, findings, and review of the angiography of previous retinal, carotid, or aortic arch disease.

o Neovascular fronds can be confirmed by fluorescein angiography.

o Ultrasonography is helpful when the vitreous is impenetrable to light.

o Vascular disease evaluation by techniques described for arterial occlusion (see VB, above).

Main differential diagnosis

o Diabetic retinopathy

o Retinal tear and detachment

o Sickle cell disease

o Coats's or Eales's disease

o Leukemia

o Others (see VIIA, 1, Main differential diagnosis, above)

References

Brown G, Shields JA: Cilioretinal arteries and retinal arterial occlusion. Arch Ophthalmol 97:84, 1979.

Hayreh SS: Pathogenesis of occlusion of the central retinal vessels. Am J Ophthalmol 72:998, 1971.

Scheie HG: Evaluation of ophthalmoscopic changes of hypertension and arteriolar sclerosis. Arch Ophthalmol 49:117, 1953.

Tomsak RL, Hanson M, Gutman FA: Carotid artery disease and central retinal artery occlusion. Cleve Clin Q 46:7, 1979.

Tomsak RL, Hanson M, Gutman FA: Carotid-artery disease and retinal-artery occlusion. Lancet 1:1084, 1979.

Willerson D Jr, Aaberg TM: Acute central retinal artery occlusion and optic disc neovascularization. Arch Ophthalmol 96:451, 1978.

C. SICKLE CELL DISEASE (Figs. 4.84-4.86; see 4.85 also in color section)

The inherited substitution of the amino acid valine for glutamic acid in the number six position on the beta chain results in an abnormal hemoglobin designated S because of curved (sickle) shape of the red blood cells. Abnormal insertion of lysine instead of glutamic acid gives rise to C hemoglobin.

In the United States, about 10 percent of the black population has these hemoglobin abnormalities. Studies differ, but about eight to 11 out of 100 have SA, two to three out of 100 have AC, one in 600 SS, one in 1,500 SC, and one in 6,000 CC hemoglobin.

The majority of sickle cell patients with ocular disease are those with SS hemoglobin (sickle cell anemia) and SC hemoglobin (SC disease).

Ophthalmoscopic findings

o Venous dilatation and tortuosity; hyperemia of the disc and exaggerated artery-vein crossing changes are usually the first retinal vascular evidence of disease.

o Transient dark red spots on the disc, suggesting plugged small vessels, occur in about 10-12 percent of SS, SC, and S-thal patients.

o Localized, dark, and sheathed veins, particularly in the temporal periphery, are often associated with microaneurysms.

o A rete of new blood vessels may initially appear as a pink "salmon" patch. They are usually far into the periphery.

o Exudates of cholesterol and hemorrhage may lie on the retina or in the vitreous.

Fig. 4.84 Small dark red spots or comma-shaped vessels (arrows) may be seen on the disc (a, left) or the conjunctiva (b, right) in patients with sickle cell disease. Fig. 4.84a from Goldbaum MH, Jampol LM, Goldberg MF: The disc sign in sickling hemoglobinopathies. **Arch Ophthalmol** 96:1597, 1978. Copyright © 1978, American Medical Association. Used with permission. Fig. 4.84b from Minatoya H, Acacio I, Goldberg M: Fluorescein angiography of the bulbar conjunctiva in sickle cell disease. **Ann Ophthalmol** 5:980, 1973. Used with permission.

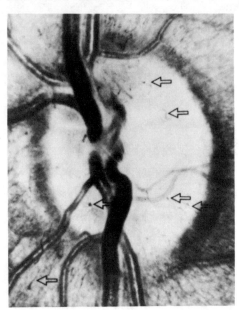
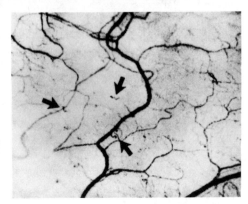

Fig. 4.85 New blood vessels on the retinal surface in a 41-year-old black female with sickle cell hemoglobinopathy (arrow). The retina distal to this "seafan" is relatively avascular. The patient had recurrent intravitreal hemorrhage. Also shown in color section.

Fig. 4.86 Black sunbursts in the retinal periphery are associated with vessel closure in sickle cell disease. From Asdourian G, Nagpal KC, Goldbaum M, et al: Evolution of the retinal black sunburst in sickling haemoglobinopathies. **Br J Ophthalmol** 59:710, 1975. Used with permission.

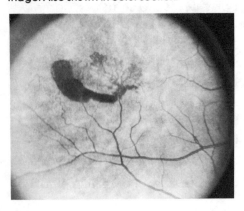
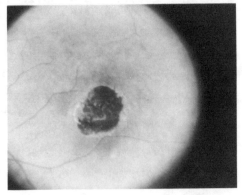

- Angioid streaks (see Chapter 6:IIID,6) extending out from the disc occur in about 6-8 percent of patients.
- Black "sunburst" scars in the choroid and retinal pigment epithelium may resemble old chorioretinitis.
- Closure of peripheral arterioles is associated with edema in the acute phase and thinning of the retina in late stages. Spontaneous regression (autoinfarction) of proliferative vessels may occur.
- Extensive gray bands involving the vitreous and retina, intravitreal hemorrhage, and retinal detachment signify a late stage of the disease (hemorrhagic glaucoma often follows).
- Central retinal artery occlusion is reported to be more common in patients with sickle cell trait and particularly those with glaucoma.
- Sickle cell retinopathy patients subjected to photocoagulation or cryotherapy will manifest the scars of that treatment.

Symptoms & signs

- Pain in abdomen, long bones, or flanks associated with hemolytic crisis are common. Pain in or around the eye occurs rarely. If the patient develops hemorrhagic glaucoma as part of the disease, specific eye pain, unrelated to a crisis, may be associated with steamy vision, cloudy cornea, and hyphema.
- Sickle cell disease rarely appears before age one year, when fetal hemoglobin has been replaced by sickle hemoglobin. Acute loss of vision in a hemolytic crisis due to central retinal artery occlusion in one or both eyes occurs rarely.
- Loss of vision from intravitreal hemorrhage or retinal detachment.
- Pallor, and segmented comma-shaped blood vessels are seen in the conjunctiva.
- Scleral jaundice as part of generalized icterus usually appears 48-72 hours after a crisis.
- Pupil responses are normal, unless visual loss or iris neovascularization (rubeosis iridis) have occurred.
- Asthenopia (ocular fatigue) and diplopia may accompany severe anemia.

Note: Sickled red cells in the anterior chamber (hyphema) following trauma or retinal detachment in a patient with sickle cell disease requires very special management. These patients should be seen by an ophthalmologist with knowledge of this disease.

Other confirming findings

o Classical sickling crises are usually well known to the patient, although subacute attacks often are ignored or misdiagnosed. A family history of similar disease aids diagnosis.

o Physical findings of hemolytic anemia, such as icterus, pallor, splenomegaly, cardiac enlargement, systolic murmurs, and skin ulcerations on the legs are a few of the manifestations.

o Laboratory evaluation of the blood for red cell sickling on smears and specific sickle preparations confirm the presence of abnormal hemoglobin. Hemoglobin electrophoresis is necessary to define the type and magnitude of abnormality. Sedimentation rate and uric acid excretion may be elevated.

o Bony rarifaction and sclerosis may be seen on roentgenogram.

o Fluorescein angiography helps define the retinal vascular disease and the effectiveness of applied treatment.

Main differential diagnosis

o Diabetic retinopathy

o Retinal vascular occlusion with compensatory neovascularization

o Coats's and Eales's disease

o Retinal tear or detachment

o Hyperviscosity states

o Other vascular diseases (see VIIA, 1, Main differential diagnosis, above)

References

Asdourian GK, Nagpal KC, Goldbaum M, et al: Evolution of the retinal black sunburst in sickling haemoglobinopathies. Br J Ophthalmol 59:710, 1975.

Goldbaum MH, Jampol LM, Goldberg MF: The disc sign in sickling hemoglobinopathies. Arch Ophthalmol 96:1597, 1978.

Minatoya H, Acacio I, Goldberg MF: Fluorescein angiography of the bulbar conjunctiva in sickle cell disease. Ann Ophthalmol 5:980, 1973.

Nagpal KC, Asdourian GK, Goldbaum M, et al: Angioid streaks and sickle haemoglobinopathies. Br J Ophthalmol 60:31, 1976.

Nagpal KC, Patrianakos D, Asdourian GK, et al: Spontaneous regression (autoinfarction) of proliferative sickle retinopathy. Am J Ophthalmol 80:885, 1975.

Powers DR: Natural history of sickle cell disease: The first ten years. Semin Hematol 12:267, 1975.

Radius RL, Finkelstein D: Central retinal artery occlusion (reversible) in sickle trait with glaucoma. Br J Ophthalmol 60:428, 1976.

Welch RB, Goldberg MF: Sickle-cell hemoglobin and its relation to fundus abnormality. Arch Ophthalmol 75:353, 1966.

Wise GN, Dollery CT, Henkind P: The Retinal Circulation. New York: Harper & Row, 1971, p 388.

D. OTHER RARE CAUSES (Figs. 4.87 - 4.89)

Neovascularization of the retina and the disc has been associated with many diseases, occasionally seen without explanation, and also reported as a dominantly inherited abnormality. In most cases, the retinal findings are not specific enough to identify the disease.

Ophthalmoscopic findings

o New blood vessels may be seen on the disc, in the peripheral retina, or, in some patients, both.

o New vessels often originate in the retina at sites of arteriolar narrowing or blood column hiding (white walls).

o New vessel growth is usually slow and often less extensive than seen in proliferative diabetic retinopathy.

o Intravitreal and preretinal hemorrhage may occur and tends to be less severe and clear more quickly than in proliferative diabetic retinopathy.

o Microaneurysms, hemorrhages, exudates, vascular sheathing, and shunting are common.

o Emboli may be suspected but rarely seen.

Fig. 4.87 Neovascularization on the disc in a 56-year-old patient with chronic myelogenous leukemia (a, left). Fluorescein angiography demonstrates poor capillary perfusion in the macula and dye leaking from the disc (b, right). The other eye was similar.

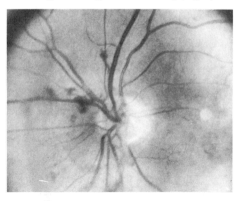
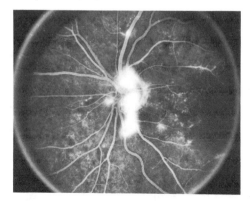

Symptoms & signs

o The ocular symptoms and signs are nonspecific and related to vascular occlusions, intravitreal hemorrhage, retinal detachment, and other disorders, all described elsewhere.

Other confirming findings

o Leukocystosis, anemia, thrombocytopenia, and bone marrow study usually define the disease. Retinal involvement is more common in myelogenous than in lymphatic leukemia. Chronic myelogenous leukemia has been the cause in most reported cases with retinal neovascularization.

o Collagen disease: Fever, rash, carditis, arthralgia, chorea, and occasionally hemiparesis in young patients with rheumatic fever, periarteritis, or lupus erythematosus may be associated with peripheral retinal neovascularization. Neovascularization is thought to follow embolic vegetations from heart valves.

o Sarcoidosis: Fever, weakness, dyspnea, uveitis, and multiple other manifestations of sarcoidosis are best reviewed in a general text of medicine. Sarcoid granulomatous perivascular infiltration is thought to be the cause for vessel obstruction and neovascularization.

Fig. 4.89 Occlusive vascular disease of the retina in a healthy eight-year-old female preceded by the acute onset of vertigo and deafness. The other eye had similar retinal vascular disease, and both suffered intravitreal hemorrhage. From Delaney WV Jr, Torrisi PF: Occlusive retinal vascular disease and deafness. **Am J Ophthalmol** 82:232, 1976. Used with permission.

Fig. 4.88 Arteriolar occlusion and neovascularization with hemorrhage in a 41-year-old female with a history of pericarditis confirmed on biopsy as periarteritis nodosa.

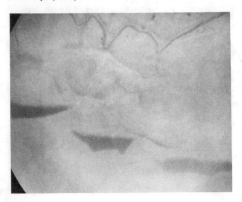

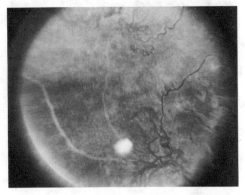

Roentgenogram, gallium scan, node biopsy, serum angiotensin converting enzyme, and exclusion of other inflammatory disease confirm the diagnosis.

o Incontinentia pigmenti (Bloch-Sulzberger and Naegeli's syndromes): Occurs mostly in full-term female infants. Hereditary nature of the disease has not been confirmed. Males may have the Naegeli form. Reticular blue-gray or brown pigmentation on the trunk or proximal extremities may be associated with spotted teeth, alopecia, or keratosis of the palms and soles. Other eye findings besides neovascularization and the multiple complications of it may include, among others, blue sclera, cataracts, nystagmus, and strabismus. Retinal dysplasia has also been found. Twenty-five to 35 percent of patients have associated eye disease.

o Retinal neovascularization and deafness: This is a rare disease reported only in females. It occurs in otherwise apparently healthy young patients. Severe hearing loss, probably due to inner ear vascular disease, may precede or accompany spontaneous retinal arteriolar occlusions. Visual loss from both vascular occlusion and intravitreal hemorrhage from new vessel fronds severely handicaps these deaf patients. There is no hereditary pattern or physical or laboratory aid to diagnosis (Fig. 4.89).

o Dominantly inherited peripheral retinal neovascularization: In one family, it has been recorded in nine members over a span of three generations.

o Eales's disease: This was originally described as a disease of young males in whom intravitreal bleeding was associated with constipation, headaches, and epistaxis. Peripheral retinal venous engorgement and cuffing may be associated with hemorrhage and exudation. Neovascularization is a late occurrence. Occasionally, central nervous system and cerebral spinal fluid pleocytosis have been reported, but generally the patients are otherwise healthy. The visual prognosis is fair with 54 percent maintaining 6/15 (20/50) or better vision.

o Radiation therapy: X-ray treatment of bones and sinuses often include the eye. Over-radiation of the eye during treatment for retinoblastoma or eyelid tumors was not uncommon in the past. A neovascular response in the retina is relatively rare with a total dose of less than 4,000 rads. At least six months and, in many cases, years pass before this manifestation is seen.

o A breakdown of diseases associated with peripheral retinal neovascularization is given in Table 4.5.

Table 4.5

DISEASES ASSOCIATED WITH PERIPHERAL RETINAL NEOVASCULARIZATION

Category	Disease	Decade of onset	Involvement	Genetic transmission
Congenital	Retinal telangiectasia	1st-3rd	Widespread, periphery and posterior pole	None
Hereditary	Peripheral retinal neovascularization (familial exudative vitreoretinopathy)	Variable	Periphery	Autosomal dominant
	Hemoglobinopathies (SC, SS, AS, S-thalassemia)	Variable	Periphery (usually temporal)	Autosomal
	Incontinentia pigmenti	1st-2nd	Periphery	Autosomal dominant (usually lethal for males)
	Angiomatous retinae (von Hippel-Lindau disease)	1st-4th	Periphery	Autosomal dominant
Vaso-occlusive syndromes	Aortic arch syndromes	2nd and older	Widespread, periphery and posterior pole	None
	Branch vein occlusion	4th and older	Area occluded vein (quadratic or segmental)	None

	Diabetes mellitus	Variable	Widespread, periphery and posterior pole	Unknown
	Retrolental fibroplasia	Birth-1st	Periphery (temporal)	None
	Eales's disease	1st-3rd	Area of involved vein(s) periphery	None
	Hyperviscosity syndromes: Polycythemia Cryoglobulinemia Macroglobulinemia Chronic myelogenous leukemia	Variable	Periphery	None
Inflammatory	Sarcoidosis	Variable	Periphery	None
	Uveitis	Variable	Usually periphery	None
	Malaria	Variable	Posterior pole and periphery	None
Iatrogenic	Radiation retinopathy	Variable	Posterior pole and periphery	None
	Postphotocoagulation	Variable	Posterior pole and periphery	None

Adapted from Gitter KA, Rothschild H, Waltman DD, et al: Dominantly inherited peripheral retinal neovascularization. Arch Ophthalmol 96:1601, 1978. Used with permission.

Main differential diagnosis

o Proliferative diabetic retinopathy

o Retinal tear or detachment

o Vascular occlusive disease of retina, carotid, or aortic arch

o Retinoblastoma

o Sickle cell disease

References

Asdourian GK, Goldberg MF, Busse BJ: Peripheral retinal neovascularization in sarcoidosis. Arch Ophthalmol 93:787, 1975.

Delaney WV Jr, Torrisi PF: Occlusive retinal vascular disease and deafness. Am J Ophthalmol 82:232, 1976.

Doxanas MT, Kelley JS, Prout TE: Sarcoidosis with neovascularization of the optic nerve head. Am J Ophthalmol 90:347, 1980.

Elliot AJ: Recurrent intraocular hemorrhage in young adults (Eales's disease). Arch Ophthalmol 61:745, 1959.

Gitter KA, Rothschild H, Waltman DD, et al: Dominantly inherited peripheral retinal neovascularization. Arch Ophthalmol 96:1601, 1978.

Kelley JS, Randall HG: Peripheral retinal neovascularization in rheumatic fever. Arch Ophthalmol 97:81, 1979.

Morse PH, McCready JL: Peripheral retinal neovascularization in chronic myelocytic leukemia. Am J Ophthalmol 72:975, 1971.

Watzke RC, Stevens TS, Carney RG Jr: Retinal vascular changes of incontinentia pigmenti. Arch Ophthalmol 94:743, 1976.

Wise GN, Dollery CT, Henkind P: The Retinal Circulation. New York: Harper & Row, 1971, p 397.

Fig. 4.90 "Dragged" retina in a child with retrolental fibroplasia. Note the gray appearance of the elevated retina in a fold (a, left) that extends to the temporal periphery (b, right). The retinal pigment is abnormal in the periphery. The macula is hidden by the blood vessels. Visual acuity was limited to finger counting at ½ meter.

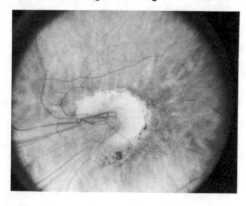 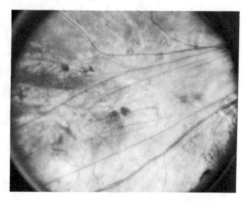

VIII. DISPLACED AND DISTORTED VESSEL COURSE

Developmental variations in the course of retinal vessels may be quite remarkable, with twisting loops rising into the vitreous before returning to the retinal plane. Intrinsic disease of the vascular walls, as in hypertension and diabetes, may alter vessel course or give that appearance, as do venous loops in diabetic retinopathy. Vessel displacement is often the most striking observation when a retinal detachment is seen for the first time. The deviation of vessels from their expected course, compared with their counterpart in another quadrant or in the other eye, gives a major clue in diagnosis.

A. RETROLENTAL FIBROPLASIA (Fig. 4.90; see also Fig. 3.22)

Retinal vascularization is just barely complete at full-term birth. The last area to receive full vascularization is the temporal retinal periphery. In the premature and an occasional full-term infant, this development must occur after birth. Our skill in managing this condition has improved considerably over the years, to the extent that retrolental fibroplasia has become preventable, or at least predictable.

Oxygen supplied to the premature infant for life-threatening cardiopulmonary disease results in oversupply to the developing retina. Withdrawal of the excess oxygen and increased nutritional demands by the developing retina and vitreous result in a deficiency that may not be met even by a rapid growth of vessels. Since the overlying vitreous derives its nourishment from the retina, it's not surprising that its usual clarity and form are affected. The scarring of the retinal pigment epithelium is less well explained and may be the result of mechanical factors, such as those seen after retinal detachment repair.

Ophthalmoscopic findings

Acute phase (usually within one to two weeks of oxygen cessation)

o   Tortuosity of the vessels as they are followed from the disc.

o   Transient acute arteriolar narrowing may be seen during or shortly after oxygen administration.

o   Neurosensory retina is gray, especially in the temporal periphery, and hides the choroidal vessels that come into view near the disc through the retinal pigment epithelium, which is typically pale in newborns. The grayness of the neurosensory retina increases in the periphery, mostly temporally, up to a ridge paralleling the ora serrata. This elevated ridge near the equator may go all around the eye, but usually is temporal.

o   Retinal blood vessels stop at the ridge and arborize. They are of irregular caliber, sometimes saccular, and loop back toward the disc.

o Vitreous over the peripheral retina is turbid.

o Both eyes are affected, although considerable difference between them is common.

Regressed phase

o Retinal vessels at the disc pass straight to the temporal retina, without the usual arching above and below the macula. Nasal vessels may pass temporally, then arch back to their normal location. The amount of vessel displacement varies, and, in many patients, one eye is more affected than the other.

o The fovea is often displaced, "dragged" out of position because of the unusual course of the retinal blood vessels.

o Pallor of the retinal pigment epithelium persists, and choroidal vessels are exposed to view as in other myopic patients.

o Patchy atrophy and pigment clumping is most noticeable temporally.

o A gray ridge persists and may be elevated slightly. Blood vessels rarely arch over it and pass on to the ora serrata.

o Bands and veils of vitreous are attached to the ridge. They are taut and do not move with ocular motion. They may extend back along retinal vessels or to the disc.

o Anterior to the ridge, the retina is often elevated, diaphanous, or both; if diaphanous, atrophic retinal pigment epithelium, choroid, and even sclera are exposed.

o Round or oval small — less than ½ disc diameter — holes may be seen along the ridge or at points of vitreous attachment.

Advanced phase

o Usually, due to a dense fibrovascular membrane behind the lens, the only view obtainable is a white pupil (leukocoria). The lens is usually clear initially. The fibrovascular membrane does not move with patient movement.

o While viewing the periphery of the pupil, you may see the ciliary processes pulled in by the membrane in a saw-tooth configuration (a point of differentiation from retinoblastoma).

o A billowing retinal detachment behind the lens may occur in less-advanced disease. It undulates with patient movement.

o Cataract, shallow anterior chamber, rubeosis iridis, hyphema, and cloudy cornea from glaucoma are common late manifestations.

Late complications

o Lattice degeneration (see Chapter 5:VIH) is common in the retinal periphery.

o Retinal detachment due to the contraction of vitreous bands usually occurs in the first five years of life. Later retinal detachment is usually associated with round or oval holes at sites of vitreous traction and may be related to periods of peak ocular growth and increasing myopia.

Symptoms & signs

o Insensitivity to light, poor pupil reactions, no response to food, dissociated eye movements, strabismus, nystagmus, eye rubbing, redness, and apparent pain in infants raise concern about vision.

o White pupil reflection.

o Visual acuity from birth may vary from no light perception to 6/6 (20/20) as corrected with glasses. Vision is often better in one eye.

o Myopia is usual.

o Loss of visual field, particularly on the nasal side.

o Cataract, rubeosis iridis, shallow anterior chamber, glaucoma, pain.

o Premature infants often have frontal bossing with a square forehead that persists in some cases throughout life.

Other confirming findings

o History of premature birth. Most victims weigh less than 2,500 grams at birth and require oxygen for cardiopulmonary disease.

o Oxygen tension above 60-90 mm Hg in the lower aorta is considered excessive by most neonatal centers. Levels are kept below this figure and discontinued as soon as no longer needed.

o Indirect ophthalmoscopy is invaluable.

o Fluorescein angiography helps define vascular abnormalities.

o Ultrasonography and radiologic studies are helpful in eyes that cannot be examined with light.

o General physical examination and indicated studies as per the differential diagnosis.

Main differential diagnosis

o Retinoblastoma

o Persistent hyperplastic primary vitreous

o Intravitreal hemorrhage

o Endophthalmitis

o Retinal dysplasia

o Hereditary high myopia

o Coloboma of disc

o Trauma with choroidal rupture

o Lowe's syndrome

o Norrie's disease

o Rhegmatogenous retinal detachment

o Coats's disease

o Familial exudative vitreoretinopathy

o 13-15 trisomy

o Incontinentia pigmenti

References

Apple DJ, Rabb MF: Clinicopathologic Correlation of Ocular Diseases: A Stereoscopic Atlas. St. Louis: Mosby, 1978.

Brockhurst RJ, Chishti MI: Cicatricial retrolental fibroplasia: Its occurrence without oxygen administration and in full-term infants. Albrecht von Graefes Arch Klin Exp Ophthalmol 195:113, 1975.

Kraushar MF, Harper RG, Sia CG: Retrolental fibroplasia in a full-term infant. Am J Ophthalmol 80:106, 1975.

Naiman J, Green WR, Patz A: Retrolental fibroplasia in hypoxic newborn. Am J Ophthalmol 88:55, 1979.

Patz A, Kalina RE, Ashton N, et al: Symposium on retrolental fibroplasia. Ophthalmology 86:1685, 1979.

Schulman J, Jampol LM, Schwartz H: Peripheral proliferative retinopathy without oxygen therapy in a full-term infant. Am J Ophthalmol 90:509, 1980.

Shahinian L Jr, Malachowski N: Retrolental fibroplasia. Arch Ophthalmol 96:70, 1978.

Tolentino FI, Schepens CL, Freeman HM: Vitreoretinal Disorders: Diagnosis and Management. Philadelphia: Saunders, 1976, p 207.

Wise GN, Dollery CT, Henkind P: The Retinal Circulation. New York: Harper & Row, 1971, p 365.

B. RETINAL VESSEL OCCLUSION

Recanalized retinal arteries and veins often have an irregular course. Comparison with other vessels in the same or other eye is essential. Vessel occlusions are discussed in detail in VB and VIA, above.

C. RETINAL DETACHMENT AND RETINOSCHISIS

Vessel displacement is part of this disease and is discussed with abnormalities of the neurosensory retina in Chapter 5: III.

D. CHORIORETINAL VESSEL ANASTOMOSIS

Retinal and choroidal circulations don't communicate, unless there's a breakdown in retinal pigment epithelium and Bruch's membrane.

E. AVULSION OF A RETINAL VESSEL (Figs. 4.91, 4.92)

The vitreous is firmly attached at its base. Weak attachments posteriorly are present at the disc and macula and along the retinal blood vessels. Commonly with the posterior vitreous separation of aging, but occasionally in the young after violent exercise or trauma, a retinal vessel may be torn from its bed by a vitreous band. Often in such cases some perivascular disease has increased vitreous adhesion to the vessel.

Ophthalmoscopic findings

o The vessel rises from the retinal plane and then returns to it more distally. A shadow of the vessel may be cast by the light of the ophthalmoscope (Fig. 4.91b).

o Intraretinal or intravitreal hemorrhage may be mild or severe. Severe hemorrhage usually indicates an arteriolar vessel is avulsed; recurrence of hemorrhage is common.

o Usually only one vessel is involved.

o The avulsed vessel is usually posterior to the equator.

o A retinal hole or tear may be present under the avulsed vessel.

Symptoms & signs

o Vision may be obscured by intravitreal or preretinal hemorrhage.

o The symptoms and signs of retinal detachment may follow, but only if a full thickness retinal break has occurred. (Remember that retinal vessels are in the superficial nerve fiber layer.)

o Scotomata may be present, but are difficult to find.

o Symptoms and signs of posterior vitreous detachment are common.

o Persistent intravitreal hemorrhage over many months may give rise to hemosiderosis of the lens, iris, and retina and occasionally cause glaucoma.

Fig. 4.91 Vitreous traction has avulsed a retinal vein from its normal location (a, below). Drawing shows the shadowcasting by the elevated vessel that can be seen with the ophthalmoscope but is difficult to photograph (b, right).

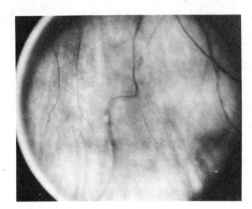

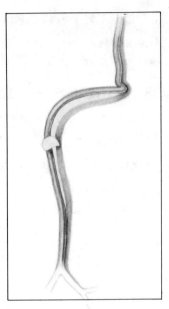

Fig. 4.92 Vitreous traction on the superior temporal vein (arrow) in a 51-year-old diabetic patient (a, left). As traction increased, the vein has been pulled out of the picture, creating a hole in the retina (arrow, b, right).

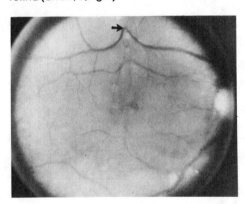

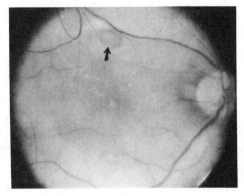

Other confirming findings

o   Diagnosis is made by ophthalmoscopic observation.

o   Fluorescein angiography is occasionally needed.

o   There may be recourse to ultrasonography if intravitreal blood obscures the view.

Main differential diagnosis

o   Retinal tear or retinal detachment

o   Proliferative diabetic retinopathy

o   All the causes of new vessel growth described in VII, above.

References

Robertson DM, Curtin VT, Norton EWD: Avulsed retinal vessels with retinal breaks. Arch Ophthalmol 85:669, 1971.

F. FABRY'S DISEASE (ANGIOKERATOMA CORPORIS DIFFUSUM UNIVERSALE)

This X-linked storage disease results from defective activity of a lysomal hydrolase, α-galactosidase A. Ceramide trihexoside accumulates, particularly in vascular endothelial cells. The eye findings are unique and often diagnostic. Severely affected hemizygous males and mildly affected heterozygous carrier females have evidence of this disease.

Ophthalmoscopic findings

o   With the ophthalmoscope as a flashlight you may see the aneurysmal dilatation corkscrew tortuosity of conjunctival vessels, whorl-like corneal opacities against the red reflex, and granular lens opacities.

o   Seventy-five percent of hemizygous males and 25 percent of heterozygous female carriers have various degrees of dilated and tortuous retinal vessels, especially veins.

o   Central retinal artery occlusion, hypertensive retinopathy, and advanced artery-vein crossing changes are common.

o   Optic atrophy and myelinated nerve fibers have been seen.

o   Papilledema and optic atrophy have been reported.

Symptoms & signs

o   Usually no visual defect.

o   Many patients are myopic.

o   Nystagmus and internuclear ophthalmoplegia have been reported.

Other confirming findings

o	All findings of the disease may occur before age 30. Hemizygous males severely affected; heterozygous females mildly.

o	Pain, burning, particularly in the hands and feet, are among the early complaints.

o	Various purple- or maroon-colored clusters of vascular skin lesions are present.

o	Cardiac disease, including congestive heart failure and arrhythmias, are part of the disease.

o	Renal disease and hypertension are common.

o	Cerebrovascular disease may present as hemiplegia, aphasia, vertigo, or collapse.

o	Each organ system needs appropriate evaluation by hematologic, radiologic, and other means.

o	Diagnosis is confirmed by measuring ceramide trihexoside in plasma or urine.

Main differential diagnosis

o	Hypertension (all causes, including pheochromocytoma)

o	Premature arteriosclerotic disease

o	Corneal drug effects, as with chloraquine (Aralen), indomethacin (Indocin), chlorpromazine

o	Papilledema due to increased intracranial pressure

o	Embolic disease of all types

o	Fucosidosis and other mucopolysaccharidoses

References

Desnick RJ, Blieden LC, Sharp HL, et al: Cardiac valvular anomalies in Fabry's disease. Circulation 54:818, 1976.

Sher NA, Letson RD, Desnick RJ: The ocular manifestations in Fabry's disease. Arch Ophthalmol 97:671, 1979.

Sher NA, Reiff W, Letson RD, et al: Central retinal artery occlusion complicating Fabry's disease. Arch Ophthalmol 96:815, 1978.

Weingeist TA, Blodi FC: Fabry's disease: Ocular findings in a female carrier. Arch Ophthalmol 85:169, 1971.

IX. ABNORMAL BLOOD COLOR

Blood color is more than the iron content of red cell hemoglobin. The relative density of red cells, plasma quality, the state of oxygenation, and even the chemical composition of hemoglobin are factors. Ocular disease, such as arteriovenous anastomosis or hemangiomas cause local alterations in the blood color. Significant color abnormalities are often bilateral and related to serious systemic disease. The color of retinal and choroidal blood is an important source of information.

A. ACUTE ANEMIA

Severe, sudden blood loss threatens the patient with perhaps permanent loss of vision.

Ophthalmoscopic findings

o General pallor of retinal and choroidal blood columns and narrow arteries.

o Splinter hemorrhages, cotton-wool spots.

o One or both discs may be pale and swollen and later develop optic atrophy.

o Usually hemorrhages and other findings are bilateral.

o In some patients, the retina is white with a cherry red spot at fovea as in central retinal artery occlusion.

Symptoms & signs

o Visual loss may be ignored initially because of the acute illness due to blood loss.

o Visual loss may be profound, with no light perception, or it may be minimal and affect one or both eyes.

o Altitudinal field loss or a central scotoma may be present in one or both eyes.

o Pupil reactions vary from normal to dilated and fixed in severe visual loss.

o Severe intraretinal or subretinal hemorrhage or edema may result in pigment deposition as healing occurs.

Other confirming findings

o Pallor, sweating, shock, collapse, and other symptoms and signs associated with severe blood loss are well described in medical texts.

o Laboratory evidence confirming the type and degree of blood loss are also well described.

Main differential diagnosis

o Diabetic retinopathy, especially in a patient with insulin shock or acidosis

o Papilledema due to increased intracranial pressure

o Pulmonary and ocular embolic disease

o Temporal (giant cell) arteritis with central nervous system involvement

o Rocky Mountain spotted fever, with collapse

References

Haye C, Bernard J, Dufier JL, et al: The ophthalmologic manifestations of acute idiopathic aplastic anemia. Arch Ophthalmol 34:793, 1974.

Merin S, Freund M: Retinopathy in severe anemia. Am J Ophthalmol 66:1102, 1968.

Rubenstein RA, Yanoff M, Albert DM: Thrombocytopenia, anemia, and retinal hemorrhage. Am J Ophthalmol 65:435, 1968.

Wise GN, Dollery CT, Henkind P: The Retinal Circulation. New York: Harper & Row, 1971, p 308.

B. LIPEMIA RETINALIS (Fig. 4.93; see also in color section)

Creamy discoloration of the blood is a startling finding rarely forgotten.

Ophthalmoscopic findings

o Generalized salmon-colored blood in retina and choroidal vessels.

o Findings are said to appear first in the more peripheral blood vessels.

o Vessel borders are indistinct.

Symptoms & signs

o Visual acuity is usually normal.

o No ocular symptoms, except asthenopia (fatigue) due to debilitation of intercurrent disease.

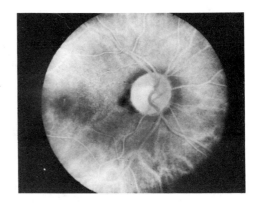

Fig. 4.93 Lipemia retinalis in a 23-year-old female diabetic in acidosis. Visual acuity was 6/6 (20/20). Blood lipid was 8,000 mg/100 ml. From O'Connor PR, Donaldson DD: Lipemia retinalis. **Arch Ophthalmol** 87:230, 1972. Copyright © 1972, American Medical Association. Used with permission. Also shown in color section.

Other confirming findings

o   History of alcoholism, diabetes mellitus, pancreatitis, liver disease, familial hyperlipidemia, or exposure to solvents such as carbon tetrachloride.

o   Diabetic patients are in acidosis.

o   Acute abdominal pain occurs in familial hyperlipidemia as well as in pancreatic and liver disease. Evaluation of acute abdominal pain is essential.

o   Triglycerides and other lipid fractions markedly elevated, perhaps 8,000 mg/100 ml.

Main differential diagnosis

o   Severe blood loss anemia

o   Advanced arteriosclerotic retinopathy

o   Central retinal artery occlusion

o   Acute leukemia

References

O'Connor PR, Donaldson DD: Lipemia retinalis. Arch Ophthalmol 87:230, 1972.

Wise GN, Dollery CT, Henkind P: The Retinal Circulation. New York: Harper & Row, 1971.

C. LEUKEMIA

Occasionally, a markedly elevated white blood cell count may result in a salmon color of the blood. Other leukemia findings in the retina and choroid are described in VIB, above.

D. MULTIPLE EMBOLI OR PARTICLE DISPERSION (see Fig. 4.51)

Multiple particles of injected foreign material or emboli from artheromatous vessel walls may reduce blood flow and give a speckled appearance to retinal blood columns.

E. POLYCYTHEMIA (see VIB, above)

Vessel distension and flow of increased number of red blood cells, many with carbaminohemoglobin, give the retina and choroid a blue discoloration (cyanosis).

F. CARBON MONOXIDE POISONING

Acute carbon monoxide poisoning results in a hemoglobin-carbon monoxide complex (carboxyhemoglobin) that prevents normal oxygen binding. Carboxyhemoglobin has a cherry red color that can be noted in the patient's skin, lips, nailbeds, and the retina.

Ophthalmoscopic findings

o Striking cherry red color of the blood in the retina and choroid of both eyes.

o Hemorrhages, marked vessel narrowing, and segmentation of blood columns may be seen.

o In chronic carbon monoxide poisoning, hemorrhages and cotton-wool infarcts may be present.

Symptoms & signs

o Patients are usually unconscious and near death.

o Pupils may be dilated and fixed.

o Roving eye movements and III, IV, or VI cranial nerve palsy may be present.

Other confirming findings

o In acute carbon monoxide poisoning, the history and findings are rarely difficult to elicit.

o Carboxyhemoglobin levels and blood gas determinations confirm the diagnosis in both acute and chronic poisoning.

Main differential diagnosis

o   Severe blood loss anemia with collapse

o   Bilateral central retinal artery occlusion

o   Lipid storage disease in children

References

Walsh FB, Hoyt WF: Clinical Neuro-Ophthalmology, vol 3. Baltimore: Williams & Wilkins, 1969.

G. TOMATO CATSUP FUNDUS (see Chapter 7: IIIA)

A diffuse choroidal hemangioma may give the whole interior of the eye a marked red color. It's unilateral, associated with skin and other hemangiomas of the Sturge-Weber syndrome.

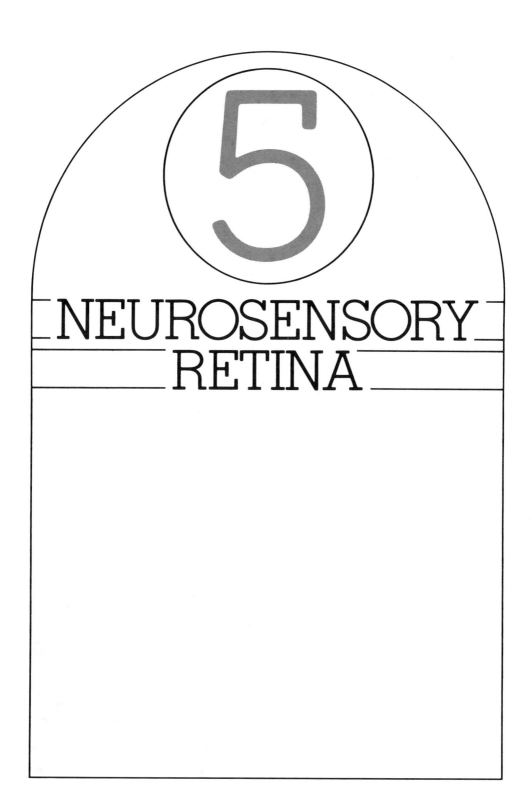

5

NEUROSENSORY RETINA

Although the neurosensory retina is never without a relationship with the overlying vitreous, the underlying retinal pigment epithelium, and its blood supply, to understand the ophthalmoscopic appearances, it's helpful to consider it separately. The neurosensory retina consists of tissues embryologically derived from the inner layer of the optic cup (see Fig. 1.6).

I. OPHTHALMOSCOPIC ANATOMY

A. THE TRANSPARENCY OF THE NEUROSENSORY RETINA

To allow maximum light transmission to the rods and cones (see Fig. 1.5) the neurosensory retina is transparent and therefore invisible to observation in its normal condition, even at high magnification. There are a few exceptions.

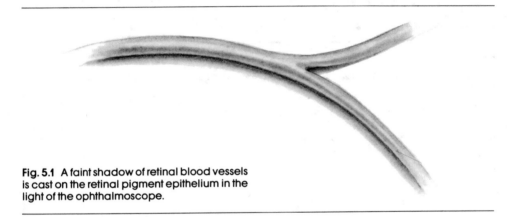

Fig. 5.1 A faint shadow of retinal blood vessels is cast on the retinal pigment epithelium in the light of the ophthalmoscope.

Fig. 5.2 Shadows cast on the retinal pigment epithelium by blood vessels as well as relative movement (parallax) give clues to retinal thickness or the elevation of vessels or other objects above the retinal plane (see Fig. 4.91).

Fig. 5.3 Yellow pigment in the fovea (macula lutea) is normal and more visible in young people.

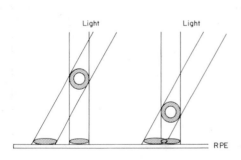

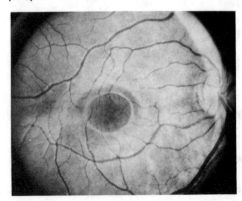

It's possible to see the normal nerve fibers near the disc, particularly when a heavily pigmented retinal pigment epithelium provides a background. The view can be enhanced by red-free light, which helps eliminate confusing reflections (see Fig. 1.33). Benign myelination of the retina makes the course and appearance of the nerve fibers more visible, and this helps in understanding the anatomy (see Fig. 3.21). Along the ora serrata, the retina is often gray; however, this is difficult to see with the monocular ophthalmoscope without pressing on the sclera to bring it into view — a maneuver that itself alters the color.

B. RETINAL THICKNESS

This is difficult to estimate with the ophthalmoscope. Some idea can be obtained by using a slit aperture available on some ophthalmoscopes, but the slit lamp and contact lens are better. Shadows cast by the retinal blood vessels on the retinal pigment epithelium (Fig. 5.1) and parallax from altering the angle of view give the best clues (Fig. 5.2). The retina is thickest at the border of the fovea (350μ) and thinnest at the foveola itself (90μ). It thins in the periphery (equator, 150μ; ora, 100μ).

C. MACULA

Histologic and ophthalmoscopic definitions of the macula often differ. In Fig. 1.13a, the commonly used ophthalmoscopic interpretation is superimposed on a photograph. The macula is roughly 2 disc diameters ($3{,}000\mu$) in all directions around the foveal light reflection. One disc diameter ($1{,}500\mu$) defines the fovea, and the foveola is the flat central part of the retina (500μ), corresponding to the avascular zone. The term umbo is used to define the area of the foveal light reflection. Standard use of this terminology facilitates communication.

The retinal vasculature at the macula has been treated in Chapter 4. The larger retinal capillaries are just within resolution and can be seen with the ophthalmoscope. There is evidence that the capillary-free zone of the adult retina is vascularized in prenatal development. A process of spontaneous obliteration results in closure of these vessels shortly before birth. The capillary-free zone enlarges slightly with age. The presence of vessels within the area is abnormal.

In addition to the larger and more deeply pigmented cells of the retinal pigment epithelium at the macula, there may be a yellow coloration, the macula lutea (Fig. 5.3). This poorly understood xanthophyllic pigment in the outer plexiform layer of the neurosensory retina is often more noticeable in young patients and may occasionally be misinterpreted as disease.

II. MISSING RETINA

Defects in the retina expose the underlying pigment epithelium to view (see Fig. 1.8). These defects may be very large or very tiny. They may be located anywhere in the neurosensory retina, but certain types of defects are characteristically in the macula, along blood vessels, or in the periphery. Retinal breaks are associated with many diseases.

A. MACULAR HOLE (Figs. 5.4, 5.5; see 5.5 also in color section)

Macular holes follow severe ocular trauma, chronic cystoid macular edema, myopic degeneration, vitreous traction, and epiretinal membrane formation. The majority are idiopathic senile macular holes of unknown etiology.

Ophthalmoscopic findings

o   A sharp, usually circular defect in the neurosensory retina, where the foveal light reflex should be, exposes the underlying retinal pigment epithelium to clear view.

o   Hole size may be the diameter of a major retinal vessel or as large as the disc.

o   A halo of gray retina may accentuate the hole and probably is due to a small neurosensory retinal detachment. In very myopic patients, a significant retinal detachment may extend to the periphery (see III, below).

Fig. 5.5 Traumatic macular hole two days after blunt trauma in a 16-year-old male. Note the subretinal blood above the macula and residual Berlin's edema around the hole. Also shown in color section.

Fig. 5.4 Spontaneous macular hole in a 67-year-old female with hypertension. Visual acuity is reduced to counting fingers.

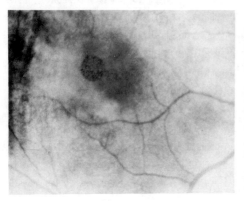

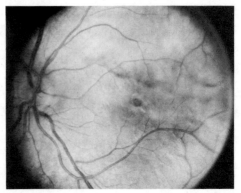

o Retinal pigment epithelium seen through or around the hole may have yellow lipofuscin granules and pigment clumping.

o Hypertensive vascular disease or myopic degeneration are frequently present.

o With careful focusing, you may see a small operculum of retinal tissue attached to the posterior hyaloid (vitreous) and suspended over the hole. It's smaller than the hole and moves slightly with eye movement. It's not present in all macular holes.

o Holes in preretinal membranes may resemble true macular holes, but can usually be distinguished by lack of a clear view of the retinal pigment epithelium through the hole and by adjacent glistening, wrinkling, and distortion of the neurosensory retina. The usual halo of neurosensory retinal detachment is absent.

o Without using the biomicroscope and contact lens, it's often difficult to distinguish macular cysts from holes. Proximal illumination sometimes reveals septae or a thin inner wall, confirming a cyst. The cyst may act as a small lens and magnify retinal pigment epithelial details.

Symptoms & signs

o Visual acuity is 6/60 (20/200) or less in a true macular hole. It is usually better—6/12 (20/40) to 6/60 (20/200)— and may even be normal in a patient with a false hole in a preretinal membrane. The patient may discover poor vision incidentally. Patients with cysts or false holes may complain of distortions or micropsia. Patients with true holes often say vision has decreased over a period of weeks or months associated with slight distortion and after-image effect. There may also be a sudden decrease to the final vision after months of gradual change.

o If a macular hole results in extensive retinal detachment, peripheral vision will be lost. But most macular holes don't cause a retinal detachment, and only central vision is affected.

o Pupil reaction to light may not be sustained in the affected or other eye (Marcus Gunn's sign).

o There's no pain with spontaneous macular holes. Traumatic macular holes are associated with severe ocular contusion. Unlike peripheral retinal holes, these patients rarely describe flashes of light (photopsia).

Other confirming findings

o Traumatic macular holes tend to occur in young active patients. Patients with idiopathic senile macular holes average 68 years of age, and 76 percent are women. Less than 10 percent have bilateral holes, and it is rare for both eyes to be affected simultaneously. Hypertension may be more prevalent in patients who develop idiopathic senile macular holes. Most retinal detachments due to macular holes are in highly myopic patients.

o   Fluorescein angiography demonstrates the nature of the defect.

o   Evidence of chronic cystoid macular edema, epiretinal membrane, and vitreous traction can be confirmed on biomicroscopic examination.

o   Causes of cystoid edema that may result in macular holes include vascular disease, hereditary disease such as retinitis pigmentosa, drug toxicity as with epinephrine drops, retinal aneurysms, and choroidal tumors. For a more complete list, see references.

Main differential diagnosis

o   Cystoid macular edema

o   Surface wrinkling retinopathy

o   Diabetic retinopathy

o   Foerster-Fuchs spot

o   Senile macular degeneration

o   Solar retinopathy

References

Gass JDM: Stereoscopic Atlas of Macular Diseases. St. Louis: Mosby, 1977, p 334.

Yannuzzi LA, Gitter KA, Schatz H: The Macula: A Comprehensive Text and Atlas. Baltimore: Williams & Wilkins, 1979, p 265.

B. RETINAL (FLAP OR OPERCULATED) TEARS
(Figs. 5.6-5.9; see 5.6 also in color section)

Full-thickness tearing of the neurosensory retina has been associated with maldevelopment, acquired and inherited vitreoretinal degenerations, and trauma. Systemic diseases linked with retinal breaks include diabetes mellitus with retinopathy, Marfan's syndrome, homocystinuria, Ehlers-Danlos syndrome, multiple inflammatory diseases that damage the retina and vitreous as part of the disease, such as toxoplasmosis, and others. The most common retinal disease associated with tears is lattice degeneration.

The vitreoretinal bond is a very weak one throughout most of the eye. Abnormal firmness of this bond, from whatever cause, predisposes to vitreous traction on the neurosensory retina with age. The term tear implies vitreous traction on the retina. The Greek word <u>rhegma</u> (rip or tear) is used to define retinal detachments, contrasting with those without a retinal break.

Not all retinal tears lead to a retinal detachment. In fact, most do not. The presence of retinal tears and holes has been found in up to 8 percent of the population while the incidence of retinal detachment is about 0.2 percent. The 8 percent prevalence includes only full-thickness neurosensory retinal tears. Partial-thickness breaks also occur.

Retinal tears vary from microscopic to giant size tears that circumvent the whole retina. They may be multiple or single, silent or symptomatic. All are associated with an ophthalmoscopically visible abnormality. Many, but not all, occur in the peripheral part of the retina, and pupillary dilation is often required to see them.

Ophthalmoscopic findings

o   Retinal pigment epithelium and choroid exposed to sharp view in the tear have a bright red appearance.

o   Margins may be gray due to early retinal detachment (see Fig. 5.12).

o   Retinal blood vessels may pass along the margin, bridge the flap, or be disrupted and hemorrhage into the retina and vitreous.

o   When the flap has torn free, it may be seen as an out-of-focus gray-white opacity in the overlying vitreous, casting a shadow on the retina.

o   Absence of retinal blood vessels may be the best clue to missing retina in very large breaks (Fig. 5.8).

Fig. 5.6 Horseshoe-shaped tear in the peripheral retina in a 61-year-old aphakic male. The retina is detached and wrinkled. The everted edges of the tear are a poor prognostic sign. Also shown in color section.

Fig. 5.7 Retinal tear in a 40-year-old diabetic with retinopathy. Note the operculum (arrow) torn from the retina.

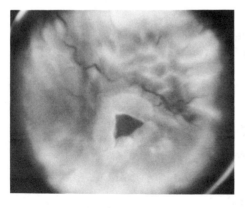

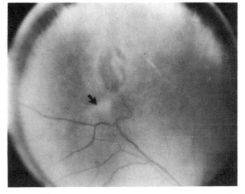

Symptoms & signs

o Vague flashes of light, especially in the peripheral field, may be associated with eye or head movement or entering a dark room.

o Floaters may be described as showers of fine black specks, "strings," or cobwebs before the affected eye.

o Visual acuity depends on the density of intravitreal blood over the macula or whether retinal detachment involving the macula has occurred. It may vary from normal to light perception.

o Loss of upper visual field may occur from severe hemorrhage settling in the inferior vitreous. Retinal detachment also causes loss of field.

o Pupil reactions are normal, unless extensive retinal detachment has occurred. Some patients may have all the symptoms and signs of iritis (miosis, photophobia, pain, ciliary flush) with a retinal tear or detachment.

o In diabetic retinopathy, retinal breaks occur along major retinal vessels posterior to the equator.

o In trauma, the break may be at the site of impact, especially at the inferior temporal or superior nasal ora serrata.

o Retinal breaks without symptoms and retinal detachment more often are round, nonoperculated (no flap), and small ($<$0.25 disc diameter). Fifty-five percent are inferiorly located, most at the equator or closer to the ora serrata.

o Retinal breaks with symptoms and retinal detachment are more often operculated, larger, superior, and multiple. They tend to be located at the equator. A rough rule puts 50 percent in the superior temporal quadrant, 25 percent in the superior nasal quadrant, 15 percent in the inferior temporal quadrant, and 10 percent in the inferior nasal quadrant. About 20 percent of retinal detachment patients have breaks in both eyes.

o Disinsertions due to trauma and disease, especially in young patients, are often in the inferior temporal quadrant.

Other confirming findings

o Historical and physical evidence of disease known to be associated with vitreoretinal abnormality, including prematurity, Marfan's syndrome, vascular disease such as sickle cell disease, trauma, infectious disease such as malaria, and collagen disease such as periarteritis nodosa.

o Aphakia, myopia, and family history of retinal detachment are predisposing factors.

Fig. 5.8 The retina has torn all around the periphery and collapsed in a roll above the disc. Note the absence of retinal blood vessels and the clear view of the retinal pigment epithelium. Courtesy of William Havener, M.D., Ohio State University.

Fig. 5.9 Retinal tear immediately after injury with a tennis ball. Note the small hemorrhages at the margins of the tear and the torn-out piece (operculum) out of focus to the right. Intravitreal blood makes the photograph hazy.

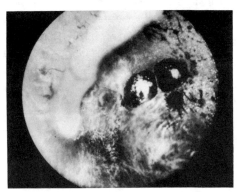

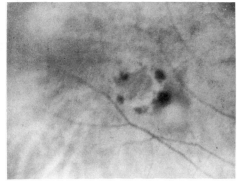

o Mean age of retinal detachment patients is 59 years, but the range extends from birth to 85 years.

o Retinal findings known to be associated with retinal tears include lattice degeneration, focal or perivascular pigmentation, chorioretinal scars, developmental retinal folds and coloboma, retinoschisis, and diabetic retinopathy.

o Indirect ophthalmoscopy with scleral depression and slit lamp biomicroscopy with a contact lens aid in diagnosis.

o Ultrasonography is helpful when intravitreal blood obscures the retina.

Main differential diagnosis

o Chorioretinal scars, as in histoplasmosis syndrome

o Photocoagulation or cryocoagulation scars

o Paving stone degeneration

o Intraretinal hemorrhage of all causes

o Localized hyper- or hypopigmentation

o Congenital developmental abnormalities

o Retinal blood vessel avulsion

References

Byer NE: Prognosis of asymptomatic retinal breaks. Arch Ophthalmol 92:208, 1974.

Smolin G: Statistical analysis of retinal holes and tears. Am J Ophthalmol 60:1055, 1965.

Tolentino FI, Schepens CL, Freeman HM: Vitreoretinal Disorders: Diagnosis and Management. Philadelphia: Saunders, 1976.

C. ROUND HOLES (Fig. 5.10; see also in color section)

Full-thickness retinal breaks may occur without vitreous traction. These holes are usually oval or round and often occur in clusters or in association with degenerative disease of the peripheral retina, as in lattice degeneration. They constitute a large proportion of routinely discovered retinal holes. It's presumed that they are the result of atrophy of the retina, since no operculum of avulsed tissue is seen. Retinal detachment may result from round holes. Both round and flap (traction) retinal breaks can occur in the same eye.

Ophthalmoscopic findings

o   Retinal pigment epithelium and choroid are exposed to view in the hole and give a bright red appearance.

o   Margins may be gray.

o   Pigmented line around the holes give evidence of where retinal detachment started and failed to progress for a period — a so-called high water mark or demarcation line.

o   Retinal blood vessels always pass around round holes.

o   They are most commonly seen in the temporal quadrants, at the equator of the globe, or further anterior. Often they are associated with lattice or other types of retinal degeneration. An exception is the macular hole.

Symptoms & signs

o   Round holes are asymptomatic unless they cause a retinal detachment. The only exception is loss of vision in the macular atrophic hole.

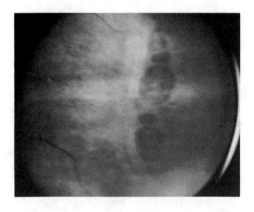

Fig. 5.10 Multiple round holes without opercula in the temporal retina of a 19-year-old male. Visual acuity was 6/4.5 (20/15) without glasses. Also shown in color section.

Other confirming findings

o Round holes cause retinal detachment more frequently in highly myopic patients.

o The confirming findings described for retinal tears (see B, above) also apply here.

Main differential diagnosis

o Chorioretinal scars, as in histoplasmosis syndrome

o Photocoagulation or cryocoagulation scars

o Paving stone degeneration

o Intraretinal hemorrhage of all causes

o Localized hyper- or hypopigmentation

o Congenital developmental abnormalities

o Retinal blood vessel avulsion

References

Byer NE: Prognosis of asymptomatic retinal breaks. Arch Ophthalmol 92:208, 1974.

Smolin G: Statistical analysis of retinal holes and tears. Am J Ophthalmol 60:1055, 1965.

Tolentino FI, Schepens CL, Freeman HM: Vitreoretinal Disorders: Diagnosis and Management. Philadelphia: Saunders, 1976.

D. RETINAL DISINSERTION (Figs. 5.11, 5.12)

Avulsion of the retina from its normal attachment at the ora serrata may result from blunt trauma to the eye at any age. It also occurs spontaneously in children. In both instances, there's a predilection for the inferior temporal quadrant of the globe. In trauma, this is probably due to lack of bony orbital protection for that area. The explanation for its spontaneous occurrence in young patients remains elusive, but its 25 percent bilaterality suggests a maldevelopment of the vitreoretinal attachments.

Retinal disinsertion in children deserves special attention, because delay in diagnosis is very common. This delay frequently results in permanent loss of central vision in eyes that could have easily been repaired surgically. The delay may be caused by the natural reticence of the child or the relative absence of symptoms (since no large blood vessels are disrupted by disinsertion). Also, the loss of upper field can go unnoticed by the patient, and parents tend to laugh off "black eyes."

Fig. 5.11 Drawing of retinal disinsertion from its anterior attachment. This type of retinal break occurs spontaneously in children and often results from trauma.

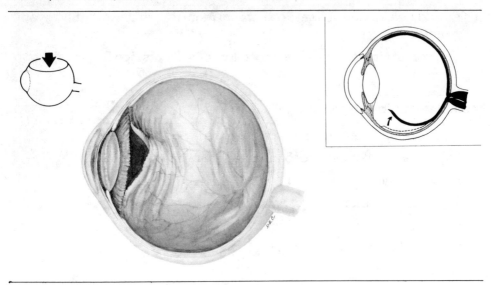

Ophthalmoscopic findings

o   Retinal blood vessels stop abruptly at the edge of a disinsertion. Inferior temporal quadrant is usually involved, but it can happen in any quadrant.

o   On the edge of disinsertion, the retinal pigment epithelium and choroid are exposed to view, giving a sharp red color.

o   Disinserted edge of retina may be rolled up, grayish in color, or avulsed with both ends still attached, like a bucket handle.

o   Some pigment or blood may be present in the vitreous, and other signs that indicate ocular trauma may also be present, such as choroidal rupture and macular hole.

o   Retinal detachment is usually already present when the patient is seen.

Symptoms & signs

o   Spontaneous retinal disinsertion in children is often so silent it isn't discovered until retinal detachment reduces vision. Traumatic macular hole or choroidal rupture may reduce visual acuity and coexist with disinsertion.

o   Signs of iritis (miosis, ciliary flush, photophobia) may occur in both traumatic and nontraumatic disinsertion.

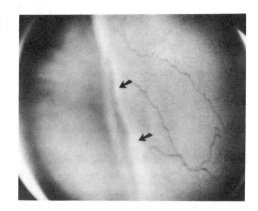

Fig. 5.12 Retinal disinsertion in an 11-year-old child. Note that the tortuous retinal vessels and gray elevated retina stop abruptly (arrows), and the retinal pigment epithelium and choroid are exposed to view at the edge of the disinsertion.

o Ecchymosis and swelling of lids after trauma are common.

o Pupil may be fixed, dilated, or irregular.

o Hyphema (blood in anterior chamber) may be present.

o Loss of upper field occurs when retinal detachment starts inferiorly.

o Usual complaints of retinal detachment, flashes and floaters, are not described by children.

Other confirming findings

o History of trauma directly to eye.

o Spontaneous retinal disinsertion does not appear inherited, related to any known birth trauma, noxious agent, or other specific diseases.

o Both traumatic and spontaneous disinsertion are more common in children who do not wear glasses — that is, who are not myopic.

o The age range of children who develop spontaneous disinsertion is 10 to 20 years, while traumatic disinsertion patients are slightly younger.

o Indirect ophthalmoscopy and scleral depression, slit lamp biomicroscopy with a contact lens, and ultrasonography are helpful aids in examination.

o Examination under anesthesia may be necessary in small and uncooperative children.

Main differential diagnosis

o Intravitreal hemorrhage

o Chorioretinal scars

o Acute toxoplasmosis

o   Toxocara canis or cati infestation

o   Eales's and Coats's diseases

o   Juvenile retinoschisis

o   Coloboma

References

Delaney WV Jr: Retinal disinsertion in children. Clin Pediatr 18:380, 1979.

Tasman W: Retinal Diseases in Children. New York: Harper & Row, 1971, p 121.

III. ELEVATION OF THE RETINA

The neurosensory retina may be either pulled or pushed from its normal position. In searching for the cause of elevation, attention must not be directed at the retina alone, but also to the vitreous, retinal pigment epithelium, choroid, sclera, and even the orbit.

For the retina to move forward requires a concomitant displacement of vitreous. Largely water, the vitreous is more condensed over gradual elevations such as tumors, and its collagen fibers are more readily seen. In rapid elevations, a pre-existing fluid space in the vitreous cavity must be present. Fluid movement to the subretinal space occurs either by flow, membrane transfer, failure of the retinal pigment epithelial pump, or all three.

Retinal elevation may be simulated by several conditions. A cataract, intravitreal blood, or asteroid hyalosis may obscure the view just enough to suggest retinal elevation when compared to more clearly seen areas of the same eye. Proliferation in retrolental fibroplasia, diabetes, sickle cell, Eales's disease, or peripheral uveitis may form elevated vascular or fibrous sheets from the retinal plane into the vitreous. True retinal elevation may occur in these diseases as well, but the membranes formed give the appearance of retinal elevation.

A. RHEGMATOGENOUS RETINAL DETACHMENT (Figs. 5.13-5.17; see also Figs. 2.60 and 8.21; see 5.14, 5.15, 2.60, and 8.21 also in color section)

The term retinal detachment, or separation, is used to indicate division of the neurosensory retina from the retinal pigment epithelium at the natural embryonic cleavage.

Detachment of the macular retina from the retinal pigment epithelium results in critical, and in many cases irreversible, loss of vision. The resulting separation of the rods and cones from their choroidal supply of oxygen and nutrition is nearly as damaging as a similar deficit in brain tissue. The uninterrupted blood flow in the central retinal vessels and choriocapillaris allows some cells to survive, if the separation is not too prolonged.

Rhegmatogenous refers to retinal detachment associated with a rip or break (rhegma) in the retina.

Ophthalmoscopic findings

o Elevation of the retina may be so high that it is visible right behind the lens, or so minimally elevated that it is difficult to detect (see B2, below); you need more than the usual plus power to focus the retinal blood vessels as you follow them peripherally from the disc into the elevated retina. Retinal detachment may be localized (Figs. 5.14 and 5.17) or total.

o Retinal vessels are usually tortuous and displaced from their normal location.

o Elevated retina is gray and normal transparency is lost, except in shallow longstanding retinal detachment or highly myopic eyes. You can best see shallow elevations by proximal illumination and by carefully noting refocusing requirements.

o Retina is wrinkled, except for a retinal cyst in longstanding retinal detachment. Contrast Fig. 5.16 with retinoschisis and retinal detachment associated with choroidal tumors.

o The retina often quivers or undulates with patient movement. This contrasts with retinal cysts, retinoschisis, and retinal detachment with tumors.

o Retinal tears or holes, including macular holes, can be found in all but about 5 percent of these retinal detachments. Most are found at the equator or anteriorly.

o Pigmented or yellow subretinal lines — demarcation lines or high water marks — at the edge of longstanding retinal detachment indicate where the retinal detachment stopped progressing for a period of four months or longer.

o Colobomata, falciform folds, staphylomata may be present.

Symptoms & signs

o Symptoms of a retinal tear, such as flashes and floaters, may precede retinal detachment.

o Central visual acuity is normal in peripheral retinal detachment that has not reached the macula, unless intravitreal blood or other macular pathology is present. An exception is the macular hole as cause of retinal detachment.

Fig. 5.13 Histologic section of a retinal detachment. Precise terminology is retinal separation, because the cleavage is between the neurosensory retina and the pigment epithelium, both retinal tissue. Courtesy of Torrence Makley, M.D., Ohio State University.

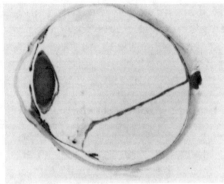

Fig. 5.14 Retinal detachment in a 50-year-old female. The superior retina hangs down over the disc. Visual acuity limited to counting fingers. Also shown in color section.

Fig. 5.15 Retinal detachment from a disinsertion (same patient as in Fig. 5.12). The retinal pigment epithelium and choroid are seen well near the superior, but not the inferior vessels. The inferior vessels are tortuous and out of focus. Also shown in color section.

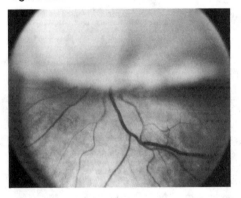

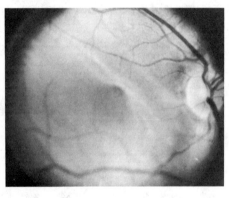

Fig. 5.16 Retinal cyst in a longstanding retinal detachment. Note the choroid can be seen magnified through the cyst (contrast with Fig. 5.17). Retinoschisis and cysts have a smooth, unwrinkled appearance.

Fig. 5.17 Total retinal detachment with the disc obscured by folds of the retina in a funnel shape.

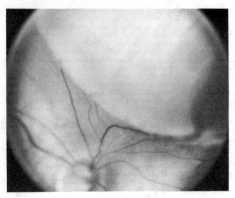

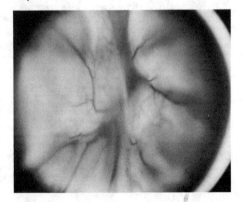

o Detachment of the macular retina is accompanied by loss of vision. The patient may describe distortions, dimness of light, loss of color vision, and, occasionally, monocular diplopia or triplopia.

o The patient may describe loss of any part of his peripheral field of vision. Any loss is opposite the affected retina. Peripheral retinal detachment may be present inferiorly for a long time, and the loss of superior field may be noted by the patient only when the other eye is covered or retinal detachment approaches the macula. Superior detachments usually have a more rapid loss of inferior field. Visual field testing confirms the defect. The loss is not total; light perception remains in the affected field, in contrast with retinoschisis.

o Afferent pupil reaction may be seen if the macula is detached.

o Cells in the vitreous, signs of iritis, and low intraocular pressure may be present.

o Retinal elevation may be acute (one to two hours) or chronic. It may progress rapidly or remain unchanged for years.

Other confirming findings

o History of familial blindness should alert you. Dominant recessive and sex-linked retinal elevations occur. Aphakic (39 percent), myopic (35 percent), and traumatized (15 percent) eyes account for most retinal detachments. The median age of rhegmatogenous retinal detachment patients is 59 years. The age range is wide, and the silent onset of retinal disinsertion in children should not be forgotten.

o Among the hereditary syndromes associated with retinal detachment, Marfan's syndrome, homocystinuria, Weill-Marchesani syndrome, pseudoxanthoma elasticum, Ehlers-Danlos syndrome, and Wagner's disease are the most common. Retinal elevation associated with advanced diabetic retinopathy may or may not be due to a retinal break.

o Visual field testing, ultrasonography, computerized axial tomography, fluorescein angiography, light adaptation, and electroretinogram aid in diagnosis.

Main differential diagnosis

o Malignant melanoma of the choroid and choroidal detachment, mostly in adults

o Retinoblastoma, mostly in children

o Proliferative diabetic retinopathy

o Macular degeneration, usually after age 50

- o   Tumors metastatic to choroid or retina, mostly in adults
- o   Retinoschisis, both adults and children
- o   Central serous choroidopathy, young adults
- o   Retrolental fibroplasia, usually in infants of premature birth
- o   Congenital falciform retinal fold, coloboma
- o   Coats's and Eales's diseases
- o   Retinal dysplasia associated with aniridia or Wilm's tumor of kidney

References

Havener WH, Gloeckner S: Atlas of Diagnostic Techniques and Treatment of Retinal Detachment. St. Louis: Mosby, 1967.

Krill AE: Krill's Hereditary Retinal and Choroidal Diseases, vol 2. Hagerstown, Md: Harper & Row, 1977.

Norton EWD: Differential diagnosis of retinal detachment. In Symposium on Retina and Retinal Surgery. New Orleans Academy of Ophthalmology. St. Louis: Mosby, 1969, pp 52-65.

Tolentino FI, Schepens CL, Freeman HM: Vitreoretinal Disorders: Diagnosis and Management. Philadelphia: Saunders, 1976.

B. NONRHEGMATOGENOUS RETINAL DETACHMENT

Separation of the neurosensory retina from the retinal pigment epithelium —by traction, subretinal accumulation of fluid, displacement by tissue swelling or tumor, or a combination of all three — without the presence of a retinal break presents an important differential diagnosis. Many diseases are associated with retinal elevation. Although the following is not exhaustive, it presents the ophthalmoscopic findings of the common causes and gives references to others.

Fig. 5.18 Advanced proliferative diabetic retinopathy with retinal detachment. Note that retinal blood vessels are missing on the right and the retina has been pulled into the fibrovascular tissue.

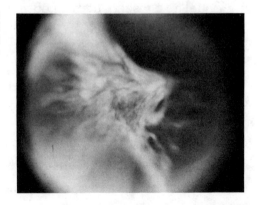

1. Proliferative diabetic retinopathy (Fig. 5.18)

Ophthalmoscopic findings

o   The evidence of advanced diabetic retinopathy can usually be found (see Figs. 4.73-4.78).

o   Retinal elevation may be localized to a particular area of traction along a vessel, it may circle the macula, be confined to the macula, or extensively pull the whole retina into a fibrovascular mass.

o   Intravitreal or preretinal blood often makes the definition of the elevation difficult.

o   Caliber of abnormal vessels may equal or exceed normal retinal vessels.

For symptons & signs, other confirming findings, main differential diagnosis, see Chapter 4: VIIA.

2. Central serous retinopathy (idiopathic central serous choroido-pathy, central angiospastic retinopathy) (Fig. 5.19)

Despite the name, this disease of young patients is more related to defective retinal pigment epithelium than either the neurosensory retina or choroid.

Ophthalmoscopic findings

o   Round or oval elevation of the neurosensory retina in or near the fovea is usual finding; there may be many elevations.

o   Elevation is usually shallow.

Fig. 5.19 Central serous retinopathy in a 38-year-old female. The retinal elevation forms a vertical oval including the whole macula (a, left). Fluorescein angiography confirms the faint spot above the fovea as the cause (b, right).

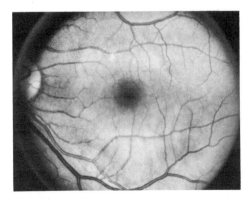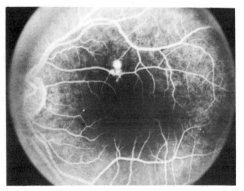

o Faint change in color, highlights from the retina, and the refocusing required help define margins; fine striae or many fine yellow dots may be present in elevation.

o Retinal pigment epithelium may be mottled or yellow in one or more areas under the neurosensory retinal elevation, usually in the upper part. One of these areas is usually the cause for the subretinal fluid.

o Size of neurosensory retinal elevation is usually 2-3 disc diameters, but several elevations of different sizes may be present in the same eye. A large elevation may extend into the inferior periphery and become quite elevated, but this is rare.

o Both eyes may become affected, but rarely at the same time.

Symptoms & signs

o Unless the macula or paramacular retina is involved, patient is asymptomatic.

o Distorted vision is the most common complaint, followed by blurred vision, after-images (flashbulb effect), micropsia, and dimness of vision.

o Visual acuity usually 6/12 (20/40) or better and can be improved with a plus lens (focusing upon the retinal elevation) or a pinhole.

o Pupil reactions normal.

o Scotoma and distorted area plotted on Amsler grid.

o Spontaneous recovery is common after weeks or months.

Other confirming findings

o Patients are usually between 20-45 years old and in good health.

o Males more often affected (10 to one over females).

o Patient usually involved in a stressful situation.

o Blacks and Orientals rarely have the disease.

o Recurrence in the same or other eye in 50 percent of patients.

o Indirect ophthalmoscopy provides additional information.

o Biomicroscopy with contact lens provides additional facts.

o Fluorescein angiography provides important information.

Main differential diagnosis

o Histoplasmosis syndrome

o Senile macular degeneration

- o Focal chorioretinitis
- o Metastatic carcinoma of choroid
- o Vitelliform macular degeneration
- o Choroidal nevus
- o Choroidal melanoma
- o Angioid streaks
- o Rhegmatogenous retinal detachment

References

Gass JDM: Bullous retinal detachment: An unusual manifestation of idiopathic central serous choroidopathy. Am J Ophthalmol 75:810, 1973.

Gass JDM: Serous detachment of the macula secondary to congenital pit of the optic nervehead. Am J Ophthalmol 67:821, 1969.

Gass JDM: Stereoscopic Atlas of Macular Diseases. St. Louis: Mosby, 1977, p 28.

Lewis ML: Idiopathic serous detachment of the retinal pigment epithelium. Arch Ophthalmol 96:620, 1978.

Meredith TA, Braley RE, Aaberg TM: Natural history of serous detachments of the retinal pigment epithelium. Am J Ophthalmol 88: 643, 1979.

Yannuzzi LA, Gitter KA, Schatz H: The Macula: A Comprehensive Text and Atlas. Baltimore: Williams & Wilkins, 1979, p 166.

3. Malignant hypertension, toxemia of pregnancy, congestive heart failure (Fig. 5.20)

These three interrelated vascular problems result in retinal detachment in a small group of the affected patients. It's possible that many more have the difficulty, but are overlooked in the gravity of their conditions.

Ophthalmoscopic findings

- o Evidence of Grade III to IV hypertensive retinopathy is always present (see Table 4.2).
- o Shallow elevation and edema both give the retina a gray translucent appearance, obscuring the view of the retinal pigment epithelium.
- o Vitreous may be cloudy from extravasated protein and hemorrhage.
- o Bullous elevation of the retina occurs in about 10 percent of patients with eclampsia. It's usually bilateral.
- o Retinal elevation may shift with changes in patient's position.

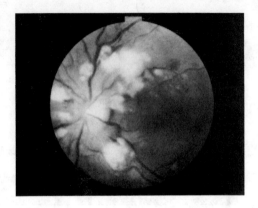

Fig. 5.20 Hypertensive retinopathy in a young woman with toxemia of pregnancy. The patient also has a shallow retinal detachment. Courtesy of William Havener, M.D., Ohio State University.

o Hypertensive and arteriosclerotic vascular disease may be seen for years after toxemia is resolved.

o Ischemic optic neuropathy or papilledema occur.

Symptoms & signs

o Loss of vision is bilateral and profound — often limited to hand motion — and occurs acutely.

o Field loss may vary with shifting of subretinal fluid.

o Pupils may be dilated and poorly reactive when there is extensive retinal detachment involving the macula.

o Visual recovery after termination of hypertensive episode may be initially rapid, but some permanent visual loss and optic atrophy are common.

Other confirming findings

o Toxemia is rarely seen before sixth month gestation. Malignant hypertension can occur in young patients, usually in third decade of life.

o Evidence of pregnancy, glomerulonephritis, pheochromocytoma, and other causes of acute hypertension are usually present.

o Diastolic blood pressure is greater than 100 and may reach 130 mm Hg.

o Generalized edema of trunk, face, and limbs may be present.

o Laboratory, roentgenogram, and other physiologic evidence to support diagnosis are described in the references.

Main differential diagnosis

o   Papilledema due to intracranial mass

o   Proliferative diabetic retinopathy

o   Bilateral rhegmatogenous retinal detachment

o   Bilateral uveal effusion

o   Bilateral retinoblastoma

References

Beeson BP, McDermott W, Wyngaarden JB, eds: Textbook of Medicine. Philadelphia: Saunders, 1979.

Duke-Elder S, Dobree JH: System of Ophthalmology, vol 10. St. Louis: Mosby, 1967, p 350.

4. Trauma (Figs. 5.21, 5.22; see 5.22 also in color section)

Shortening of preretinal or subretinal scar tissue induced by hemorrhage or foreign material may gather the retina in elevated folds even if there is no retinal break.

Ophthalmoscopic findings

o   Hemorrhage, hemolyzed blood remnants, or foreign materials present at or near the elevated retina.

o   Irregular depigmentation and pigment proliferation at the site of trauma.

o   Alteration of the normal course of retinal blood vessels and anastomosis with the choroid.

Fig. 5.21 Contusion resulted in a large choroidal rupture nasal to the disc (a, left). Note how the blood vessels are swept toward the defect and fovea is displaced (arrow) almost to the disc (b, right). Visual acuity was 6/15 (20/50). Courtesy of Paul Torrisi, M.D., Syracuse, New York.

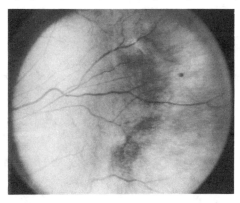 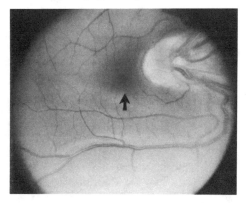

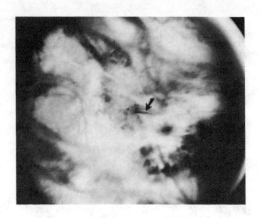

Fig. 5.22 Ruptured globe and elevated, gray retinal folds caused by a BB injury. An eyelash is imbedded in the retina (arrow). Also shown in color section.

o Hiding of retinal blood vessels, disc, or macula by retinal folds or preretinal bands.

o Vitreous condensations attached to the elevated retina.

Symptoms & signs

o Loss of vision depends on the locality and extent of retinal damage.

o Distal retinal elevation may, together with loss of vision, cause traction on macula.

o Loss of visual field corresponds to the area of retinal elevation.

Other confirming findings

o History of injury.

o External, biomicroscopic, indirect ophthalmoscopic evidence of ocular contusion or penetration.

o Roentgenographic, ultrasonographic, computerized axial tomographic or fluorescein angiographic evidence of injury.

Main differential diagnosis

o Congenital retinal malformations, such as falciform fold

o Rhegmatogenous retinal detachment

o Proliferative diabetic retinopathy

o Toxocara canis infestation

o Coats's disease

References

Freeman H, ed: Ocular Trauma. New York: Appleton-Century-Crofts, 1979.

Havener WH, Gloeckner SL: Atlas of Diagnostic Techniques and Treatment of Intraocular Foreign Bodies. St. Louis: Mosby, 1969.

5. Retrolental fibroplasia (see Chapter 4: VIIIA)

This vascular disease of newborns has effects that vary from mild peripheral retinal scarring to devastating bilateral blindness. Retinal detachment due to contracture of the vitreous with or without retinal breaks can occur, usually in the first two to three decades of life. In patients with limited vision from the initial disease, the further loss becomes readily apparent to them. Because the temporal retinal periphery is most severely affected by the initial disease, subsequent retinal detachment usually starts in that area, resulting in a loss of nasal visual field. The patients rarely complain of floaters or flashes so often described by patients with retinal tears.

6. Congenital falciform fold, posterior hyperplastic primary vitreous, and retinal dysplasia (Fig. 5.23)

Persistence of the primary vitreous is a developmental anomaly nearly always in microphthalmic eyes.

Attachments of the primary vitreous to the sensory retina may exist at any site. Shrinkage of the fibroglial elements results in a tent-rope elevation of the retina that may extend from the disc to the periphery, widening as it goes. The retina in the fold is often dysplastic.

Ophthalmoscopic findings

o White pupil (leukocoria) may prevent a view of retina.

o Vitreous membranes are always present, usually extending from disc to midperiphery.

o Retinal fold can be in any quadrant.

o Remnants of hyaloid artery system are often present.

o Intravitreal hemorrhage and rhegmatogenous retinal detachment may occur.

o Lens may be clear but subluxated and later cataractous.

o Unilateral in 83 percent of cases.

o Most eyes microphthalmic and/or microcorneal (corneal diameter often < 10 mm).

Fig. 5.23 Congenital falciform fold in a young man who developed a retinal detachment.

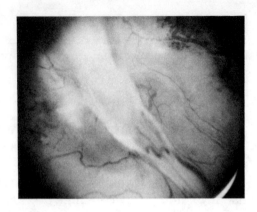

Symptoms & signs

o   Visual acuity ranges from 6/7.5 (20/25) to light perception.

o   Strabismus and nystagmus common.

o   Dilated fixed pupil in presence of retinal detachment, severe intravitreal hemorrhage, and low visual acuity.

o   Defective visual field corresponding with retinal fold.

Other confirming findings

o   Family history negative; most cases are sporadic.

o   Full-term gestation, no oxygen therapy in history.

o   Average age at diagnosis six years.

o   Negative roentgenogram for occult foreign body; eosinophile count and Toxocara ELISA test are normal.

o   Indirect ophthalmoscopic, biomicroscopic, and ultrasonic examination confirmatory.

o   Surgical intervention, when indicated, provides tissue for pathologic diagnosis.

Main differential diagnosis

o   Occult intraocular foreign body

o   Parasitic infection, such as Toxocara canis

o   Retrolental fibroplasia

o   Incontinentia pigmenti

o   Sickle cell disease

References

Haddad R, Font RL, Reeser F: Persistent hyperplastic primary vitreous: A clinicopathologic study of 62 cases and review of the literature. Surv Ophthalmol 23:123, 1978.

Peyman GA, Sanders DR, Goldberg MF, eds: Principles and Practice of Ophthalmology. Philadelphia: Saunders, 1980.

Pruett RC, Schepens CL: Posterior hyperplastic primary vitreous. Am J Ophthalmol 69:534, 1970.

C. RETINOSCHISIS (SPLIT RETINA)

Splitting of the neurosensory retina into one or more layers is an entity distinct from separation of the neurosensory retina from the retinal pigment epithelium, or retinal detachment. It occurs commonly in the peripheral retina with aging and less commonly at birth in a sex-linked hereditary form. The appearance and clinical course is different for each. The cleavage usually starts in the outer plexiform retinal layer, but may be at the nerve fiber layer in the reticular type.

1. Senile (adult) retinoschisis (Figs. 5.24-5.27)

Cystoid and reticular retinoschisis are discussed together.

Ophthalmoscopic findings

o   Nearly always bilateral; may be more advanced in one eye.

o   Starts peripherally, usually in the inferior temporal quadrant or superior temporal quadrant, rarely nasally.

o   Sharp posterior border where blood vessels suddenly elevate from retinal plane; in some patients, pigment (demarcation line) is present at the border, and retinal pigment epithelium often shows clumping or atrophy throughout the whole schisis area.

o   Border is usually smooth and resembles a large cyst with choroid visible through it.

o   Posterior border location is variable; very common to see small areas along ora; extension to the macula is uncommon.

o   Large retinal breaks in the outer layer are often posteriorly located and multiple. The anterior edge of the breaks is often difficult to define. Retinal vessels pass over the breaks without distortion. Smaller breaks may be seen in the inner layer; they are usually more peripheral than outer layer breaks and difficult to see, because retinal pigment epithelial atrophy decreases the contrast.

Fig. 5.24 Splitting of the neurosensory retina (retinoschisis). The retina is artificially elevated. Courtesy of Torrence Makley, M.D., Ohio State University.

Fig. 5.25 Senile cystoid retinoschisis in a 50-year-old male. A retinal vessel arches over the elevated inner layer of the retinal split. The other eye was similar.

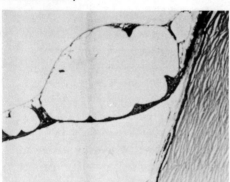
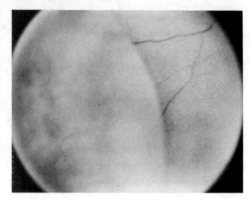

o   Elevated retina is smooth and may have white glistening highlights; it doesn't move with patient movement.

o   When detachment occurs, the elevated retina becomes translucent and the choroid cannot be seen as well.

o   Spontaneous collapse of retinoschisis may occur, leaving a pale retinal pigment epithelium with clumps of pigment and sometimes a demarcation line.

Symptoms & signs

o   Rarely symptomatic; if retinal detachment occurs, vision drops precipitously; visual recovery after successful surgery is often 6/60 (20/200) or less. In some patients, macula is involved in retinoschisis, and vision is reduced to light perception.

o   Pupil reaction is normal when light is directed on the nasal retina, but poor on retinoschisis area.

o   Loss of peripheral vision is rarely noted by the patient.

o   Usual flashes, floaters are not reported by these patients, even when retinal detachment occurs. Because the upper field is usually affected, the patient is unaware of loss until the macula is involved; patient may become aware of visual difficulty only on covering the other eye.

o   Dark adaptation and color vision remain normal unless the macula is involved.

o   Visual field loss is absolute — no light perception because the rods and cones are disconnected from the ganglion cells by the retinal split.

Fig. 5.26 Triangular retinal hole in the flat outer layer of reticular retinoschisis appears darker than the rest of the retina. The anterior edge of these holes may be difficult to see.

Fig. 5.27 Cystoid retinoschisis in a 37-year-old female has a beaten silver appearance near the ora serrata (to the right). The other eye was similar.

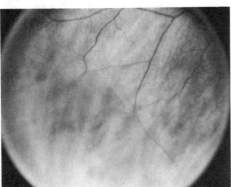 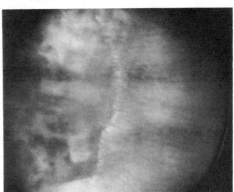

Other confirming findings

o Affects both sexes equally.

o Rarely seen in patients younger than 50.

o No hereditary pattern.

o May be more common in patients with diminished ocular blood flow, as in carotid artery stenosis.

o Indirect ophthalmoscopy with scleral depression and biomicroscopy are usually diagnostic.

o Electroretinogram may have an absent b-wave in extensive disease.

o Ultrasonography, fluorescein angiography.

o Diagnostic photocoagulation.

Main differential diagnosis

o Retinal detachment, either rhegmatogenous or nonrhegmatogenous

o Choroidal melanoma or metastatic tumor

o Retinal cyst in longstanding retinal detachment

o Hereditary vitreoretinal degeneration

o Juvenile retinoschisis

References

Goettinger W: Senile Retinoschisis. Stuttgart: Thieme, 1978.

Tolentino FI, Schepens CL, Freeman HM: Vitreoretinal Disorders: Diagnosis and Management. Philadelphia: Saunders, 1976.

Fig. 5.28 Juvenile retinoschisis in a 25-year-old male. Note how the color of the choroid can be seen distal to the edge (arrow) through the thin, elevated inner layer (a, left). Involvement of the macula is associated with poor vision and may be present without the peripheral retinoschisis (b, right).

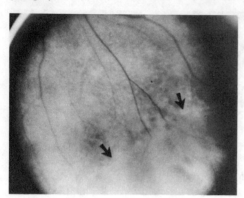 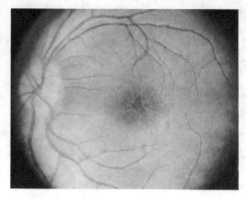

2. Juvenile (sex-linked or x-linked) retinoschisis (Fig. 5.28)

The plane of cleavage in juvenile retinoschisis is in the nerve fiber layer. This contrasts with senile retinoschisis. Because the elevated inner layer is so thin, retinal blood vessels seem suspended, which leads to the term vascular veils to describe the appearance.

Ophthalmoscopic findings

o Always bilateral.

o Ophthalmoscopic focus to follow blood vessels may require high plus lenses, and vessels may be right behind the lens.

o Vessels may be present in inner layer or may cross the schisis cavity beneath the surface of the innermost retinal layer.

o Plicated spoke-like foveal retina in both eyes is pathognomonic and nearly always present.

o Intravitreal or intracavity hemorrhage may occur. Fluid levels of unclotted blood may be created by positioning.

o Retinal pigment epithelium may show irregular atrophy and hyperpigmentation, even at macula. Demarcation line may be present.

o Inferior temporal retina most often affected early, but eventually all quadrants may be involved.

o Retinal detachment may occur, but is rare.

o Silver-gray patches, arborizing sheets, and perivascular cuffs may develop.

o Vitreous bands and veils may traverse the cavity.

Symptoms & signs

o   Visual acuity may be normal, but usually 6/15 (20/50) to 6/60 (20/200) early in life, gradually decreasing with age. Sudden visual loss may occur with hemorrhage.

o   Usually, the patients are farsighted and astigmatic.

o   Peripheral field loss in superior nasal quadrant or general constriction with relative central scotoma can be detected.

o   There may be acquired red-green color blindness.

o   Dark adaptation slow.

Other confirming findings

o   X-linked in males; present from birth. Carrier females have no evidence of disease.

o   May be a predilection for male children to occur in these families.

o   This disease has been seen in all races.

o   The gene has high penetrance.

o   Fluorescein angiography shows delayed circulation time and pigment defects in macula in late stages.

o   Electroretinogram, subnormal; electro-oculogram, normal.

Main differential diagnosis

o   Retinal detachment, inferior disinsertion of the young

o   Cystoid macular edema, as in peripheral uveitis (pars planitis)

o   Vitreoretinal degeneration of Goldmann-Favre.

o   Wagner's vitreoretinal dystrophy

o   Chorioretinitis

o   Stargardt's disease

o   Dominant cystoid macular edema

o   Traumatic macular cyst and photic cyst

References

Deutman AF: The Hereditary Dystrophies of the Posterior Pole of the Eye. Springfield, Ill: Thomas, 1971.

Krill AE: Krill's Hereditary Retinal and Choroidal Diseases, vol 2. Hagerstown, Md: Harper & Row, 1977, p 1044.

3. Goldmann-Favre disease (see Fig. 5.28)

This rare nightblindness disease resembles juvenile retinoschisis, becoming symptomatic between the ages of 10 and 20 years. It's a progressive disorder.

Ophthalmoscopic findings

o Optic atrophy, vessel attenuation, and pigmentation often indistinguishable from retinitis pigmentosa (rod-cone dystrophy).

o Coarse microcystic changes in the macula.

o Peripheral retinoschisis, often with large holes in the inner layer, involves mostly the temporal retina.

o Bilateral.

Symptoms & signs

o Visual acuity decreases between ages of 10 and 20 years.

o Nightblindness is noted about same time as decreased vision.

o Color vision is defective when visual loss is severe.

o Ring scotoma resembles retinitis pigmentosa.

o Dark adaptation very restricted.

o Complicated cataracts develop.

Other confirming findings

o Inheritance is autosomal dominant.

o Electroretinogram usually unrecordable.

o Fluorescein angiography distinguishes the microcystic macular disease from leaking capillary disease.

Main differential diagnosis

o X-linked juvenile retinoschisis

o Wagner's disease

o Retinitis pigmentosa

References

Krill AE: Krill's Hereditary Retinal and Choroidal Diseases, vol 2. Hagerstown, Md: Harper & Row, 1977, p 1062.

IV. WRINKLING OF THE RETINA

Distortion of the retinal surface creates highlights and shadows under the ophthalmoscope's light, allowing a view of this usually transparent tissue. Diseases in contiguous tissue or the retina itself may disrupt the smooth surface. Usually the wrinkling is localized.

Wrinkles may result from displacement of the retina—as in retinal detachment or papilledema. Wrinkles caused by contraction of tissue may radiate like the spokes of a wheel. Contraction wrinkles may be on the inner or under surface of the neurosensory retina.

A. DISPLACEMENT WRINKLES

1. Retinal detachment (see IIIA, above)

2. Papilledema (see Chapter 3: VIIB, 7c)

3. Choroidal elevation (see Chapter 7: VI)

4. Choroidal folds (see Chapter 6: VIB)

5. Cystoid macular edema (Fig. 5.29)

Accumulation of fluid in Henle's layer of the macular retina highlights the fibers and appears in a stellate pattern in the neurosensory retina centered at the fovea. It indicates severe and often permanent visual loss. It's a nonspecific finding associated with a number of systemic and ocular diseases and treatments and is occasionally dominantly inherited. We don't know why the macular retina responds in this particular manner to ocular diseases.

Ophthalmoscopic findings

o   Fine, clear spaces in an otherwise slightly translucent central retina.

o   Fine cysts may be of various sizes and arranged in rows, giving appearance of wrinkles.

o   May be very subtle and discernible only by proximal illumination.

o   Disc and retinal blood vessels, particularly veins, may be dark, dilated, and tortuous. In some patients, splinter hemorrhages or microaneurysms are present in macular arcades.

o   Larger cysts at the foveola may resemble a macular hole.

o   Retinal pigment epithelium appears smudged, and abnormal pigment gives a yellow color (lipofuscin).

Fig. 5.29 Cystoid macular edema in a 16-year-old female with chronic venous stasis (a, left). Visual acuity was 6/30 (20/100). The other eye is normal. Intravenous fluorescein pools in the cystic spaces (b, right).

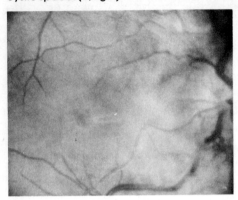 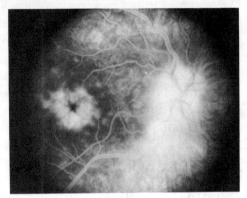

o Retinal vascular disease or peripheral retinal or intravitreal inflammatory disease may be present.

o Macular hole may be present in other eye.

Symptoms & signs

o Decreased vision is present, varying from 6/9 (20/30) to counting fingers; patient may note vision is better with eccentric fixation.

o Patient may see far away but not read.

o Central vision is burred, distorted, "too small," or "tilted," and recovery of vision after bright light exposure is delayed. Peripheral vision is normal.

o Vision may vary a few lines on eye chart day to day.

o Pupil reactions are usually normal.

o Central scotoma found on field testing.

Other confirming findings

o Some systemic and ocular diseases and treatments known to be associated at times with cystoid macular edema are listed in Table 5.1.

o Fluorescein angiography is confirmatory.

Main differential diagnosis

o Macular hole

o Drusen

Table 5.1

DISEASES, CONDITIONS, AND TREATMENTS
ASSOCIATED WITH CYSTOID MACULAR EDEMA

Aphakia (50% of cataract surgery patients have cystoid macular edema, usually transiently in the first six weeks after surgery)

Behcet's disease

Branch or central vein occlusion or stasis

Choroidal hemangioma

Choroidal melanoma

Choroidal metastatic tumor

Diabetes mellitus with retinopathy involving the macular capillaries

Dominantly inherited macular disease

Epinephrine used topically in glaucoma treatment

Epiretinal membrane

Goldman-Favre disease

Hereditary nightblindness

Juvenile retinoschisis

Peripheral uveitis (pars planitis)

Retinal detachment (if the macular retina has been detached longer than four weeks, the macula may show cystoid changes, even after successful reattachment)

Retinal telangiectasis

Retinitis pigmentosa

Sarcoid uveitis

Sun gazing (solar retinopathy)

Sympathetic ophthalmia

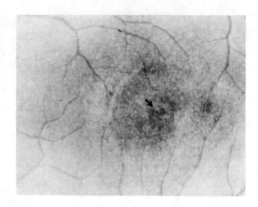

Fig. 5.30 Tiny cyst (arrow) in the fovea of a 15-year-old male thought to be due to excessive exposure to sunlight. Visual acuity was 6/15 (20/50).

o Stargardt's disease and fundus flavimaculatus

o Vitelliform degeneration (Best's disease)

o Embolic retinal artery occlusion

o Solar retinopathy (Fig. 5.30)

o Drug-induced cystic macular edema

References

Deutman AF, Pinckers AJ, Aan de Kerk AL: Dominantly inherited cystoid macular edema. Am J Ophthalmol 82:540, 1976.

Gass JDM: Stereoscopic Atlas of Macular Diseases. St. Louis: Mosby, 1977, p 250.

Yannuzzi LA, Gitter KA, Schatz H: The Macula: A Comprehensive Text and Atlas. Baltimore: Williams & Wilkins, 1979.

6. Hypotony (see Chapter 3: VIIB, 2b)

Low intraocular pressure (hypotonia) follows loss of ocular contents or the failure of the eye to produce adequate aqueous.

B. CONTRACTION WRINKLES

1. Diabetic retinopathy (see Chapter 4: VIIA)

Fibrovascular proliferation on the retinal surface is a common and often visually disastrous complication of diabetic retinopathy.

2. Inflammatory disease of retina and vitreous (see V, below)

3. Epiretinal membranes

a) CONGENITAL PRERETINAL MACULAR FIBROSIS (Fig. 5.31)

Epiretinal membranes are occasionally found in children with normal vision or on routine examination for minimally decreased vision. The primary vitreous separates from the retina at the gestational 13-mm stage. Incom-

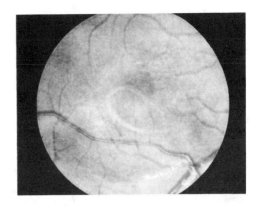

Fig. 5.31 Congenital epiretinal membrane in a 12-year-old female with poor vision from birth. The retinal blood vessels are not distorted. Visual acuity was 6/60 (20/200).

plete separation from the internal limiting membrane results in preretinal membrane before retinal vessels and differentiation of the fovea occur at the 100-mm stage. This explains the lack of vasculature or visual disturbance in most patients.

Ophthalmoscopic findings

o   Membranes may be translucent or opaque.

o   Wrinkles in the retina radiate from membrane.

o   Retinal blood vessels are not tortuous or distorted by the wrinkles.

o   Vitreous is clear.

o   Retinal pigment epithelium appears normal.

o   Unilateral in almost every patient.

o   Remnants of hyaloid artery system may be present.

Symptoms & signs

o   Unless the opaque part of the membrane covers the fovea, visual acuity is normal.

o   Other symptoms and signs are rare.

Other confirming findings

o   Ocular and system review and familial history are rarely contributory.

o   Most patients are discovered on routine examination.

o   Eye is normal size and/or equal to other eye.

o   Fluorescein angiography confirms normal vasculature.

o   Electroretinogram normal.

Main differential diagnosis

o Proliferative diabetic retinopathy

o Surface wrinkling retinopathy

o Cystoid macular edema

o Inflammatory vitreoretinal membranes

o Posterior hyperplastic primary vitreous, retinal dysplasia

References

Wise GN: Congenital preretinal macular fibrosis. Am J Ophthalmol 79:363, 1975.

Wise GN: Relationship of idiopathic preretinal macular fibrosis to posterior vitreous detachment. Am J Ophthalmol 79:358, 1975.

b) SURFACE WRINKLING RETINOPATHY (PRERETINAL MACULAR FIBROSIS, CELLOPHANE MACULOPATHY) (Fig. 5.32; see also in color section; see also Fig. 4.76)
Surface wrinkling retinopathy is an acquired disease. Most patients are older than 40 years. Its spontaneous occurrence in eyes with previously good visual acuity usually brings the patient to the physician.

Ophthalmoscopic findings

o Distortions of the retinal blood vessels exaggerate fine plications in the neurosensory retina.

o Surface membrane may be visible or only suspected by glistening highlights, like reflections from crumpled cellophane.

o Striae (fine wrinkles) often extend 2-3 disc diameters from the central membrane in a spoke-like, frequently asymmetric fashion.

o Defect most often comes to attention when it involves the macula, but can be seen in other areas, usually not far from the disc.

o Veins may be dark and dilated. Small microaneurysms are sometimes present.

o Hypertensive retinopathy and/or arteriosclerotic retinopathy are usually present.

o Majority of patients have only one eye affected.

o Slow progression or regression may occur, but most patients have little change from the findings noted at discovery. A pseudomacular hole may develop in the membrane. It can be distinguished from a true macular hole by biomicroscopic examination.

Fig. 5.32 Spontaneous surface wrinkling retinopathy in a hypertensive 23-year-old male. Visual acuity was 6/9 (20/30). Note the tortuosity of the inferior vessels. Also shown in color section.

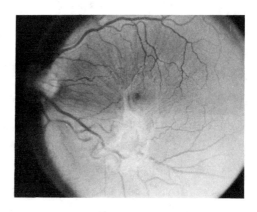

Symptoms & signs

o Many patients are unaware of visual loss or other symptoms until their eyes are tested or they happen to cover the unaffected eye.

o Visual acuity varies from 6/7.5 (20/25) to 6/60 (20/200) but is usually 6/9 (20/30) to 6/15 (20/50).

o The patient who is aware of visual defect reports double, bent, blurred, or smaller than normal vision.

o Only with difficulty can a scotoma be found on field testing.

o Progressive visual loss is unusual, and in most patients, the vision stays at the discovery level. Visual acuity rarely improves, but patients seem to adapt to the distortions after about six months.

Other confirming findings

o Rarely presents as a unilateral birth defect causing poor vision and strabismus.

o Most cases occur spontaneously after age 40. Some follow retinal detachment, photocoagulation, or other ocular surgery.

o Hypertension and arteriosclerosis are usually present.

o Posterior vitreous detachment from the retina is often present.

o Indirect ophthalmoscopy and biomicroscopic examination with contact lens are indicated.

o Fluorescein angiography helps define the disease.

o Medical evaluation with particular emphasis on vascular disease is appropriate.

Main differential diagnosis

o   Irvine-Gass vitreous traction maculopathy

o   Cystoid maculopathy

o   Branch or central retinal vein occlusion

o   Retinal detachment

o   Macular hole

o   Juvenile retinoschisis

o   Congenital preretinal macular fibrosis

o   Hamartoma of the retinal pigment epithelium

References

Gass JDM: Stereoscopic Atlas of Macular Diseases. St. Louis: Mosby, 1977, p 355.

Wise GN, Dollery CT, Henkind P: The Retinal Circulation. New York: Harper & Roe, 1971, p 403.

Yannuzzi LA, Gitter KA, Schatz H: The Macula: A Comprehensive Text and Atlas. Baltimore: Williams & Wilkins, 1979.

c) HAMARTOMA OF THE RETINAL PIGMENT EPITHELIUM AND RETINA (see Chapter 3: VF, 6)

V. RETINAL OPACITIES AND HAZY VITREOUS

You can roughly localize a retinal opacification by seeing whether it obscures the major retinal blood vessels, since they traverse the superficial ganglion cell layer. Cellular response to an acute inflammatory focus in the retina may cause an exudate and hemorrhage in the pigment epithelium or the overlying vitreous. Retinal opacification may at one phase be clearly visible and later obscured by vitreous cells and protein.

A single small lesion in the retina may be associated with a surprising cellular and exudative reaction in the overlying vitreous. It may not even be possible to find the offending locus until clearing occurs. Indirect ophthalmoscopy is invaluable, because it allows a better view through cloudy vitreous. The differential diagnosis of cloudy vitreous is described in Chapter 8. All such eyes shouldn't be immediately considered infected.

A. TOXOPLASMOSIS (Figs. 5.33-5.35; see 5.35b also in color section)

Toxoplasma gondii is acquired in utero and occasionally by ingestion. It has a predilection for central nervous system and retinal tissue in humans. It's

Fig. 5.33 Toxoplasmosis presumed to be congenital because of the early onset and asymmetry. Note the circumpapillary scarring, attenuated retinal vessels, optic atrophy, and choroidal destruction.

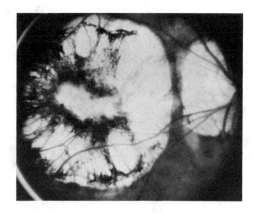

destructive and in congenital infection may have severe sequelae — not just for the eye, but survival. Infections acquired in the adult are milder, but threaten vision.

Ophthalmoscopic findings

Old lesions

o   Old lesions may be large, single, or multiple. Multiple scars are usually adjacent to one another.

o   Destruction of retina and choroid may expose sclera to view.

o   Scars are more common in posterior retina, and the macula is frequently involved.

o   Scars may be bilateral.

o   Pigment hyperplasia results in patches of heavy pigmentation, often at the margins of the scar.

o   Consecutive optic atrophy and retinal vessel narrowing result from severely scarred areas.

o   Occasional retinochoroidal vessel anastomosis can be seen.

o   Overlying vitreous is usually clear by this stage, but veil-like strands are common.

o   There may be a posterior vitreous detachment, with bands attached to scarred areas.

Active lesions

o   View may be hazy or almost obscured.

o   New lesion usually occurs at or near the margin of an old scar.

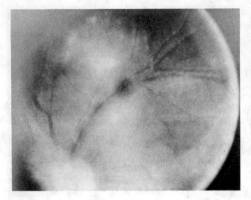

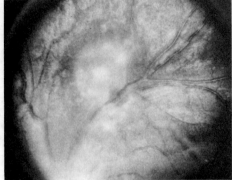

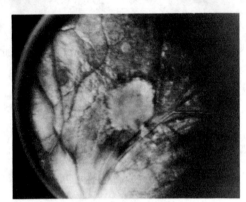

Fig. 5.34 Active toxoplasmosis. Note how the vitreous has cleared between Fig. 5.34a (above left) and 5.34c (right). The active lesion has occurred at the upper margin of an old pigmented scar; toxoplasmosis titer 1:128. Fig. 5.34a: July 6, 1977; 5.34b (above right): August 2, 1977; 5.34c: October 12, 1977. The only treatment was topical medication for associated iritis.

o Activity begins to subside in four to six weeks, and pigmentation occurs within one year.

o Small hemorrhages may be present near active lesions.

o Serous elevation of the neurosensory retina may surround lesion.

o In some patients, retinal tears occur at the margin of necrotic areas, followed by a retinal detachment.

o Retinal arterial occlusion at the inflammatory site has been reported.

Symptoms & signs

o Vision depends on the degree of vitreous opacification and on foveal or optic nerve destruction. Usually, visual acuity is in the 6/12 (20/40) to 6/60 (20/200) range, but lesions in the fovea may reduce visual acuity to counting fingers. Improvement with vitreous clearing usually begins in three to four weeks. No improvement of visual acuity can be expected with a foveal lesion.

o Floaters are a common complaint.

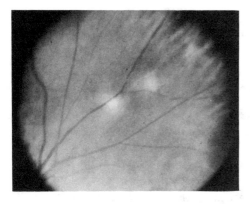

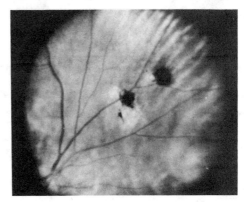

Fig. 5.35 Acquired toxoplasmosis. Two active lesions November 1975 (a, above left) in a patient with hazy vitreous, toxoplasmosis titer of 1:16, and no other lesions in either eye. New lesion occurred in February 1978 at the border of the scar (b, above right). New lesion was inactive by March 1978 without treatment and pigmented by June 1978 (c, right). Repeat toxoplasmosis titer 1:64. Fig. 5.35b also shown in color section.

o Aching pain, photophobia, circumcorneal flush from iritis may accompany active retinal disease.

o Edema of macula by a nearby lesion may cause complaints of distortion of images.

o Pupil reaction varies with the amount of retina and optic nerve destruction.

o Absolute scotomata corresponding to retinal scars are found on field testing.

Other confirming findings

o Toxoplasmosis early in gestation usually results in fetal death. Infection later in pregnancy may result in delivery of a newborn with neonatal jaundice, splenohepatomegaly, interstitial pneumonitis, anemia, and leukopenia. Seizures, hydrocephalus, and mental retardation may follow. X-rays can show calcification of a particular curvilinear type. Calcifications are localized in the hemispheres, as distinct from involvement of the choroidal plexus in cytomegalic inclusion.

o There may be a history of exposure to animals — particularly cats — and ingestion of raw meat. Inhalation of oocytes infects animals and possibly humans.

o Best tests available are Sabin-Feldman dye, hemagglutination, precipitin, indirect fluorescent antibody. There is no correlation between level of test response and activity of ocular disease. A positive test, even in undiluted serum, is significant in the presence of a clinically compatible lesion.

o Dye-test-positive women or those with clinical evidence of the disease don't pass it to their offspring. There is a 14 percent chance that women who convert from dye-test negative to dye-test positive in the first trimester will give birth to children with the disease.

Main differential diagnosis

o Luetic necrotizing retinochoroiditis

o Tuberculous necrotizing retinochoroiditis

o Candida and Aspergillus endophthalmitis

o Toxocara canis and other parasitic ocular granulomas

o Cytomegalic inclusion virus retinitis

o Herpes simplex retinitis

References

Desmonts G, Couvreur J: Congenital toxoplasmosis. N Engl J Med 290:1110, 1974.

Gass JDM: Stereoscopic Atlas of Macular Diseases. St. Louis: Mosby, 1977, p 294.

O'Connor GR: Manifestations and management of ocular toxoplasmosis. Bull NY Acad Med 50:192, 1974.

Teutsch SM, Juranek DD, Sulzer A, et al: Epidemic toxoplasmosis associated with infected cats. N Engl J Med 300:695, 1979.

Fig. 5.36 Presumed candida endophthalmitis in a 32-year-old diabetic. Patient had two exploratory laparotomies and postoperative hyperalimentation for fever of unknown cause. Also shown in color section.

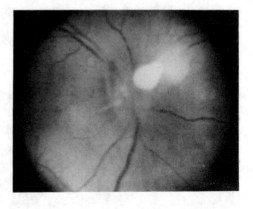

B. EMBOLIC RETINAL ABSCESS

(Figs. 5.36-5.37; see also in color section)

Bacterial or fungal organisms entering the bloodstream may be carried to the eye. Culturing the offending organism from the eye to fulfill Koch's postulates is a difficult task.

Ophthalmoscopic findings

o   Foci may be single, multiple, and bilateral.

o   White or gray mildly elevated avascular mass, rarely larger than 1 disc diameter, may be multilobed.

o   Overlying vitreous is hazy, with strands and clouds of cells emanating from the lesion.

o   Surrounding retina and optic disc are swollen, vessels tortuous.

o   Hemorrhages and Roth's spots nearby.

o   Stress lines may radiate from lesion.

o   May heal with a pigmented scar or little evidence of the acute disease.

o   Vitreous veils may remain over healed lesion.

Symptoms & signs

o   Patients are often acutely ill, and ocular symptoms may be ignored, even though early treatment is the most successful.

o   Visual acuity varies, depending on proximity of lesions to disc or macula and intensity of cellular reaction.

o   Pupil reactions vary with the magnitude of retinal and optic nerve damage.

Fig. 5.37 Roth's spots in a 39-year-old male diabetic with pneumococcal septicemia. The inferior retina is elevated. Also shown in color section.

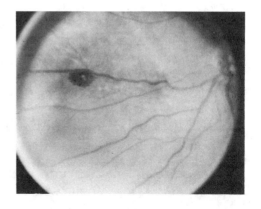

o   Photophobia, aching pain, and ciliary flush indicate accompanying iritis.

o   Usually, an absolute scotoma corresponds to the infected area.

Other confirming findings

o   History of acute febrile illness involving the bloodstream, such as endocarditis. Fungal endophthalmitis may follow a debilitating illness requiring antibiotic therapy and intravenous feeding. Drug addicts may introduce either bacteria or fungi by unclean injection techniques.

o   Blood cultures are indicated.

o   Aqueous and vitreous obtained surgically for culture may be the only way to identify the organism.

Main differential diagnosis

o   Toxoplasmosis

o   Toxocara canis and other larval parasites

o   Intraocular foreign body

o   Sarcoidosis

o   Tuberculosis

o   Syphilis

o   Cytomegalic inclusion virus retinitis

o   Herpes simplex retinitis

o   Retinoblastoma

o   Myelogenous leukemia

References

Edwards JE, Foos RY, Montgomerie JZ, et al: Ocular manifestations of candida septicemia: Review of 76 cases of hematogenous candida endophthalmitis. Medicine 53:47, 1974.

Gass JDM: Stereoscopic Atlas of Macular Diseases. St. Louis: Mosby, 1977, p 355.

Meyers SM: The incidence of fundus lesions in septicemia. Am J Ophthalmol 88:661, 1979.

C. TOXOCARA CANIS (see Chapter 3: VE)

D. RETAINED INTRAOCULAR FOREIGN BODY
(Figs. 5.38, 5.39; see also Fig. 5.22)

Prolonged retention of copper-containing foreign bodies in the eye may deposit particles in the neurosensory retina and vitreous (chalcosis). Ocular

Fig. 5.38 Chalcosis of the macular retina in a 19-year-old male five years after an exploding shell casing penetrated the eye (a, left). Removal of the copper foreign body resulted in clearing of the metallic deposits (b, right). The patient's vitreous was green. Visual acuity was 6/6 (20/20) throughout. From Delaney WV Jr: Presumed ocular chalcosis: A reversible maculopathy. Ann Ophthalmol 7:378, 1975. Used with permission.

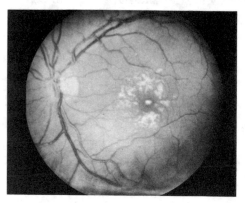
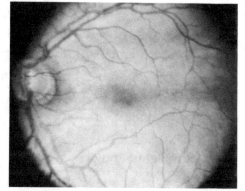

Fig. 5.39 Metallic foreign body on the retina in a 28-year-old male. The patient felt something hit his eye while waiting in his auto at an intersection. Also shown in color section.

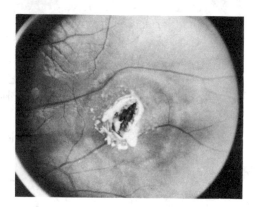

destruction by copper is greatest from the pure metal. Intraretinal copper has a distinct appearance. Ferrous metals cause black particle deposition (see Chapter 6: IIID, 2; see also Fig. 3.66 in color section)

Ophthalmoscopic findings

o Yellow deposits in the retina are concentrated at the macula.

o Blood vessels may be slightly narrowed and show yellow deposits along their course.

o The vitreous is green or yellow and liquid.

o Scars and other evidence of the original trauma and surgical intervention may be visible.

Symptoms & signs

o Loss of vision in the affected eye is the usual complaint after the acute, painful initial injury has passed. Patient may describe overall dimness of light in affected eye.

o Vision varies from no light perception to 6/6 (20/20).

o Central scotoma or general constriction of field may be found.

o Pupil reactions are often sluggish, and iris is discolored — green in copper, yellow in iron.

o Color vision is often defective.

Other confirming findings

o History of trauma from an explosion, metal hitting on metal, or the like can usually be elicited. Ophthalmoscopic and radiologic studies may have failed to reveal the foreign body, especially if it's near the front of the eye.

o Radiologic study often does not find a small foreign body retained long after the injury. Computerized axial tomography is not better than standard radiologic study for diagnosis, but aids localization once found. Glass, wood, and plastic do not show well on either radiologic study.

o Indirect ophthalmoscopy with scleral depression is an excellent aid in diagnosis.

o Electroretinogram is helpful in both diagnosis and prediction of retinal function.

o Ultrasonography helps find and localize a foreign body.

Main differential diagnosis

o Recurrent uveitis or retinitis, as in toxoplasmosis

o Toxocara canis or other larval infestation

o Intravitreal hemorrhage (all causes)

o Endophthalmitis

References

Delaney WV Jr: Presumed ocular chalcosis: A reversible maculopathy. Ann Ophthalmol 7:378, 1975.

Havener WH, Gloeckner SL: Atlas of Diagnostic Techniques and Treatment of Intraocular Foreign Bodies. St. Louis: Mosby, 1969.

E. RETINOBLASTOMA (see VIB, 1, below)

F. TUBERCULOSIS (see Chapter 7: VG, 1b)

G. SYPHILIS (see Chapter 6: IVB, 1)

H. LEPROSY (see Chapter 4: IXC)

I. LEPTOSPIROSIS (see Chapter 7: VG, Table 7-1)

J. ROCKY MOUNTAIN SPOTTED FEVER (Fig. 5.40)

This acute rickettsial infection is a severe debilitating illness frequently involving the retina as part of the disease.

Ophthalmoscopic findings

o   Retina and optic disc are edematous and white.

o   Veins are engorged, and perivenous hemorrhages are common.

o   Cotton-wool (soft) exudates, usually near the disc.

o   Occlusions of retinal arteries may occur.

o   Permanent scars of the retinal pigment epithelium may remain as edema subsides.

Symptoms & signs

o   Visual acuity usually good, but may be severely impaired in both eyes.

o   Lid swelling as part of a generalized skin rash.

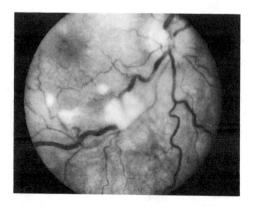

Fig. 5.40 Rocky Mountain spotted fever in a nine-year-old patient. From Smith TW, Burton TC: The retinal manifestations of Rocky Mountain spotted fever. Am J Ophthalmol 84:259, 1977. Used with permission.

o Pupil reactions usually normal, but may be abnormal in severe central nervous system disease.

o Blind spots enlarged, and quadrantal field loss may be present in severe central nervous system disease.

o Esotropia and ocular muscle palsies may develop.

Other confirming findings

o Disease is not confined to rural areas and is widespread throughout U.S.A. and Central America.

o Ticks transmit Rickettsia to humans. Several types of ticks are known to carry it; wood tick and dog tick are most common. Crushing ticks with fingers has been known to inoculate people.

o Incubation period three to 12 days.

o Prodrome of malaise, headache, anorexia, and nosebleeds may precede the rash, high fever, and joint and muscle pains that more clearly indicate the onset of disease.

o Laboratory findings of elevated white blood count. Agglutinins against Proteus vulgaris OX-19 above 1:320 are usually found, as well as positive complement fixation tests.

Main differential diagnosis

o Typhus
o Meningococcemia
o Measles
o Typhoid fever
o Acute necrotizing retinitis of herpes simplex or cytomegalic inclusion virus

References

Murray ES: Rocky Mountain spotted fever: A life-saving diagnostic problem. Clinical Medicine August 1976, p 9.

Presley GD: Fundus changes in Rocky Mountain spotted fever. Am J Ophthalmol 67:263, 1969.

Smith TW, Burton TC: The retinal manifestations of Rocky Mountain spotted fever. Am J Ophthalmol 84:259, 1977.

Vaughan VC, McKay RJ, Behrman RE, eds: Nelson Textbook of Pediatrics. Philadelphia: Saunders, 1979.

K. ACUTE NECROTIZING RETINITIS (CYTOMEGALIC INCLUSION VIRUS, HERPES SIMPLEX, SUBACUTE SCLEROSING PANEN-CEPHALITIS) (Fig. 5.41; see also in color section)

Severe bilateral visual loss may result from cytomegalic inclusion disease and the herpes simplex virus in newborns or adults whose resistance is weakened by other illness or drugs. The neurosensory retina is the principal site of infection in the eye.

Ophthalmoscopic findings

o In the acute phase, the view of the retina is hazy, due to serum-like vitreous protein and cells. Some red blood cells may be present, but intravitreal hemorrhage is not prominent.

o Large yellow patches appearing to be conglomerations of smaller defects start near the disc and extend into the mid-peripheral retina. The retinal pigment epithelium is hidden from view in these areas.

o Hemorrhage is often present on the surface of the yellow patches.

o Exudative retinal detachment may occur.

o Retinal vessels may be attenuated.

o In the healing phase, the yellow-red patches resolve gradually from the periphery and leave a scalloped border of retinal pigment epithelial atrophy.

o Retinal pigment epithelium healing results in patches of exposed choroid and pigment hyperplasia.

o Retinal vessel narrowing and optic atrophy follow.

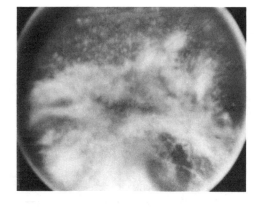

Fig. 5.41 Cytomegalic inclusion virus retinopathy in a 56-year-old renal transplantation patient. Visual acuity both eyes was 6/60 (20/200). Also shown in color section.

Symptoms & signs

o Bilateral loss of central vision is rapid, usually within a week; one eye may be more advanced than the other, and unilateral involvement has been reported, especially in herpes simplex infection.

o Central scotomata are common.

o Pupils are often dilated, and sustained light response is poor.

o Iritis may be present with photophobia, aching pain, ciliary flush, and miosis.

Other confirming findings

o Infection of newborns with cytomegalic inclusion disease virus is associated with pneumonitis, fever, anemia, thrombocytopenia, jaundice, and hepatosplenomegaly. Skull roentgenogram shows calcifications at the choroidal plexus. Afflicted children have motor and mental difficulties. Diagnosis can be confirmed by recovering virus in the urine and is presumed by finding a rising complement-fixation titer. Adults are usually debilitated from lymphoma, multiple myeloma, leukemia, anemia, or have had a renal transplant requiring prolonged steroid and immunosuppressive therapy. Retinal cytomegalic inclusion disease infection occurs in renal transplantation patients without immune titers prior to surgery. Histologic studies have confirmed the marked destruction of the retina and adjacent tissues.

o Newborns with meningoencephalitis due to herpes simplex virus usually die in infancy. Inclusion bodies and veins may be found in the urine.

o Subacute sclerosing panencephalitis (subacute inclusion body encephalitis) is usually diagnosed at autopsy. Giant cells, fungus spore-like inclusions, and other evidence suggest measles virus as the cause.

Main differential diagnosis

o Toxoplasmosis

o Embolic retinal abscess

o Miliary tuberculosis

o Syphilis

o Rocky Mountain spotted fever

o Sarcoidosis

o Toxocara canis or cati

References

Astle JN, Ellis PP: Ocular complications in renal transplant patients. Ann Ophthalmol 6:1269, 1974.

Berger BB, Weinberg RS, Tessler HH, et al: Bilateral cytomegalovirus panuveitis after high-dose corticosteroid therapy. Am J Ophthalmol 88:1020, 1979.

Boniuk I: The cytomegaloviruses and the eye. Int Ophthalmol Clin 12:169, 1972.

Cogan DG, Kuwabara T, Young GF, et al: Herpes simplex retinopathy in an infant. Arch Ophthalmol 72:641, 1964.

Green SH, Wirtschafter JD: Ophthalmoscopic findings in subacute sclerosing panencephalitis. Br J Ophthalmol 57:780, 1973.

L. LEUKEMIA (see Chapter 4: IXC)

M. RETICULUM CELL SARCOMA

Acute necrotizing lesions in the retina have been described in this disease, but the vitreous seems most involved (see Chapter 8: IVC, 5)

N. SARCOIDOSIS (BOECK'S SARCOID) (see Fig. 3.40)

This granulomatous disease of immune complex etiology affects many organs, and the eye is commonly involved. Original descriptions of the disease emphasized iritis, and this is the most frequent ocular manifestation. Additional experience has shown that the retina, choroid, optic nerve, lacrimal gland, and conjunctiva can be involved in some patients.

Ophthalmoscopic findings

o   Aqueous and vitreous inflammatory reaction may make retinal examination difficult. Gray vitreous snowballs occur.

o   Swelling of disc from granulomata may resemble papilledema.

o   Scattered, light-colored nodules, especially along veins in the inferior retina, may appear to drip like wax. They frequently remain for years.

o   Sheathing of veins and neovascularization may occur and can be accompanied by hemorrhage.

o   Nodules described above may affect the choroid.

o   Disease is usually bilateral.

Symptoms & signs

o   Iritis with photophobia, redness, and pain occurs in about 8 percent of patients with ocular sarcoidosis. Iris-lens adhesions (posterior synechiae) are common.

- Reduced tear production from lacrimal gland involvement results in dry-eye symptoms.
- Decreased vision may be from iritis, synechiae, cataract, vitreous opacity or from retinal, choroidal, or optic nerve granulomata.
- Iritis, fever, and parotitis constitute Heerfordt's disease.
- Glaucoma from chronic iritis occurs.
- Pupil may be fixed or irregular from synechiae.
- Epiphora (tearing) from obstructed tear passages rare.

Other confirming findings

- Some kind of ocular involvement in sarcoidosis occurs in about 28 percent of patients.
- Females and blacks are affected a little more frequently than males and whites.
- Age of onset usually 25 to 34 years.
- Thoracic disease only occurs in 44 percent; chest roentgenogram and gallium scan aid diagnosis.
- Central nervous system disease occurs in 6 percent.
- Conjunctival biopsy positive in 17 percent.
- Serum angiotensin-converting enzyme is positive in 80-83 percent of patients.

Main differential diagnosis

- Toxoplasmosis
- Chorioretinitis (unknown cause)
- Intraocular foreign body
- Bacterial or fungal endophthalmitis
- Parasitic infection
- Reticulum cell sarcoma

References

Gass JDM: Stereoscopic Atlas of Macular Diseases. St. Louis: Mosby, 1977, p 302.

Gass JDM, Olson CL: Sarcoidosis with optic nerve and retinal involvement. Trans Am Acad Ophthalmol Otolaryngol 77:739, 1973.

Karma A: Ophthalmic changes in sarcoidosis. Acta Ophthalmol [Suppl] 141:1, 1979.

O. SUBACUTE NEURORETINITIS AND VITRITIS (WIPE-OUT SYNDROME) (Fig. 5.42)

Unilateral profound unexplained loss of vision in patients averaging 10 years of age appears to affect retina, retinal pigment epithelium, and optic nerve. It is uncommon.

Ophthalmoscopic findings

o   Edema of disc initially, followed by pallor.

o   White edematous retina, resembling vascular occlusion.

o   Arteries are narrow.

o   Vitreous contains many cells.

o   Mottled depigmentation and pigment clumping occurs later.

o   Macula may be spared.

Symptoms & signs

o   Visual acuity varies from 6/21 (20/70) to light perception in affected eye.

o   Other eye is normal.

o   Pupil reaction to light may be poor in extensive disease.

o   Constricted field or scattered scotomata.

Other confirming findings

o   In some patients, there is a history of a preceding chicken pox or flu-like illness.

o   Family history is negative for similar disease.

Fig. 5.42 Diffuse unilateral subacute neuro-retinitis and vitritis (wipe-out syndrome) in a 17-year-old black male. Visual acuity was 6/120 (20/400). Note the marked narrowing and sheathing of the retinal arteries, pallor of the disc, and generalized mottling and depigmentation. The other eye was normal. From Gass, J. Donald M. : Stereoscopic atlas of macular diseases, ed. 2, St. Louis, 1977, The C. V. Mosby Co. Used with permission.

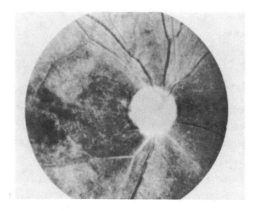

- Normal ophthalmodynamometry findings.
- Occasional patient has an elevated serum glutamic oxalacetic transaminase and lactic acid dehydrogenase.
- The disease may be called unilateral retinitis pigmentosa in end stages.

Main differential diagnosis

- Leber's optic atrophy
- Rubella retinopathy
- Unilateral retinitis pigmentosa
- Behcet's disease
- Vogt-Koyanagi-Harada disease

References

Gass JDM: Stereoscopic Atlas of Macular Diseases. St. Louis: Mosby, 1977, p 226.

P. PARS PLANITIS (CHRONIC CYCLITIS, PERIPHERAL UVEITIS) (Fig. 5.43)

Exudative material on the peripheral retina and pars plana, mostly in young patients, is a distinct disease of unknown cause.

Ophthalmoscopic findings

- The disease is nearly always bilateral, although one eye frequently has more activity.
- It's confined to the lower half of the eye. In rare patients, however, the inflammation extends superiorly along the ora serrata.
- "Puffballs" of inflammatory cells lie on the peripheral retina or are suspended in the vitreous.
- Yellow, irregular exudate obscures the inferior ora serrata and pars plana.
- There is sheathing and engorgement of inferior veins, and in late stages of the disease, some may enter the yellow material and appear to cross the ora serrata.
- Retinal detachment may occur inferiorly without a retinal hole or tear. A retinal tear adjacent to scars may lead to retinal detachment as the disease subsides and vitreous shortening occurs.

o Intravitreal hemorrhage, cells, and veils may be present, especially inferiorly, and, except for hemorrhage, often persist for years.

o Cystic macular edema is common in acute disease.

o Hyperemia and, in some patients, neovascularization of the disc are present in acute phase.

o Retinal pigment epithelial hyperplasia near the inferior ora is a common sequela.

Symptoms & signs

o Blurred or distorted vision in one eye is the usual chief complaint.

o Patient is rarely aware that the other eye is involved.

o Floaters are occasionally described.

o Mild aching, discomfort, and photophobia when iritis accompanies the disease.

o Pupil reactions are usually normal, unless iritis occurs.

o If cystic macular edema develops, relative central scotoma will follow.

o Loss of peripheral field is found, usually superiorly, especially if retinal detachment occurs.

Other confirming findings

o With most patients, personal and family history and review of systems don't contribute to the diagnosis.

o While occasionally seen in patients over the age of 40, the majority of patients are between eight and 30 years.

Fig. 5.43 Cloudy vitreous and edematous inferior retina in the left eye of a 10-year-old female. The other eye was similar, and both eyes had retinal hemorrhages and exudate on the pars plana.

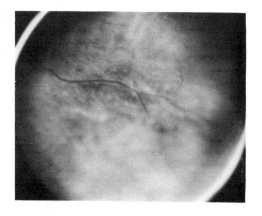

- Characteristic nature and location of the pathology, bilateral presentation, frequent uncomplicated resolution, and the generally good visual prognosis — 73 percent with 6/15 (20/50) or better — are best diagnostic criteria.
- Laboratory and other testing, including vitreous aspiration, provide no diagnostic or etiologic clues at present.
- Cataracts and retinal detachment are the most common complications.
- Iritis, if present, usually is mild and nongranulomatous.

Main differential diagnosis

- Toxoplasmosis
- Peripheral uveitis of unknown cause
- Subacute neuroretinitis and vitritis
- Vogt-Koyanagi-Harada disease
- Behcet's disease
- Sarcoidosis

References

Hogan MJ, Kimura SJ, O'Connor GR: Peripheral retinitis and chronic cyclitis in children. Trans Ophthalmol Soc UK 85:39, 1965.

Smith RE, Godfrey WA, Kimura SJ: Chronic cyclitis: 1. Course and visual prognosis. Trans Am Acad Ophthalmol Otolaryngol 77:760, 1973.

Yannuzzi LA, Gitter KA, Schatz H: The Macula: A Comprehensive Text and Atlas. Baltimore: Williams & Wilkins, 1979, p 349.

Q. VOGT-KOYANAGI-HARADA DISEASE (see Chapter 6: IIC)

While retina and vitreous are involved in this disease, the pigmented uveal retinal tissue are primarily affected.

R. BEHCET'S DISEASE (see Chapter 4: VD)

Vascular occlusion is the prominent feature of this disease.

S. AMYLOIDOSIS (see Chapter 7: VID, I, and Chapter 8: IVC, 2)

Amyloid deposition in the eye involves the vitreous but the choroid, orbit, and, in some patients, the retina may be affected.

VI. RETINAL OPACITIES AND CLEAR VITREOUS

This section considers local or generalized losses of retinal transparency when the view is not impeded by cloudy vitreous. A clear view of retinal opacities doesn't mean the vitreous is uninvolved in the disease. Clarity of the vitreous may vary considerably in two patients with the same disease, or in one patient in different stages of a disease.

A. MYELINATED NERVE FIBER LAYER

This usually benign and incidental finding may occasionally be associated with poor vision (see Fig. 3.21).

B. TUMORS OF THE RETINA

1. Retinoblastoma (Figs. 5.44-5.46; see 5.46 also in color section)

This congenital tumor may arise in several sites in one or both eyes. It's highly malignant, metastisizing by direct extension, blood, and lymphatics. It's almost invariably fatal without treatment. It usually remains confined to the eye for a relatively long time, and cure is possible by early detection. The vitreous is usually clear in children with this malignant tumor. Vitreous seeding, however, may be present.

Ophthalmoscopic findings

o White "cat's eye reflection" of the ophthalmoscope's light may fill the pupil or be seen only in a specific direction of gaze. (Parents may bring in photographs of their children that demonstrate this appearance. The white reflection and the tendency to esotropia or exotropia may account for parents' complaints that the children have a strange expression.) The red reflection should be examined from all directions.

o Thirty percent have both eyes involved.

o Seventy-five percent of the tumors arise in the peripheral retina. (Dilated pupil and general anesthesia may be needed for ophthalmoscopy.)

o Eighty-four percent have more than one tumor in an involved eye.

o Exophytic tumors are usually associated with a retinal detachment (see Fig. 5.14).

o Endophytic tumors have creamy, pink color. Early endophytic tumors show as tiny, gray mounds with slightly abnormal retinal vascular pattern and faint color change at the border of the lesion.

o   Telangiectatic, microaneurysmal vessels on the surface of tumors. Major retinal vessels are dilated and may resemble those of angiomatosis retinae (see Figs. 4.33-4.35). Large draining vein may exit from the tumor substance. (Veins larger than expected in the peripheral retina of a patient require careful evaluation for tumor at the ora serrata.)

o   Hemorrhage may be present on the tumor surface, and exudate may surround the base of large vascular tumors.

o   Gray, feathery opacities in the vitreous are often localized over retinal tumors. They may be more discrete and calcified after radiation. Gray opaque tumor tissue may break off and float in vitreous following

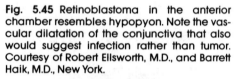

Fig. 5.44 Subretinal retinoblastoma in a child has displaced the retina into the mid-vitreous. Courtesy of Robert Ellsworth, M.D., and Barrett Haik, M.D., New York.

Fig. 5.45 Retinoblastoma in the anterior chamber resembles hypopyon. Note the vascular dilatation of the conjunctiva that also would suggest infection rather than tumor. Courtesy of Robert Ellsworth, M.D., and Barrett Haik, M.D., New York.

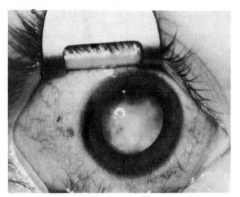

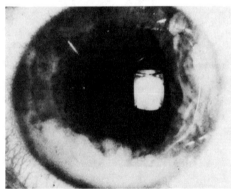

Fig. 5.46 Retinoblastoma in the left eye of a two-year-old male. The other eye had multiple tumors. Radiation arrested growth of the tumor (a, left) and resulted in calcification (b, right). The "fish flesh" (arrow) of regressing tumor remains. Also shown in color section.

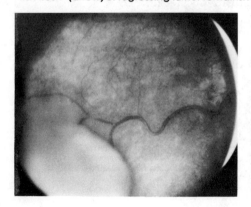

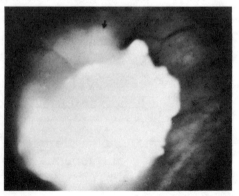

irradiation. Occasional implantation of seeds on the retina survive treatment and form flat, gray membranes that later develop into pink, solid tumors.

o Flecks of calcium are dense white spots, sometimes with iridescence, within tumor.

o Gray "fish flesh" at base or "cottage cheese" on the surface indicate regressing tumors.

o Recurrence of retinoblastoma after initial successful treatment is more common in the inferior peripheral retina.

Symptoms & signs

o Table 5.2 lists in order of frequency by percentage the presenting signs in patients with retinoblastoma.

o Spontaneous necrosis may produce severe inflammatory response resembling endophthalmitis and orbital cellulitis with obvious pain, swelling, and redness.

o "Crossed eye" is a common parental complaint about the child. The parent may also note accompanying poor vision.

o Dilated, fixed pupil, the presence of hyphema, discolored iris, or a "steamy" cornea may be complaints.

o Involved eyes are normal size; microphthalmos is rare. Phthisical eye in child may indicate spontaneously regressing retinoblastoma.

o Meningeal symptoms and signs occur in central nervous system extension.

o Radiation-induced and other new primary tumors have been reported in retinoblastoma patients, and symptoms and signs of these tumors should be evaluated.

Other confirming findings

o Average age at diagnosis, 18 months; range, birth to 62 years.

o No sex or race predilection.

o Bilateral in 30 percent of patients.

o Family history: Survivors with bilateral disease transmit retinoblastoma to 50 percent of their children. Sporadic unilateral survivors transmit disease to 10-20 percent of their children. Dominant inheritance, perhaps one in 17,000 births. Chance that normal parents with one retinoblastoma child will have another is 4 percent.

o Ultrasonography aids diagnosis when there is no ophthalmoscopic view.

o Fluorescein angiography occasionally helpful (dose of fluorescein adjusted to patient weight).

o Radiograph for calcification; computerized axial tomography probably best and also allows assessment of orbit, optic nerves, and brain.

o Homovanillic acid, vanillylmandelic acid, total metanephrines, and catecholamines do not aid diagnosis.

o Plasma carcinoembryonic antigen and alpha fetoprotein may be elevated, but are not diagnostic; levels fall after treatment.

o Lactic acid dehydrogenase in aqueous humor is elevated with retinoblastoma in the anterior chamber and erratically in posterior tumor.

o Immune complexes (Raji cell radioimmunoassay) often elevated.

Table 5.2

FREQUENCY OF PRESENTING SIGNS IN PATIENTS WITH RETINOBLASTOMA

Presenting sign or problem	Percentage
White, or "cat's eye," reflex	56
Strabismus	20
esotropia 11%	
exotropia 9%	
Red, painful eye with glaucoma	7
Poor vision	5
Routine examination	3
Orbital cellulitis	3
Unilateral mydriasis	2
Heterochromia irides	1
Hyphema	1
"Strange expression"	0.5
Nystagmus	0.5
White spots on iris	0.5
No appetite, failure to thrive	0.5

From Ellsworth RM: The practical management of retinoblastoma. Trans Am Ophthalmol Soc 67:462, 1969. Used with permission.

PHYSICIANS' GUIDE TO OCULOSYSTEMIC DISEASES

o ^{57}Co-bleomycin scintigraphy may aid diagnosis, particularly in metastatic disease.

o Retinoblastoma has been associated with D-chromosome deletion (13q) anterior polar cataracts, 13qXp chromosome translocation, Down's syndrome.

Main differential diagnosis

o Toxocara canis or cati

o Retinal astrocytoma (Mulberry tumor)

o Congenital retinal detachment or falciform fold

o Juvenile retinoschisis

o Von Hippel-Lindau disease

o Coats's disease

o Norrie's disease

o Hemorrhagic diseases of newborn

o Battered-child syndrome

o Persistent hyaloid artery

References

Abramson DH, Ronner HJ, Ellsworth RM: Second tumors in nonirradiated bilateral retinoblastoma. Am J Ophthalmol 87:624, 1979.

Char DH, Christensen M, Goldberg L, et al: Immune complexes in retinoblastoma. Am J Ophthalmol 86:395, 1978.

Ellsworth RM: The practical management of retinoblastoma. Trans Am Ophthalmol Soc 67:462, 1969.

Felberg NT, Michelson JB, Shields JA: CEA family syndrome. Cancer 37: 1397, 1976.

Howard GM, Ellsworth RM: Findings in the peripheral fundi of patients with retinoblastoma. Am J Ophthalmol 62:243, 1966.

Krill AE: Krill's Hereditary Retinal and Choroidal Diseases, vol 2. Hagerstown, Md: Harper & Row, 1977, pp 1173-1187.

Michelson JB, Felberg NT, Shields JA: Fetal antigens in retinoblastoma. Cancer 37:719, 1976.

Orlowski JP, Levin HS, Price RL, et al: Normal urinary excretion of catecholamine catabolites in children with retinoblastoma. Med Pediatr Oncol 4:343, 1978.

Ozawa H, Tanaka Y, Tamura S, et al: Retinoblastoma and d-chromosome deletion (13q-). Jpn J Ophthalmol 22:320, 1978.

Piro PA, Abramson DH, Ellsworth RM, et al: Aqueous humor lactate dehydrogenase in retinoblastoma patients. Arch Ophthalmol 96:1823, 1978.

Tanaka H, Minami M, Tsuchida T: ^{57}Co-bleomycin scintigraphy for diagnosis of retinoblastoma. Jpn J Ophthalmol 22:412, 1978.

2. Astrocytoma (astrocytic hamartoma) (Fig. 5.47; see also in color section; see also Fig. 3.32)

These nonmetastasizing neoplasms represent anomalies of tissue maturation and formation. They arise in tissues normally found at that location and do not represent cellular proliferation of previously normal tissue. They are, therefore, hamartomas.

Astrocytic cells make up a large part of the retinal tumors seen in neurofibromatosis (Recklinghausen's disease) and tuberous sclerosis (Bourneville's disease), two of the mother-spot diseases (phakomatoses). The tumors may be indistinguishable in the two diseases. The absence of growth and the other clinical findings confirm the benign tumor diagnosis. Early diagnosis and careful observation are essential to avoid overlooking retinoblastoma.

Table 5.3

OCULAR LESIONS ASSOCIATED WITH TUBEROUS SCLEROSIS

Ocular tissue	Lesions
Eyelid	Adenoma sebaceum, vitiligo, poliosis, ptosis, epicanthal folds, facial weakness
Conjunctiva	Pedunculated gray-white nodules
Cornea	Keratoconus
Anterior chamber angle	Iris processes, secondary glaucoma
Iris	Rubeosis iridis, iridocyclitis, coloboma
Ciliary body	Neoplasm
Lens	Subluxated lens, cataract
Pupil	Third-nerve paresis
Vitreous	Phakoma buds and fragments, massive invasion by pseudoglioma
Globe	Enophthalmos, myopia, phthisis bulbi
Extraocular muscles	Strabismus, third- or sixth-nerve paresis, nystagmus, involuntary movements (rolling of eyes)
Retina and optic disc	Phakomas
Choroid	Atrophy, angiomas

From Krill AE: Krill's Hereditary Retinal and Choroidal Diseases, vol 2. Hagerstown, Md: Harper & Row, 1977. Used with permission.

Astrocytic tumors of the retina may occur as isolated findings (see Fig. 3.32) unassociated with tuberous sclerosis. Table 5.3 lists lesions associated with tuberous sclerosis according to the ocular tissue involved.

Ophthalmoscopic findings

o Translucent, knobby, reflective, relatively flat tumor that may be white or golden (Mulberry tumor).

o In some patients, it may be elevated, very vascular, and lift the neurosensory retina.

o Sometimes it's associated with fibrous proliferation that distorts blood vessels, but usually vessels can be seen passing through the tumor unaffected or only slightly altered in course.

o Tumors may be multiple and bilateral or single and isolated.

o Disc and macula may be involved (see Chapter 3: VF, 6, and VII; see also Fig. 3.32).

o Café-au-lait spots and nevi of the skin may be present.

o Choroidal neurofibromas more common than retinal.

Other confirming findings

o Hamartomas of the retinal pigment epithelium and retina and isolated retinal astrocytomas are rare. No inheritance patterns are known, and associated systemic disease is an inconsistent finding.

o Findings in neurofibromatosis (Recklinghausen's disease) are outlined in Table 5.4.

o Findings in tuberous sclerosis (Bourneville's disease) are outlined in Table 5.5.

Fig. 5.47 Mulberry-like astrocytoma of the peripheral retina. Courtesy of Richard Freeman, M.D., Auburn, New York. Also shown in color section.

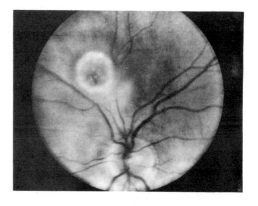

Table 5.4

OCULAR AND SYSTEMIC FINDINGS IN NEUROFIBROMATOSIS

Incidence	One in 2,500 to 3,300 live births
Inheritance	Autosomal dominant, varying expression
Race	No predilection
Orbit	Neurofibromas, defects in bony walls, pulsating exophthalmus, rare malignant change to neurilemoma, meningioma
Eyelids	Ptosis, neurofibromas, nevi, hemangiomas
Lacrimal apparatus	Aberrant or enlarged gland
Conjunctiva	Neurofibromas, angioma, nevi
Cornea	Increased visibility of corneal nerves, nodules
Sclera	Neurofibroma along intrascleral course of ciliary nerves
Optic nerve	Glioma, atrophy, swollen disc, meningioma
Ocular muscles	Nystagmus, strabismus
Globe	Myopia, phthisis bulbi
Iris	Neurofibromas, melanoma, sector atrophy, heterochromia, ectropion uveae
Ciliary body	Neurofibromas
Anterior chamber	Glaucoma
Lens	Cataract, dislocated lens
Skin	Café-au-lait, multiple neurofibromas
Gastrointestinal	Macroglossia and macrocheilia, esophagus, stomach, ileum, colon, anal canal
Central nervous system	Acoustic neuroma, meningiomas, schwannoma, spinal ependymomas
Bony lesions	Kyphoscoliosis, orbital defects, box-like enlargement of sella tursica
Endocrine	Pheochromocytoma, acromegaly, myxedema, hypopituitarism

Adapted from Krill AE: Krill's Hereditary Retinal and Choroidal Diseases, vol 2. Hagerstown, Md: Harper & Row, 1977. Used with permission.

Table 5.5

SYSTEMIC FINDINGS IN TUBEROUS SCLEROSIS

System or organ	Disorder	Finding
Central nervous system	Mental retardation, psychopathic tendencies, epilepsy	Abnormal EEG and X-ray studies
Skin	Adenoma sebaceum, depigmented nevi, café-au-lait shagreen patches	Butterfly distribution on face
	Vitiligo, poliosis, hypertrichosis	Face and lids
	Subungual fibromas	Toes
	Port-wine veins, lipomata	Face
Kidney	Hypernephroma and other tumors, polycystic, horseshoe kidney	Hematuria, uremia, abnormal intravenous pyelogram
Lungs	Pulmonary cysts, "honeycomb" lungs Glomangioma, adenoma, leiomyoma	Hemoptysis, recurrent pneumothorax
Bone	Periosteal thickening, sclerosis, cystic lesions	Flat bones, skull
	Osteoporosis	Hands
Heart	Subendocardial, endocardial fibrosis	Heart failure, ECG changes

Adapted from Krill AE: Krill's Hereditary Retinal and Choroidal Diseases, vol 2. Hagerstown, Md: Harper & Row, 1977. Used with permission.

Main differential diagnosis

o Retinoblastoma

o Myelinated nerve fibers

o Pseudoglioma, as with retinal dysplasia, Coats's disease, posterior hyperplastic primary vitreous, Toxocara canis, toxoplasmosis

o Metastatic tumor

o Meningioma or glioma of optic disc

o Von Hippel-Lindau disease

o Drusen of the disc

o Hemangioma of the disc

References

Cotlier E: Café-au-lait spots of the fundus in neurofibromatosis. Arch Ophthalmol 95:1990, 1977.

Hoyt CS: The ocular findings in infantile spasms. Ophthalmology 86:1794, 1979.

Krill AE: Krill's Hereditary Retinal and Choroidal Diseases, vol 2. Hagerstown, Md: Harper & Row, 1977.

Ramsay RC, Kinyoun JL, Hill CW, et al: Retinal astrocytoma. Am J Ophthalmol 88:32, 1979.

Turek M: Retinal tumors in neurofibromatosis. Can J Ophthalmol 12:68, 1977.

Yannuzzi LA, Gitter KA, Schatz H: The Macula: A Comprehensive Text and Atlas. Baltimore: Williams & Wilkins, 1979, p 325.

3. Vitelliform degeneration (Best's disease) (see Chapter 6: IIIC, 1b).

This disease looks like what a retinal tumor is expected to be, but is a degenerative disease.

4. Metastatic tumor to retina (see Chapter 7: VIC).

Tumors metastatic to the retina are extremely rare. This is not surprising since 77 percent of ocular blood flow is to the choroid.

References

Young SE, Cruciger M, Lukeman J: Metastatic carcinoma to the retina: Case report. Ophthalmology 86:1350, 1979.

C. TRAUMA (BERLIN'S EDEMA, COMMOTIO RETINAE)
(Fig. 5.48; see also in color section; see also Fig. 5.5)

Contusion injuries of the eye, both penetrating and nonpenetrating, but particularly the latter, produce a gray-white loss of transparency of the neurosensory retina that was first described by Berlin. It's also been seen in patients after nearly fatal electric shock.

Ophthalmoscopic findings

o   Diffuse gray-white appearance of the neurosensory retina, with many highlights. The striations of the nerve fiber layer are visible.

o   It usually involves the posterior eye in blunt injury, but may also be localized at the site of impact.

o   It may be associated with underlying choroidal rupture, intravitreal hemorrhage, or retinal tears or disinsertion.

o   Retinal blood vessels are not hidden.

o   Fades within a few days.

Symptoms & signs

o   Vision may be reduced to counting fingers. (When poor vision is associated solely with Berlin's edema, observation may reveal a macular hole, hidden choroidal rupture, and flat retinal detachment as edema subsides.)

o   Pain from iritis, miosis, other effects of trauma.

o   Pupil may be fixed and dilated or irregular with iridodonesis.

o   Distance visual acuity may be good, but near vision poor (paralysis of accommodation).

o   Field loss corresponds to edematous retina.

o   Lens subluxation or dislocation (see Chapter 2) may be present.

o   Enophthalmos, double vision, or both suggest blow-out fracture of the orbit.

Other confirming findings

o   History of trauma, usually from a blunt object

o   Indirect ophthalmoscopy with scleral depression aid examination of the peripheral retina.

o   Slit lamp evidence of trauma is commonly found.

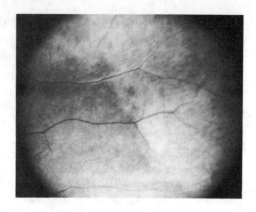

Fig. 5.48 Glistening edema of the peripheral retina in a 16-year-old female hit by a soccer ball. The normal color returned in two weeks. Also shown in color section.

o   Ultrasonography aids diagnosis in patients with intravitreal blood.

o   Computerized axial tomography and other radiographic studies for foreign body or orbital fracture.

Main differential diagnosis

o   Myelinated nerve fiber layer

o   Lipid storage disease

o   Central or branch retinal artery occlusion

o   Carotid artery occlusion

References

Duke-Elder S: Text-book of Ophthalmology, vol 6. St. Louis: Mosby, 1954, p 5840.

Sipperley M O, Quigley HA, Gass JDM: Traumatic retinopathy in primates. Arch Ophthalmol 96:2267, 1978.

D. DIABETIC RETINOPATHY AND OTHER VASCULAR DISEASES

The gray membrane opacities on or under the retina from proliferative vascular disease, such as proliferative diabetic retinopathy, are discussed in Chapter 4.

E. MACULAR DEGENERATION

Senile macular degeneration is perhaps the most common cause of visual loss. It results in opacities in and around the macula easily misinterpreted as retinal in origin. The retina is involved, but the process begins in the retinal pigment epithelium or choroid.

F. GANGLION CELL STORAGE DISEASE (LIPOIDOSES OF TAY- SACHS DISEASE, SANDHOFF'S DISEASE, GM₁ GANGLIOSIDOSIS, NIEMANN-PICK DISEASE, MUCOLIPIDOSIS I, METACHROMATIC LEUKODYSTROPHY, AND JUVENILE MUCOLIPIDOSIS) (Fig. 5.49)

The cherry-red spot classically described in Tay-Sachs disease results from deposition in and destruction of the retinal ganglion cells by deposits of phospholipids, cholesterol, and protein. The pathognomonic deposit is a sphingolipid, called ganglioside GM_2, which is due to a failure of an enzyme (hexosaminidase A) to break down the normal brain and retinal lipid in the infant.

The cherry-red spot is also seen in Niemann-Pick disease and GM_1 gangliosidosis. The ophthalmoscopic appearance results from the white discoloration of the retina by lipid deposits in ganglion cells surrounding the thin, ganglion-cell-free fovea, accentuating the normal red reflex located there. Other lipid storage diseases involve principally the retinal pigment epithelium and are discussed in Chapter 6.

Ophthalmoscopic findings

o   White, opaque retina in the macula, surrounding a contrasting bright red fovea.

o   Opaque retina may extend to mid-periphery, but disappears in fluffy edges as the ganglion cell population decreases.

o   Retina is flat.

o   Disc pallor (optic atrophy) is common.

o   Incidence of cherry-red spot noted in Table 5.6.

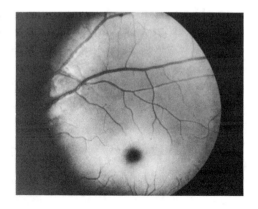

Fig. 5.49 Cherry-red spot in a child with Tay-Sachs disease. Courtesy of J.D.M. Gass, M.D., Miami, Florida.

Table 5.6

INCIDENCE OF CHERRY-RED SPOT IN SOME
GANGLION CELL STORAGE DISEASES

Disease	Incidence in percentage of cases
GM$_1$ gangliosidosis	100
Juvenile mucolipidosis	100
Sandhoff's disease	100
Tay-Sachs disease	90-95
Mucolipidosis I	50
Niemann-Pick disease	50
Metachromatic leukodystrophy	rare

Symptoms & signs

o   Horizontal pendular nystagmus.

o   Strabismus.

o   Progressively poor vision.

o   Corneal clouding.

Other confirming findings

o   See Table 5.7.

Main differential diagnosis

o   Central retinal artery occlusion

o   Berlin's edema (traumatic retinopathy, battered-child syndrome)

o   Leber's amaurosis congenita

o   Oguchi's disease

References

Brady RO: Ophthalmologic aspects of lipid storage diseases. Ophthalmology 85:1007, 1978.

Kirkham TH, Coupland SG, Guitton D: Sialidosis: The cherry-red spot — myoclonus syndrome. Can J Ophthalmol 15:35, 1980.

Krill, AE: Krill's Hereditary Retinal and Choroidal Diseases, vol 2. Hagerstown, Md: Harper & Row, 1977, p 1137.

Sogg RL, Steinman L, Rathjen B, Tharp BR, et al: Cherry red spot — myoclonus syndrome. Ophthalmology 86: 1861, 1979.

Table 5.7.

NONOCULAR FINDINGS IN GANGLION CELL STORAGE DISEASES

Disease	Age at onset	Heredity	Race	Clinical	Laboratory	X-ray
GM₁ gangliosidosis	6 months-5 years	Autosomal recessive	Multi-racial	Frontal bossing, saddle nose, low-set ears, large tongue, hypertrophy of gums, mild corneal clouding, mild hepatosplenomegaly	Liver, skin, leukocytes decreased B-galactosidase	Vertebrae beaked, shoe-like sellae, Hurler-like kyphosis
Juvenile mucolipidosis	4-10 years	Autosomal recessive, consanguinity common	unknown	Mild CNS signs, no hepatosplenomegaly	Normal or elevated liver acid hydrolases, decreased skin B-galactosidases	Hurler-like kyphosis
Metachromatic leukodystrophy	6 months	autosomal recessive, consanguinity common	multi-racial	CNS signs	Arylsulfase-A deficient in leukocytes, urine, and skin fibroblasts	Normal
Mucolipidosis I	6 months	unknown	multi-racial	CNS signs milder, may be no hepatosplenomegaly	Normal or elevated liver acid hydrolases	Hurler-like kyphosis
Niemann-Pick disease	6 months	Autosomal recessive	Jewish & multi-racial	CNS disease, hepatosplenomegaly	bone marrow foam cells, decreased sphingomyelinase in leukocytes	Hurler-like kyphosis
Sandhoff's disease	3-12 months	Autosomal recessive	Multi-racial	Similar to Tay-Sachs, plus mild hepatosplenomegaly	Serum leukocytes decreased, total hexosaminidase	Normal
Tay-Sachs disease	3-12 months	Autosomal recessive	Jewish	"Beautiful baby": fine hair, pink coloring, long eye-lashes; motor weakness, startle reaction, convulsions, macrocephaly	Serum leukocytes decreased, hexosaminidase A	Normal
Sialidosis	(see references)					

Adapted from Krill AE: Krill's Hereditary Retinal and Choroidal Diseases, vol 2. Hagerstown, Md: Harper & Row, 1977. Used with permission.

G. TAMOXIFEN (NOLVADEX) TOXICITY OR DEPOSITION (Fig. 5.50)

This chemotherapeutic agent used in breast cancer results in particle deposition in the neurosensory retina at certain dosages.

Ophthalmoscopic findings

o Small, irregular refractile particles around macula.

o Particles superficial to retinal blood vessels.

o Patient may have macular edema.

Symptoms & signs

o Decreased vision, but usually better than 6/60 (20/200).

o Visual loss may be worse in one eye than the other.

o Probably progressive.

o Slurred speech, hearing loss, tremor, swaying gait, peripheral neuropathy may be present.

Other confirming findings

o History of breast carcinoma.

o Treatment of 60-100 mg/M^2 of tamoxifen over one year.

o Whorl-like corneal opacities.

o Electroretinogram and electro-oculogram.

o Fluorescein angiography.

o Sudden hypercalcemia may occur with fatal consequences.

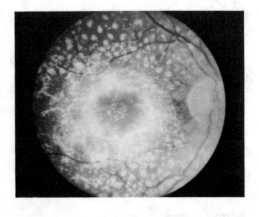

Fig. 5.50 Fundus of left eye with multiple tiny, refractile, intraretinal lesions and larger, granular areas at the level of the retinal pigment epithelium in a patient on tamoxifen therapy for breast carcinoma. Courtesy of Mano Swartz, M.D., Salt Lake City, Utah.

Main differential diagnosis

o   Chloroquine retinopathy

o   Hereditary maculopathies

o   Oxalosis

o   Talc emboli

o   Cystinosis

o   Gyrate atrophy of choroid

References

Beck M, Mills PV: Ocular assessment of patients treated with tamoxifen. Cancer Treat Rep 63:1833, 1979.

Kaiser-Kupfer MI, Lippman ME: Tamoxifen retinopathy. Cancer Treat Rep 62:315, 1978.

McKeown CA, Swartz M, Blom J, et al: Tamoxifen retinopathy. Br J Ophthalmol 65:177, 1981.

Spooner D, Evans BD: Tamoxifen and life-threatening hypercalcaemia. Lancet 2:413, 1979.

H. LATTICE, SNAIL-TRACK, AND SNOWFLAKE DEGENERATION (Figs. 5.51-5.53)

These peripheral vitreoretinal degenerations predispose the patient to retinal detachment. Once discovered, the patient should be observed regularly, with warnings to report symptoms promptly. The three are clinically distinctive in appearance, but their existence as separate diseases is not well established.

Ophthalmoscopic findings

Lattice

o   Found between the equator and ora serrata.

o   More common on the temporal side.

o   Lies parallel to the equator, but sometimes obliquely with posterior end along retinal vessels behind the equator.

o   May be multilevel elliptical patches in same eye, with normal-appearing retina between, or may fill area from equator to ora serrata.

o   Vitreous strands may be attached to the margins.

o   Various degrees of pigmentation, thinning, and lattice-like white lines are seen.

Fig. 5.51 Peripheral vitreoretinal disease, sometimes called lattice or snail-track degeneration. Variable amounts of pigmentation may be present. Tears or holes in the retina (see Figs. 5.6, 5.10) are often associated with this type of degeneration.

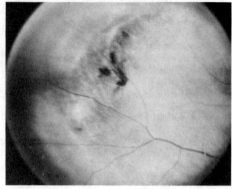

Fig. 5.52 Snail-track peripheral vitreoretinal degeneration. Patients with this disorder are slightly predisposed to retinal detachment.

Fig. 5.53 Snowflake degeneration of the retina in a 24-year-old. It extended 360° around the periphery.

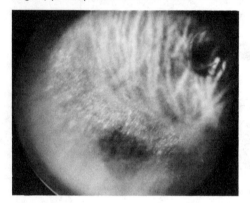
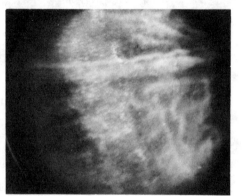

o Small round holes without opercula (see Fig. 5.10) occur within the patches, and tears are usually at the ends or include a whole patch of lattice in the operculum.

o Nearly always bilateral.

Snail track

o White, frost-like lines at the equator.

o Sharply demarcated.

o Usually there are single continuous lines that may be found to extend all around the eye.

o Vitreous adhesions are at the margins.

o Round holes without opercula occur within the track.

Snowflake

o At early stages, only a whitening of the peripheral retina is present.

o Later, crystalline yellow-white spots appear in the superficial retina from the equator to the ora serrata.

o Sheathing of the retinal vessels is followed by their disappearance from view and by increased pigmentation throughout the area.

o Round holes without opercula and tears may occur.

Symptoms & signs

o There are no specific symptoms, unless retinal tears or retinal detachment occur.

o Most patients are seen because of myopia or vitreous floaters.

Other confirming findings

o Lattice degeneration with and without myopia has been inherited in an autosomal dominant pattern; snail track is probably autosomal recessive, snowflake autosomal dominant.

o Cleft palate, arthropathy, and cataract, as well as myopia of prematurity or febrile illness early in life, have been associated with lattice degeneration.

o Indirect ophthalmoscopy with scleral depression is invaluable.

o Biomicroscopy and contact lens provide further detail.

Main differential diagnosis

o Wagner's vitreoretinal degeneration

o Goldmann-Favre disease

o Syphilitic retinopathy

o Malarial, typhoid, scarlet fever retinopathy

o Senile retinoschisis

o Juvenile retinoschisis

References

Hirose T, Wolf E, Schepens CL: Retinal functions in snowflake degeneration. Ann Ophthalmol 12:1135, 1980.

Krill, AE: Krill's Hereditary Retinal and Choroidal Diseases, vol 2. Hagerstown, Md: Harper & Row, 1977, p 1093.

Straatsma BR, Allen RA: Lattice degeneration of the retina. Trans Am Acad Ophthalmol Otolaryngol 66:600, 1962.

Tolentino FI, Schepens CL, Freeman HM: Vitreoretinal Disorders: Diagnosis and Management. Philadelphia: Saunders, 1976.

Fig. 5.54 Wagner's vitreoretinal degeneration with bands in the vitreous seen here causing traction on the retina and small hemorrhages (a, left). Patients with this disorder are likely to have a myopic crescent on the nasal side of the disc (b, right). They have an increased risk of retinal detachment.

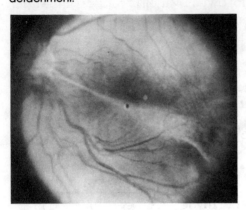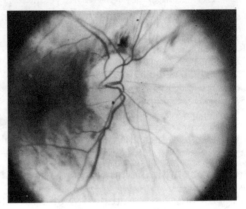

I. WAGNER'S DISEASE (Fig. 5.54)

In 1938, Wagner reported vitreoretinal degeneration in 13 members of one family. Further recognition of patients with this disease has emphasized its importance as a cause of retinal detachment.

Ophthalmoscopic findings

o   Vitreous degeneration results in watery pockets crossed by dense bands. There may be large holes in the vitreous.

o   Gray preretinal, nonvascular filamentous bands may circle the eye at the equator.

o   Multiple peripheral patches of black hyperpigmentation circle the eye from equator to ora serrata, often with tongues of pigmentation extending posteriorly along the vessels.

o   Situs inversus of the disc is common, with blood vessels entering temporally and a myopic crescent on the nasal side.

o   Fine, shiny, white dots may sheath peripheral vessels. Lattice degeneration may be present.

o   Paving stones (punched out retinal pigment epithelial plaques) are common peripherally.

Symptoms & signs

o There are no symptoms specifically related to the disease. Most patients are seen because they have myopic astigmatism, cataracts, or retinal detachment after age 10 and often before age 40.

o A variant of the disease is also dominantly inherited and includes pedigrees with cleft or high arched palates, flattened nasal bridge, high cheek bones, and prominent jaw.

o Dark adaptation and color vision are normal.

o Concentric narrowing of visual field occurs.

o Strabismus may occur.

o Chronic open-angle glaucoma occurs in 30 percent of patients.

Other confirming findings

o Autosomal dominant inheritance with a penetrance of nearly 100 percent. Discovery of the disease is usually between ages of five and 20.

o Indirect ophthalmoscopy with scleral depression is valuable.

o Biomicroscopy with contact lens aids vitreous examination.

o Electroretinogram and electro-oculogram often slightly abnormal.

o Ultrasonography confirms retinal detachment in eyes with opaque cataracts.

o General medical evaluation for associated findings.

Main differential diagnosis

o Goldmann-Favre disease

o Retinitis pigmentosa

o Retrolental fibroplasia

o Juvenile retinoschisis

References

Delaney WV Jr, Podedworny W, Havener WH: Inherited retinal detachment. Arch Ophthalmol 69:44, 1963.

Krill AE: Krill's Hereditary Retinal and Choroidal Diseases, vol 2. Hagerstown, Md: Harper & Row, 1977, p 1068.

Maumenee IH: Vitreoretinal degeneration as a sign of generalized connective tissue diseases. Am J Ophthalmol 88:432, 1979.

J. FAMILIAL EXUDATIVE VITREORETINOPATHY (Fig. 5.55)

This rare vitreoretinal degeneration was first described in 1969.

Ophthalmoscopic findings

o   Peripheral retina is gray-white, especially on the temporal side, and faint vitreous bands may be seen.

o   Retinal vessels become tortuous in the temporal periphery and run up to the ora serrata at larger than normal caliber before turning to traverse along it.

o   Yellow-white subretinal exudate resembling Coats's disease develops in the periphery and may extend posteriorly to reach the macula.

o   Organization of the exudate produces a fibrovascular retinal scar in the periphery that may drag the retina as in retrolental fibroplasia.

o   Retinal detachment may follow the retinal distortion.

Symptoms & signs

o   Progressive loss of previously normal vision occurs usually in the first or second decade of life, although late mild disease has been seen up to age 50.

o   Retinal detachment, cataracts, iris atrophy, and glaucoma are late-stage findings.

o   Color vision is normal.

o   Field loss is associated with retinal detachment.

Other confirming findings

o   Autosomal dominant inheritance affects males and females nearly equally. Penetrance approaches 100 percent.

o   Indirect ophthalmoscopy with scleral depression aids diagnosis.

o   Fluorescein angiography may be helpful.

o   Biomicroscopy and contact lens examination provide details of the vitreous.

o   General medical evaluation for associated findings.

Main differential diagnosis

o   Retrolental fibroplasia

o   Retinitis pigmentosa with a "Coats's response"

o   Coats's disease

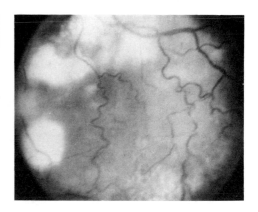

Fig. 5.55 Familial exudative retinopathy in a 34-year-old male whose brother and cousin have similar disease. Visual acuity was 6/60 (20/200).

o   Peripheral uveitis (pars planitis)

o   Retinoblastoma

o   Sickle cell disease

o   Incontinentia pigmenti

References

Gow J, Oliver GL: Familial exudative vitreoretinopathy: An expanded view. Arch Ophthalmol 86:150, 1971.

K. PAVING STONE DEGENERATION (Fig. 5.56)

Chorioretinal atrophy in the periphery along the ora serrata takes its name from the side-by-side patches. It's very common and may be an aging change.

Ophthalmoscopic findings

o   Yellow-white circular or oval patches of retinal pigment epithelial atrophy, often with a black pigment border.

o   Choroidal vessels may be absent or sparse in patches.

o   More common in the inferior temporal quadrant along the ora serrata.

o   Usually clustered and coalescent.

o   Nearly always bilateral.

Symptoms & signs

o   There are no symptoms, and the disease is generally considered benign.

o   Retinal detachment may be slightly more common in these patients.

Fig. 5.56 Paving-stone degeneration in the peripheral retina of a 78-year-old man.

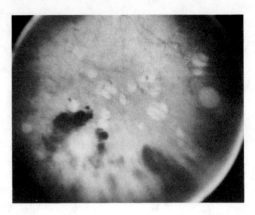

Other confirming findings

o   There is no known inheritance pattern.

o   Patients often have arteriosclerosis, hypertension, or other vascular disease.

o   Most patients are older than 50 years.

Main differential diagnosis

o   Choroidal scars from inflammation

o   Myopic degeneration

o   Degeneration from ocular trauma

References

O'Malley CC: Genetics of cobblestone degeneration of the retina. In Retinal Disease (Kimura SJ, Caygill WM, eds), pp 197-199. Philadelphia: Lea & Febiger, 1966.

O'Malley P, Allen RA, Straatsma BR, et al: Paving-stone degeneration of the retina. Arch Ophthalmol 73:169, 1965.

Straatsma BR, Allen RA, O'Malley P, et al: Pathologic and clinical manifestations of paving-stone degeneration of the retina. In New and Controversial Aspects of Retinal Detachment (McPherson A, ed), pp 76-99. New York: Harper & Row, 1968.

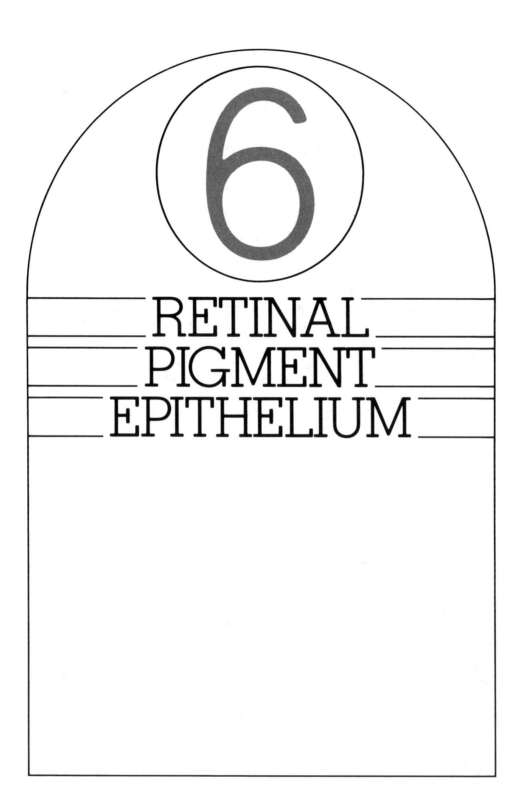

6

RETINAL PIGMENT EPITHELIUM

Only a single cell layer thick, the retinal pigment epithelium is of vital importance to ocular function. Fully exposed to ophthalmoscopic view by the transparency of the neurosensory retina, it can be studied in detail with the ophthalmoscope at 15 times magnification.

I. OPHTHALMOSCOPIC ANATOMY

There are two pigmented coats of the eye. The mesodermally derived uvea consists of the choroid, ciliary body, and anterior leaf of the iris. The pigment of these tissues is histologically distinct from that of the retinal pigment epithelium, arising from the neuroectoderm of optic cup. The two layers can be distinguished by their colors. The melanin of the uvea is gray or brown, while that of retinal pigment epithelium is jet black. Strictly speaking, there's a third pigmented layer, the localized luteal pigment of the neurosensory retina at the fovea. This yellow pigment is best seen in young patients. The uveal pigment of the choroid is discussed in Chapter 7.

There's a natural cleavage between the rods and cones, derived from the inner layer of the invaginating optic cup, and the retinal pigment epithelium. The retinal pigment epithelium adheres firmly to Bruch's membrane, to which it contributes (see Fig. 1.6).

Health of the retinal pigment epithelium is critical to the visual process. In addition to maintenance of its own metabolism, it provides the proper chemical environment, including vitamin A, for the rods and cones. A single retinal pigment epithelial cell may ingest 4,000 cast-off discs from the rods and cones a day. By absorbing incoming light, the retinal pigment epithelium prevents back-scatter into the neurosensory retina, which would blur the visual image.

Fig. 6.1 Fundus of Caucasian (a, left), fundus of black (b, right). Also shown in color section.

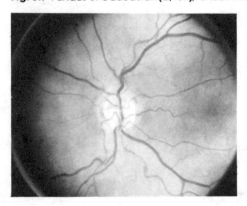 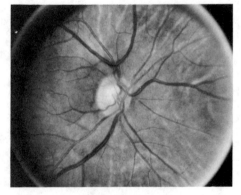

This thin sheet of pigmented cells lying on the very vascular choroid provides the orange-red glow of the fundus reflection (see Chapter 2). Not only skin and hair, but also ocular pigmentation, vary between people (Fig. 6.1; see also in color section) and in the same person with age (Fig. 6.2). The retinal pigment epithelium and choroid increase in pigmentation in the first decade of life. Pigmentation at the macula, even in very blonde patients, may hide large choroidal vessels that are easily visible elsewhere in the eye (Fig. 6.3; see also color section). The retinal pigment epithelium is still only one cell layer thick at the macula, but the cells are taller (columnar) and contain more pigment granules. It's not unusual for pigmentation to vary moderately within the same eye or to be variegated (Fig. 6.4; see also in color section). This appearance has been called tigroid or tessellated (squared).

The absence of pigment doesn't mean the absence of retinal pigment epithelial cells, it's due to the absence of intracellular pigment granules.

Fig. 6.2 Reticular pigment hyperplasia in the peripheral retinal pigment epithelium is common with age.

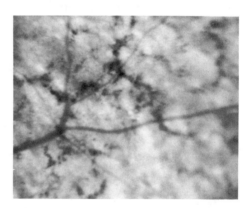

Fig. 6.3 Variations in pigmentation of the retinal pigment epithelium nasal to disc (left) and at the macula (a, left). In the periphery near a vortex vein ampulla, similar variations are common (b, right). Also shown in color section.

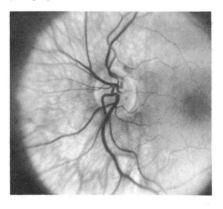
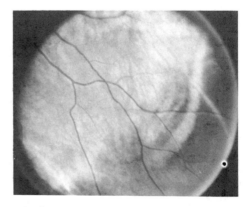

Fig. 6.4 Tigroid or tessellated pigmentation, a variation of normal. Also shown in color section.

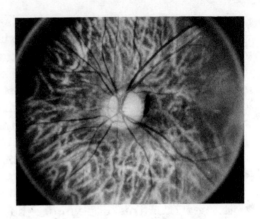

Reduced pigmentation is compatible with good vision, as demonstrated by many myopic patients with blonde retinal pigment epithelium but 6/6 (20/20) vision (properly corrected with lenses). Heavy pigmentation seems to be protective in some diseases. For example, senile macular degeneration is rare in Orientals and blacks.

Interposed between the retinal pigment epithelium and the inner layer of the choroid (choriocapillaris) is a thin, glass-like membrane. This non-cellular layer, the product of adjacent retinal pigment epithelium and choriocapillaris cells, is called Bruch's membrane.

II. SKIN, HAIR, AND EYE PIGMENT DISEASE

Too little or too much pigmentation may be localized to one or both eyes. Both effects may be associated with ocular or systemic disease, congenital and acquired. Pigment abnormality described here does not involve only the retinal pigment epithelium, but the choroid and iris as well.

A. ALBINISM AND WAARDENBURG'S SYNDROME
(Figs. 6.5-6.7; see 6.5-6.7a also in color section)

This abnormality, known since ancient times, may involve the eye and skin, the eye alone, or the skin alone. The specific type is related to absence, deficiency, or ineffectiveness of the enzyme tyrosinase, which is essential to the conversion of the amino acid tyrosine to melanin. Albinism involves only the eye in an X-linked disease in which the female carrier shows minor pigment abnormalities. It's also inherited in an autosomal recessive pattern — occasionally dominant — with eye and skin features combined. The purely cutaneous disease is dominantly inherited.

Ophthalmoscopic findings

o   Yellow-white color of the exposed choroid and sclera may be seen throughout the eye, localized to a segment, or involve only one eye and not the other. Choroidal vessels are exposed to view.

o   Usually, more pigmentation at the macula gives an orange-red color; the foveal light reflex may be absent, as well as the usual highlights around the fovea. The luteal pigment, usually seen in young patients in red-free light, is absent.

o   Pigmentation increases with age, and by the time he's 20 years old, it may be difficult to distinguish an otherwise normally dark-skinned albinotic from a blonde person without the disease.

o   Female carriers may have only slightly less pigment than normal patients.

o   Patients with pure cutaneous albinism usually have no eye findings, except in Waardenburg's syndrome and other rare conditions.

Symptoms & signs

o   Photophobia and decreased visual acuity — 6/9 (20/30) to 6/90 (20/300) — correlate with the pigment deficit. Those with the greatest pigment deficit have the worst light sensitivity and visual acuity. Ocular albinism patients are generally less afflicted than those with oculocutaneous disease.

o   Photophobia may decrease and visual acuity improve as pigmentation increases with age.

o   Head nodding or nystagmus early in life associated with poor vision may improve with increased pigmentation. Some female carriers are mildly affected.

o   Extremes of myopia, hyperopia, and astigmatism are common.

o   Strabismus, especially exotropia, and amblyopia are frequent.

o   Light reflects back through the iris.

o   Central scotomata may be found on field testing.

o   Color vision is normal, unless there is associated optic atrophy, maculopathy, or inherited color vision abnormality.

Other confirming findings

o   Ocular albinism: blue iris that transilluminates, pale retinal pigment epithelium and uvea. In X-linked inheritance, there may be a brief period in infancy of pale skin and snow-white hair.

o Oculocutaneous albinism: pale irides, snow-white hair, pale retinal pigment epithelium and uvea persisting through life. In imperfect form, pigmentation increases with age. Mostly autosomal recessive, occasional dominant inheritance.

o Cutaneous albinism (leukism, prebaldism, white forelock): patchy hypopigmentation of skin and hair is autosomal dominant.

Table 6.1

CONDITIONS ASSOCIATED WITH ALBINISM

Disease	Findings
Chédiak-Higashi syndrome	Incomplete, universal albinism
	Large eosinophilic, peroxidase-positive inclusion bodies, myeloblasts and pro-myelocytes of bone marrow, and leuko-cytes and mononuclear cells of peripheral blood
	Lymphoid-histiocytic cell infiltration of liver and spleen (hepatosplenomegaly), lymph nodes (lymphadenopathy), and central nervous system
	Neutropenia, anemia, thrombocytopenia
	Susceptibility to infection
	Unusual malignant lymphoma
	Death in first decade of life
	Autosomal recessive inheritance
Cuna Indian albino syndrome	Universal albinism
	Excess growth of fine, straight, white hair on forearms, limbs, and body
	Blepharochalasis
	Short stature
Deafness and universal albinism	Universal albinism
	Deaf-mutism
	Autosomal recessive inheritance
Hermansky's syndrome (albinism with hemorrhagic diathesis and pigmented reticuloendothelial cells)	Universal albinism
	Prolonged bleeding time
	Pigmented reticular cells of bone marrow, lymph nodes, and liver pigment in wall of small blood vessels

PHYSICIANS' GUIDE TO OCULOSYSTEMIC DISEASES

o   Electroretinogram may show supernormal response.

o   Plucked hair bulbs incubated in solutions containing tyrosine have been successfully used in chemical diagnosis and differentiation of types of albinism.

o   For findings in associated conditions, see Table 6.1.

Table 6.1

CONDITIONS ASSOCIATED WITH ALBINISM

Disease	Findings
Oculocerebral syndrome with hypopigmentation	Incomplete albinism, skin and hair of universal albino
	Severe mental deficiency
	Spastic diplegia
	Microphthalmos
	Small opaque cornea (no view of retina)
	Spastic entropion
	Possible aniridia
	Total blindness
	Autosomal recessive inheritance
Waardenburg's syndrome	Irregular leukism of forehead, hair, and body
	Premature graying of hair
	Heterochromia of irides — total, partial or sector
	Albinotic eye grounds often corresponding in location and degree to iris
	Hypochromia (both irides whitish blue)
	Lateral displacement of medial canthi and lacrimal punctae
	Medial eyebrows often meet
	Broad, high nasal bridge
	Irregular autosomal dominant inheritance
X-linked deaf-mutism and cutaneous albinism	Leukism
	Deaf-mutism
	Vestibular disturbance
	Segmental or total heterochromia
	Pigment clumps in the retina
	Hearing impairment in female carriers

Adapted from Krill AE: Krill's Hereditary Retinal and Choroidal Diseases, vol 2. Hagerstown, Md: Harper & Row, 1977. Used with permission.

Fig. 6.5 Ocular albinism in a 15-year-old male. Visual acuity was 6/15 (20/50). Also shown in color section.

Fig. 6.6 Iris heterochromia in the left eye of a patient with Waardenburg's syndrome. The right eye was normal. From Bard LA: Heterogeneity in Waardenburg's syndrome. **Arch Ophthalmol** 96:1193, 1978. Copyright © 1978, American Medical Association. Used with permission. Also shown in color section.

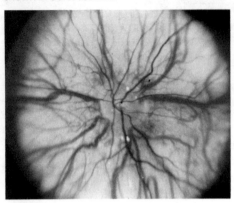 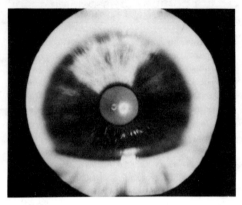

Fig. 6.7 Waardenburg's syndrome with an absent foveal light reflection, hypopigmentation (a, left) and peripheral segmental hypopigmentation (b, right). From Bard LA: Heterogeneity in Waardenburg's syndrome. **Arch Ophthalmol** 96:1193, 1978. Copyright © 1978, American Medical Association. Used with permission. Fig. 6.7a also shown in color section.

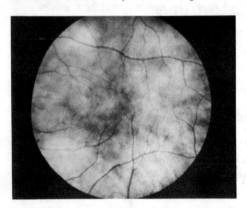 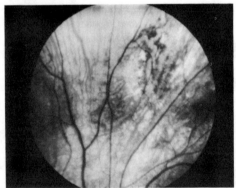

Main differential diagnosis

o   Normals with light pigmentation in early life

o   High myopia

o   X-linked nightblindness and myopia

o   Associated conditions listed in Table 6.1.

References

Bard LA: Heterogeneity in Waardenburg's syndrome. Arch Ophthalmol 96:1193, 1978.

Delleman JW, Hageman MJ: Ophthalmological findings in 34 patients with Waardenburg syndrome. J Pediatr Ophthalmol Strabismus 15:341, 1978.

Francois J: Albinism. Ophthalmologica 178:19, 1979.

Krill AE: Krill's Hereditary Retinal and Choroidal Diseases, vol 2. Hagerstown, Md: Harper & Row, 1977, p 645.

Spencer WH, Hogan MJ: Ocular manifestations of Chédiak-Higashi syndrome. Am J Ophthalmol 50:1197, 1960.

B. VITILIGO (Fig. 6.8; see 6.8a also in color section)

This patchy destruction of melanocytes of the skin results in depigmented areas that may enlarge slowly. It's known to occur in one percent of the population, and there is increasing evidence to link it with serious disease, particularly thyroid conditions, diabetes mellitus, adrenal insufficiency, and pernicious anemia.

Ophthalmoscopic findings

o Subtle, patchy chocolate-brown ragged pigmentation of retinal pigment epithelium and choroid occurs in 39 percent of patients.

o Exposure of choroidal vessels between areas of pigmentation suggests ocular albinism.

o Pigment changes may be bilateral or unilateral.

o Heavier pigment clumping may be seen in periphery.

o Macula is usually spared.

o Localized multiple depigmented areas resemble healed chorioretinitis, especially around the disc.

o Superimposed findings of related diseases.

Symptoms & signs

o Visual acuity usually 6/9 (20/30) or better; may be worse if chorioretinitis-like lesions involve fovea or superimposed disease, such as diabetic retinopathy, supervenes.

o Nightblindness is occasionally reported.

o Vitiligo of eyelids is present in 50 percent of patients.

o Eyebrow and eyelash depigmentation is common.

Fig. 6.8 Vitiligo in a 22-year-old diabetic female (a, left). Similar chocolate-brown blotches of depigmentation can be seen in the skin (b, right). Fig. 6.8a also shown in color section.

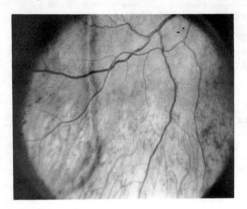 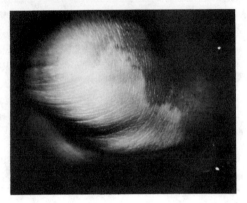

o Iris transilluminates in some patients and may be unilateral or be present in a sector heterochromia of iris that progresses with age.

o Patchy, chocolate-brown skin alternating with white areas of depigmentation.

o Whitening of hair in patches.

Other confirming findings

o Age range, 12 to 78 years; average age, 45 years.

o No social predilection.

o May be more common in females.

o Associated conditions: thyroid disease, skin melanoma, diabetes mellitus, hypadrenalism, severe food and drug allergy, retinitis pigmentosa, cholecystitis, others (see references).

Main differential diagnosis

o Rubella syndrome

o Radiation retinopathy

o Sympathetic ophthalmia

o Vogt-Koyanagi-Harada disease

o Albinism, including Waardenburg's syndrome

o Uveitis, unknown cause

o Fuchs's heterochromic iridocyclitis

References

Albert DM, Nordlund JJ, Lerner AB: Ocular abnormalities occurring with vitiligo. Ophthalmology 86:1145, 1979.

C. VOGT-KOYANAGI-HARADA DISEASE (Fig. 6.9)

Vogt-Koyanagi syndrome was originally described as anterior uveitis associated with alopecia, whitening of the hair, vitiligo, meningeal irritation, and deafness. A similar disease involving posterior uveitis (Harada's disease) with increased protein and lymphocytes in the cerebral spinal fluid suggests a common, but still unknown, etiology.

Ophthalmoscopic findings

Acute phase

o Media hazy.

o Multiple yellow defects in the retinal pigment epithelium, usually less than ¼ disc diameter in size.

o Bullous retinal detachment, which shifts with patient position, may already be present when patient is first seen.

o Both eyes usually involved simultaneously.

o Disc hyperemic.

o Choroid appears thickened and elevated.

Late phase

o Media clear slowly, leaving many vitreous veils and bands.

o The retinal vessels are attenuated.

Fig. 6.9 Vogt-Koyanagi-Harada disease in a 49-year-old woman has left patchy areas of depigmentation in both eyes.

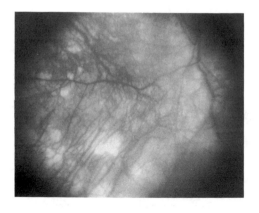

o Patchy but generalized retinal pigment epithelial atrophy and pigment clumping remain.

o Choroidal vessels are attenuated.

o Retina and choroid are thin (no shadow casting).

o Cataracts often follow.

Symptoms and signs

o Headache, nausea, vomiting, stiff neck often precede the onset.

o Rapid bilateral loss of vision, often decreased to counting fingers, due to nonrhegmatogenous retinal detachment. Retinal detachment improves in four to six weeks, but full recovery of vision is rare.

o Anterior uveitis (iritis) with photophobia, alopecia, vitiligo, hearing loss develops in some patients or may occur alone.

o Patients are often very depressed and irritable, more than expected from loss of vision; suicidal tendencies occur.

o Intraocular pressure is often low ($<$15mm Hg)

Other confirming findings

o More common in black, Oriental, or deeply pigmented white patients. No sex predilection.

o As part of general history and physical examination, whitening of hair, brows, lashes, and skin have to be sought out, since some patients hide these defects.

o Neurological evaluation, including cerebral spinal fluid protein and lymphocyte analysis, and computerized axial tomography or radioactive scan.

o Fluorescein angiography discloses vascular deficiencies in the retina.

o Electroretinogram and electro-oculogram confirm retinal malfunction.

Main differential diagnosis

o Metastatic carcinoma to the choroid

o Leukemia

o Reticulum cell sarcoma

o Posterior necrotizing scleritis

o Behcet's disease

o Sympathetic ophthalmia

References

Gass JDM: Stereoscopic Atlas of Macular Diseases. St. Louis: Mosby, 1977, p 118.

Shimizu K: Harada's, Behcet's, Vogt-Koyanagi syndromes: Are they clinical entities? Trans Am Acad Ophthalmol Otolaryngol 77:281, 1973.

Yannuzzi LA, Gitter KA, Schatz H: The Macula: A Comprehensive Text and Atlas. Baltimore: Williams & Wilkins, 1979, p 350.

D. OGUCHI'S DISEASE (Fig. 6.10)

Most patients with this unusual form of congenital nightblindness are Oriental or darkly pigmented.

Ophthalmoscopic findings

o In light-adapted state, the retinal pigment epithelium has a golden-yellow or greenish appearance, accentuating the normal blood vessels by contrast.

o Coloration may be in posterior pole, more peripheral, or both.

o Color of arteries and veins may be nearly identical.

o After 30 minutes to one hour in the dark or with an eye patch, the abnormal retinal color disappears (Mizuo phenomenon). On exposure to light, color starts to reappear in 10 minutes.

Fig. 6.10 Oguchi's disease in a 46-year-old black female with normal visual acuity. The golden color of the fundus in the light-adapted state (a, left) has disappeared after one hour in the dark (b, right). From Gass, J. Donald M. : Stereoscopic atlas of macular diseases, ed. 2, St. Louis, 1977, The C. V. Mosby Co. Used with permission.

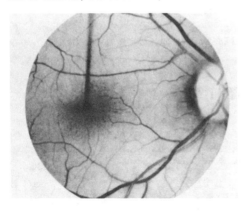
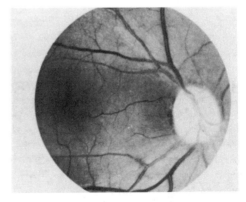

Symptoms and signs

o Visual acuity is usually normal or slightly decreased — 6/15 (20/50).

o Nightblindness from birth that may reverse after prolonged dark adaptation.

o Normal color vision.

o Visual field is normal, except in reduced illumination.

Other confirming findings

o Autosomal recessive inheritance with history of consanguinity in 60 percent of patients.

o In electroretinogram, photopic and scotopic curves are similar, unlike the normals, whose implicit time when dark-adapted is twice the light-adapted state. Carriers may show mildly abnormal electroretinogram.

o Electro-oculogram is variable.

o Findings in Oguchi's disease and stationary congenital nightblindness patients without fundus abnormality are physiologically similar, but in the latter, recessive, dominant, and X-linked inheritance are reported.

Main differential diagnosis

o Fundus albipunctatus

o Congenital stationary nightblindness

o Vitamin A deficiency

o Retinitis punctata albescens (progressive nightblindness)

o Doyne's honeycomb dystrophy (familial drusen)

References

Gass JDM: Stereoscopic Atlas of Macular Diseases. St. Louis: Mosby, 1977, p182.

Krill AE: Krill's Hereditary Retinal and Choroidal Diseases, vol 2. Hagerstown, Md: Harper & Row, 1977, p 391.

III. BLACK AND WHITE DEFECTS IN THE POSTERIOR EYE

Disturbances of the retinal pigment epithelium often result in localized loss of the pigment granules from the cells, with dispersion into adjacent tissues, total disappearance, or both. Pigment granules may be carried to nearby veins by phagocytes. Stimulated cells may produce more than the adjacent cells and become hyperpigmented. All these effects may be present in and around retinal pigment epithelial cell injury, disease, or developmental abnormalities. In some diseases, a combination of localized and generalized retinal pigment epithelial abnormality exists. For example, some patients with retinitis pigmentosa (generalized retinal pigment epithelium disease) have maculopathy (localized retinal pigment epithelium disease), even though the macula is spared in most patients until late in the disease.

This section deals with isolated defects of local areas that occur while the remainder of the retinal pigment epithelium appears normal.

A. HYPERPLASIA OF THE RETINAL PIGMENT EPITHELIUM (GROUP PIGMENTATION, BEAR-TRACK PIGMENTATION)
(Fig. 6.11; see also in color section)

Ophthalmoscopic findings

o   Black pigment contrasts sharply with its depigmented border.

o   Black spots may be multiple and grouped. Sometimes there is a pattern resembling a bear's paw print.

o   Lesions are flat; they do not elevate retinal blood vessels or disturb the neurosensory retina.

o   They are often seen posterior to the equator, but may be in any quadrant.

o   The margins and pigmentation may change slightly with age.

Symptoms and signs

o   None; the pigment is usually a finding of routine ophthalmoscopy. They are present at birth, but probably become pigmented in the first decade of life.

o   Occasionally, a scotoma may be plotted on careful field examination.

o   In rare hereditary involvement of the macula, the patient has slightly decreased vision and notes distortions.

Other confirming findings

o   There is no known hereditary pattern, although one report of sisters with typical group pigmentation in the macula has been reported.

o   Fluorescein angiography helps define the location and vascularity of the pigment.

o   A number of diseases associated with group pigmentation have been reported. All seem to be fortuitous.

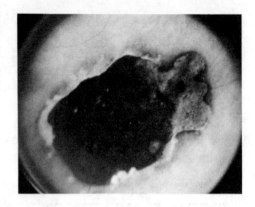

Fig. 6.11 Hyperplasia of retinal pigment epithelium. Note the black color and the border of depigmentation. Contrast with a choroidal nevus (Fig. 7.13) and hamartoma of the retinal pigment epithelium (Fig. 3.34). Also shown in color section.

Main differential diagnosis

o   Retinal pigment hyperplasia secondary to trauma, inflammation, or "fallout" after cryotherapy

o   Nevus of choroid

o   Malignant melanoma of the choroid

o   Melancytoma of the optic disc and retina

o   Rubella retinopathy

o   Toxic retinopathy, as with thioridazine (Mellaril)

o   Nevus of Ota and ocular melanosis

o   Waardenburg's syndrome

References

Blair NP, Trempe CL: Hypertrophy of the retinal pigment epithelium associated with Gardner's syndrome. Am J Ophthalmol 90:661, 1980.

Duke-Elder S: System of Ophthalmology, vol 3, part 2. St. Louis: Mosby, 1964, p 801.

Krill AE: Krill's Hereditary Retinal and Choroidal Diseases, vol 2. Hagerstown, Md: Harper & Row, 1977, pp 730-736.

B. ISCHEMIC ATROPHY OF THE RETINAL PIGMENT EPITHELIUM
(Fig. 6.12; see also in color section)

Depigmentation, atrophy, and degeneration of the retinal pigment epithelium may coexist and accompany many ocular diseases. The photographs of pure retinal pigment epithelial atrophy should be compared with the dissection shown in Fig. 1.9. It's unusual to find retinal pigment epithelial

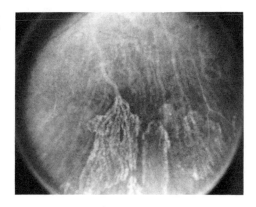

Fig. 6.12 Atrophy of the retinal pigment epithelium in a patient with carotid artery occlusion. Also shown in color section.

atrophy without compounding disease in the choroid or neurosensory retina (see Fig. 7.14).

Ophthalmoscopic findings

o   The margins are irregular.

o   Usually, the atrophic area is linear in the direction of choroidal arterial perfusion.

o   Mid-periphery is the most common site.

o   The fine choroidal vessels are exposed to view (compare with Fig. 7.14).

o   Pigment proliferation and clumping may be present, if retinal pigment epithelial cells are still viable.

o   Often multiple patches extend in a spoke-like pattern outward from the posterior pole of the eye.

o   Central retinal artery occlusion or narrowing may be present.

Symptoms and signs

o   Symptoms and signs are those of the specific diseases causing the atrophy, such as carotid artery stenosis or occlusion, hypertension, and embolic disease.

o   Visual acuity is poor, if retinal pigment epithelial atrophy involves the macula.

o   Scotomata correspond to areas of atrophy.

Other confirming findings

o   Historical or physical evidence suggesting poor arterial blood flow to the head and eyes.

o Fluorescein angiography is very useful to determine choroidal blood flow.

o Supporting laboratory, angiographic, radionuclear, ultrasonic, and plethysmographic studies help confirm the diagnosis.

Main differential diagnosis

o Congenital retinal pigment epithelial hypoplasia

o Coloboma

o Regional choroidal atrophy

o Senile macular degeneration

o Sector retinitis pigmentosa

o Choroideremia

o Paving stone degeneration

References

Wise GN, Dollery CT, Henkind P: The Retinal Circulation. New York: Harper & Row, 1971, p 309.

Zinn KM, Marmor MF, eds: The Retinal Pigment Epithelium. Cambridge, Mass: Harvard University Press, 1979, p 247.

C. INHERITED MACULAR DEGENERATION

This broad topic covers a multitude of hereditary and metabolic diseases. Many, when they are better understood, may be found to have been included here in error. Clinical classification suffers from the lack of the specificity of symptoms and the variability of ophthalmoscopic appearance. The macular pathology is often the center of attention, and yet disease of the periphery coexists.

To help you sort out this complex group of diseases, attention is directed here to those in which the macula seems to be principally involved. They are grouped, within known limits, by age of onset.

1. Onset usually before age 40

a) FUNDUS FLAVIMACULATUS, STARGARDT'S DISEASE, AND DOMINANT PROGRESSIVE FOVEAL DYSTROPHY (Fig. 6.13; see 6.13b and 6.13c also in color section)

Fundus flavimaculatus may involve only retinal pigment epithelium away from the macula, include the macula, or affect the macula alone. Therefore, some investigators feel fundus flavimaculatus and Stargardt's disease are the same condition. Some distinguish dominant progessive foveal dystrophy from both of the above on the basis of dominant inheritance and minor difference in the clinical course; its appearance, however, can't be distinguished from Stargardt's disease.

Ophthalmoscopic findings

o Visual loss may precede ophthalmoscopically visible lesions.

o Faint doughnut-shaped depigmentation and pigment stippling surround the central foveal pigment. Both eyes are very similar in appearance. Usually this precedes the transient yellow defects.

o Opaque yellow or yellow-white deposits in the retinal pigment epithelium usually are round, but often linear. Their margins are sharp, but often one end is indistinct and drawn out, resembling a fish tail.

o They may be paramacular only, but sometimes extend nearly to the equator, ending with a sharp demarcation line where the normal retinal pigment epithelium begins. This phase may be transient — two to five years — beginning in the second decade, be unassociated with loss of vision, and go undetected, unless macular lesions result in loss of vision.

o In late stages, there is pigment clumping and a golden or silver sheen; exposure of the larger choroidal vessels to view may show them to be pale or even white (choroidal sclerosis).

Symptoms & signs

o Loss of visual acuity, rarely poorer than 6/60 (20/200) starts in first two decades of life and may be more advanced in one eye than other, but usually both are affected at the same time. Complaints about vision often precede detectable macular pathology.

o Central scotomas are found after macular involvement.

o Photophobia is a rare complaint.

o Slow dark adaptation is described by some patients.

o Color vision may become defective with progressive maculopathy.

Other confirming findings

o Inheritance is autosomal recessive (few pedigrees of dominant inheritance are known).

o There are no known associated systemic diseases.

o Fluorescein angiography aids in defining the nature and extent of the retinal pigment epithelial disease.

o Electroretinogram and electro-oculogram are usually normal.

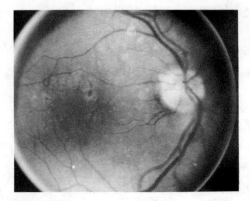

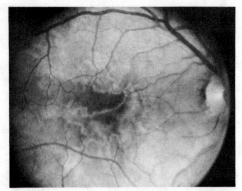

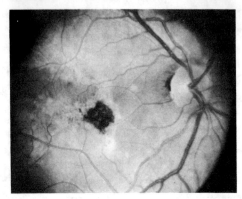

Fig. 6.13 Fundus flavimaculatus (a, above left). In addition to pigment remodeling in the fovea, there are subtle irregular yellow defects in the retinal pigment epithelium. Their location near the disc is unusual. Stargardt's maculopathy in a 26-year-old male (b, above right). Visual acuity 6/24 (20/80). The appearance one year later (c, right) with a visual acuity of 6/21 (20/70). The other eye was similar. Fig. 6.13b and 6.13c also shown in color section.

o   Dark adaptation is usually normal.

o   Color vision may be defective in severe macular disease.

Main differential diagnosis

o   Familial drusen (Doyne's honeycombed dystrophy)

o   Fundus albipunctatus

o   Retinitis punctata albescens

o   Cone and juvenile macular degeneration

o   Vitelliform macular degeneration (late stage)

o   Pericentral retinitis pigmentosa

References

Krill AE: Krill's Hereditary Retinal and Choroidal Diseases, vol 2. Hagerstown, Md: Harper & Row, 1977, pp 636-643, 749-787.

Yannuzzi LA, Gitter KA, Schatz H: The Macula: A Comprehensive Text and Atlas. Baltimore: Williams & Wilkins, 1979, pp 267-276.

b) VITELLIRUPTIVE MACULAR DYSTROPHY (VITELLIFORM DEGENERATION, BEST'S DISEASE) (Fig. 6.14; see 6.14a also in color section)

The appearance of the classical form of this disease is unforgettable. Careful observation of families over many years have provided us with knowledge of the less characteristic appearances.

Ophthalmoscopic findings

o Egg-yolk (vitelliform), subretinal cyst-like defect at the fovea occasionally contains a fluid level.

o The lesion has a yellow or yellow-white color.

o It does not disturb surrounding neurosensory retina or vessels at this stage.

o Size may be different in each eye, but both eyes are involved at the same time.

o Clumping of the contents of the cyst, possible rupture, pigment atrophy and proliferation, subretinal hemorrhage, and fibrosis may occur with age, usually before age 40, but these do not always occur in both eyes at the same time.

o Single cysts confined to the macula of both eyes is the usual presentation, but some patients have multiple lesions elsewhere in the posterior retinal pigment epithelium.

o Rarely only one eye is involved.

Fig. 6.14 Vitelliform (egg-yolk) dystrophy of the macula in a 23-year-old white female. Right (a, left) and left (b, right) eyes. Fig. 6.14a also in color section.

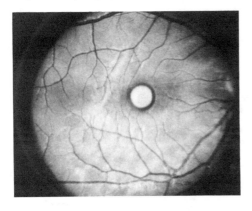 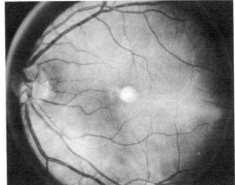

Symptoms & signs

o Mild visual loss — vision 6/12 (20/40) or better — at cyst stage.

o Amblyopia in one eye may occur in children with early onset of the disease.

o Severe loss of central vision — 6/12 (20/40) to counting fingers — follows subretinal hemorrhage and scarring.

o Some patients describe distortions of images.

o Central scotoma can be plotted on field testing.

o Children may present with crossed eyes (esotropia).

o With destruction of macula, color vision may be affected.

o Dark adaptation is normal.

Other confirming findings

o Dominant inheritance with variable penetrance, sometimes skipping generations.

o Age of onset is usually three to 15 years, with a reported range of one week to 74 years.

o Pedigrees have been reported in which all affected members had blue irides and nonaffected members brown irides.

o Many patients are farsighted (hyperopic).

o Fluorescein angiography and special photographs aid definition of stages of the disease.

o Electroretinogram and electro-oculogram are often diagnostic. Diagnosis of disease has been made by these tests in patients without visible lesions.

Main differential diagnosis

o Retinoblastoma

o Toxoplasmosis

o Senile macular degeneration

o Drusen of the retinal pigment epithelium

o Central serous choroidopathy

o Subhyaloid hemorrhage

o Coats's disease

o   Central areolar choroidal dystrophy

o   Pericentral retinitis pigmentosa

References

Deutman AF: The Hereditary Dystrophies of the Posterior Pole of the Eye. Assen, The Netherlands: Van Gorcum, 1971, p 198.

Krill AE: Krill's Hereditary Retinal and Choroidal Diseases, vol 2. Hagerstown, Md: Harper & Row, 1977, p 665.

Yannuzzi LA, Gitter KA, Schatz H: The Macula: A Comprehensive Text and Atlas. Baltimore: Williams & Wilkins, 1979, p 269.

c) CONE DEGENERATIONS AND JUVENILE MACULAR DEGENERATION (Fig. 6.15)

Bilateral pigment dystrophy in young patients can no longer simply be called hereditary or juvenile macular degeneration. Better testing methods and pedigree analysis separate the cone degeneration patients.

Ophthalmoscopic findings

o   Bull's-eye disturbance of retinal pigment epithelium around the foveola may be readily apparent or very subtle.

o   Foveola appears uninvolved and red.

o   Stippled pigmentation-atrophy band surrounding red foveola may be narrow or broad and often does not have a distinct peripheral border.

o   Second most frequent finding is a diffuse spotty pigmentation. Pigmentation may be very fine initially, forming larger clumps later.

o   Some patients may have heavy pigmentation at the fovea without a bull's-eye lesion (this has been described as inverse retinitis pigmentosa).

o   An occasional patient has a tapetal (green-white)reflex from the retina.

o   Optic atrophy may develop.

Symptoms & signs

o   Visual acuity loss seems to be more severe and more rapid, the earlier the onset of the disease. Both eyes are usually the same. Visual acuity may reach 6/120 (20/400) and stabilize.

o   Color vision may decrease even before visual acuity loss, but usually becomes evident when vision reaches 6/12 (20/40) or less.

o   Red light appears dim and green light bright (reversal of Purkinje shift).

Fig. 6.15 Progressive loss of vision and color discrimination from cone dystrophy in a 20-year-old male, starting at age 14. There is a subtle bull's-eye pigmentation at the fovea. Visual acuity was 6/18 (20/60). The other eye was similar.

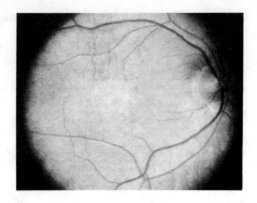

o   Photophobia is common. Excess light decreases the patient's vision.

o   Nystagmus may develop as vision decreases.

o   Central scotomas can be found on field testing.

o   Dark adaptation is usually normal, unless, which is rare, retinitis pigmentosa is associated.

Other confirming findings

o   Inheritance is autosomal dominant, although occasional recessive pedigrees have been reported.

o   Age of onset is usually before 20 years, although it's been seen at age 70.

o   Fluorescein angiography defines the extent of retinal pigment epithelium disease.

o   Photopic (mostly cone function) electroretinogram is classic.

Main differential diagnosis

o   Toxic maculopathy, as with chloroquine (Aralen) and phenothiazine

o   Stargardt's disease

o   Inverse retinitis pigmentosa (rod-cone dystrophy)

o   Achromatopsia (total color blindness: rod vision, normal-appearance)

References

Deutman AF: The Hereditary Dystrophies of the Posterior Pole of the Eye. Assen, The Netherlands: Van Gorcum, 1971, p 181.

Krill AE: Krill's Hereditary Retinal and Choroidal Diseases, vol 2. Hagerstown, Md: Harper & Row, 1977, p 421.

O'Donnell FE, Schatz H, Reid P, et al: Autosomal dominant dystrophy of the retinal pigment epithelium. Arch Ophthalmol 97:680, 1979.

d) BUTTERFLY AND RETICULAR DYSTROPHY (Fig. 6.16; see also in color section)

These two rare dystrophies are considered separate entities by nature of their inheritance. Visual acuity is not severely affected in either disease. The names describe their clinical appearance.

Ophthalmoscopic findings

o Stellate or butterfly pigmentation at the fovea involves only that area in butterfly dystrophy.

o In reticular dystrophy, a pigmented net-like appearance involves the macula and the posterior eye, even nasal to the disc.

o Some patients may have yellow or pigmented dots in the periphery.

o Disc and vessels are normal.

Symptoms & signs

o Slight decrease in visual acuity.

o Distortions sometimes described by patients.

o Strabismus may be present.

o Fields and color vision are normal.

o Dark adaptation is normal.

Fig. 6.16 Butterfly dystrophy in father (a) and daughter (b). Visual acuity was 6/7.5 (20/25) in 29-year-old daughter and the 55-year-old father. The other eye was similar in both. Also shown in color section.

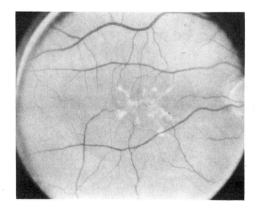
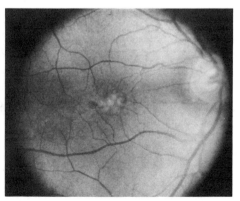

Other confirming findings

o   Butterfly dystrophy onset is as early as 11 years of age; reticular dystrophy as early as five years of age. Butterfly dystrophy is autosomal dominant; reticular dystrophy is autosomal recessive.

o   Fluorescein angiography defines the pigment layer defects.

Main differential diagnosis

o   Stargardt's disease

o   Cone dystrophy

o   Toxic maculopathy, as with phenothiazine

o   Pericentral retinitis pigmentosa

References

Deutman AF: The Hereditary Dystrophies of the Posterior Pole of the Eye. Assen, The Netherlands: Van Gorcum, 1971, pp 324, 340.

e) OTHER RARE DYSTROPHIES OF THE MACULA

(1) Dominant macular drusen and juvenile foveal dystrophy
The drusen, other findings, and course are not unlike adult-onset drusen. They are distinguished principally by early onset.

(2) Juvenile disciform degeneration
This hereditary dystrophy resembles the adult variety, but must be distinguished in children from larval infestation (Toxocara canis) and degenerating vitelliform cysts (vitelliform dystrophy).

(3) Macular pigmentation and psychomotor retardation
See Table 6.2.

2. Onset usually after age 40 (senile macular degeneration)

An aging retina is not necessarily diseased, and poor visual acuity cannot be attributed to age alone. The rods and cones are unaffected by age, as far as we know. In contrast, the retinal pigment epithelium shows failure of renewal of cell functions with age. Separating manifestations of this failure, such as drusen and lipofuscin accumulation, from the pathology of senile macular degeneration has only been begun.

Senile macular degeneration may affect as much as 3 percent of the white population. The National Advisory Eye Council estimated in 1976 that 250,000 people had severe visual impairment from macular degeneration and related diseases, and another 66,000 were legally blind. Blacks and Orientals seem relatively spared of this disease.

The hereditary nature of senile macular degeneration is not established. It's discussed here because many believe it is inherited. Because of the late onset, with patients' parents and siblings deceased or widely scattered, pedigrees are difficult to establish.

Senile macular degeneration may be several diseases. Certainly, it has various ophthalmoscopic presentations. Many factors may have significance. For example, preliminary studies indicate there is a six-to-one chance that senile macular degeneration patients are also on treatment for hypertension, compared to age- and sex-matched controls. Similarly, there is a three-to-one chance that the senile macular degeneration patient is farsighted (hyperopic).

Table 6.2

RARE DISEASES WITH EARLY MACULAR DEGENERATION

Disease	Age at onset	Macular change	Optic atrophy	Clinical signs	Laboratory
Late infantile amaurotic idiocy (Batten's disease)	2-8	Pigment	Yes	CNS	Multilamellar cytosomes and fingerprint inclusions on electromicroscopy. Normal hexosaminidase A
Juvenile GM_2 gangliosidosis	2-6	Retinitis pigmentosa	Yes	CNS	Partial serum hexosaminidase A deficiency
Sea-blue histiocyte syndrome	25	Yellow granules	No	Hepatosplenomegaly	Vacuolated histiocytes stained blue with Giemsa solution
Lactosyl ceramidosis	3	Red macula	No	CNS	RBC or cultured fibroblasts have increased lactosylceramide
Farber's lipogranulomatosis	1-3	Gray macula	No	CNS, swollen joints	Liver, spleen have increased ceramide and sphingosine

Adapted from Krill AE: Krill's Hereditary Retinal and Choroidal Diseases, vol 2. Hagerstown, Md: Harper & Row, 1977. Used with permission.

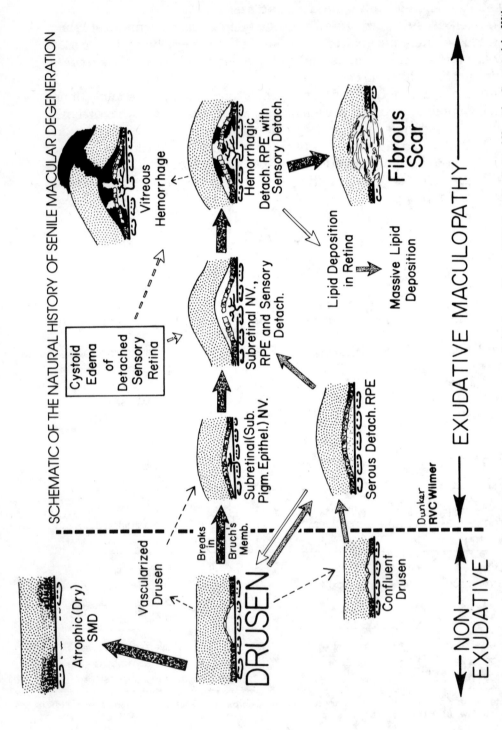

SCHEMATIC OF THE NATURAL HISTORY OF SENILE MACULAR DEGENERATION

Atrophic (Dry) SMD

Vascularized Drusen

DRUSEN

Confluent Drusen

Breaks in Bruch's Memb.

Subretinal (Sub. Pigm. Epithel.) NV.

Serous Detach. RPE

Subretinal NV., RPE and Sensory Detach.

Cystoid Edema of Detached Sensory Retina

Vitreous Hemorrhage

Hemorrhagic Detach. RPE with Sensory Detach.

Lipid Deposition in Retina

Massive Lipid Deposition

Fibrous Scar

Dunkar RVC Wilmer

NON EXUDATIVE

EXUDATIVE MACULOPATHY

From Patz A, Fine SL, Orth DH: Sights and Sounds in Ophthalmology. vol 1. St. Louis: Mosby. 1976. From the Retinal Vascular Center of the Wilmer Institute; Amalie Dunker, illustrator. Used with permission.

What follows is a general description of all types of senile macular degeneration in increasing order of severity, as roughly measured by their effect on visual acuity. It's not intended as a classification, but as an ophthalmoscopic guide. The experienced observer has seen many patients with regard to whom the findings described are out of order.

a) DRUSEN (FAMILIAL DRUSEN, DOYNE'S HONEYCOMBED DYSTROPHY, CRYSTALLINE RETINAL DEGENERATION) (Fig. 6.17; see 6.17a also in color section)

The term drusen (glands) has been used to describe smooth, globular structures in the optic disc. This has led to some confusion with drusen of Bruch's membrane and the retinal pigment epithelium. The glass-like Bruch's membrane between the choriocapillaris and retinal pigment epithelium is a noncellular product of both at their interface. Localized thickening of Bruch's membrane (drusen) displaces the overlying retinal pigment epithelial cells, causing some to be stacked up at their margins and thinned out at the apex. The result is a central area with little or no pigment and a circle of apparent hyperpigmentation.

Ophthalmoscopic findings

o   Fine yellow, white, and round or oval dots clustered in and around the macula or the whole posterior eye.

o   Size of dots varies from width of a small arteriole to width of the central retinal vein.

Fig. 6.17 Familial drusen in a 50-year-old male with 6/15 visual acuity (a, left). The other eye was nearly identical. On fluorescein angiography, many more drusen are evident (b, right). Fig. 6.17a also shown in color section.

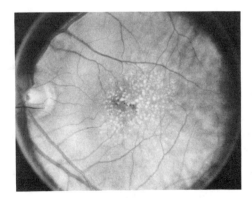 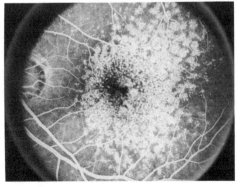

o They may coalesce, especially at the fovea.

o Some have a partial or complete black pigment circle.

o In late stages, highlights resemble crystals.

o Serous detachment of the retinal pigment epithelium, subretinal neovascularization, hemorrhage, and pigmentation of neurosensory retina may occur.

o The disease is always bilateral.

Symptoms & signs

o Decrease in visual acuity, rarely before age 40, may occur abruptly, if hemorrhage or retinal pigment epithelial detachment develops. Difficulty reading is the most common patient complaint. Visual loss in one eye may precede other by weeks to years.

o The patient experiences distortions, if neurosensory retina is elevated by blood or retinal pigment epithelial detachment.

o Central scotoma can be plotted, if visual acuity is decreased, but usually not with patients who have observable retinal pigment epithelial disease but no visual loss.

Other confirming findings

o Autosomal dominant inheritance is often discovered.

o Appearance of visible drusen in family members occurs after age 20, but the earliest so far described is at age eight.

o Fluorescein angiography helps define the extent of disease.

Main differential diagnosis

o Fundus flavimaculatus and Stargardt's disease

o Retinitis punctata albescens

o Fundus albipunctatus

o Cone dystrophy

o Toxic maculopathy, as with chloroquine (Aralen)

References

Krill AE: Krill's Hereditary Retinal and Choroidal Diseases, vol 2. Hagerstown, Md: Harper & Row, 1977, p 825.

b) COLLOID DRUSEN (Fig. 6.18)

The separation of these drusen from those previously described is based on ophthalmoscopic appearance. There is no histologic evidence to indicate they are different. Some observers consider them more likely to result in visual loss.

Ophthalmoscopic findings

o Globular yellow spots of various sizes, often with the largest at the fovea where they tend to coalesce. With proximal illumination, they appear as clusters of semitransparent circles.

o Foveal light and red reflection often obliterated.

o Macular pigmentation may be accentuated around drusen.

o Atrophy of retinal pigment epithelium, serous retinal pigment epithelial detachment, subretinal neovascularization, subretinal hemorrhage may develop more often in patients with this type of drusen.

o Always bilateral.

Symptoms & signs

o Visual acuity may not be diminished even if the drusen are under the fovea. Rapid deterioration occurs as in familial drusen with serous retinal pigment epithelial detachment, subretinal neovascularization, or hemorrhage or may be gradual with atrophy of the retinal pigment epithelium. Visual acuity may reach counting fingers in each eye.

o Visual loss in one eye often precedes loss in the other, and this varies from a few weeks to many years.

Other confirming findings

o Inheritance patterns very difficult to establish — probably autosomal dominant with incomplete penetrance.

o The onset usually after age 40. The disease may be accelerated in patients with hypertension.

o Fluorescein angiography helps define the extent and stage of the disease.

Main differential diagnosis

o Vitelliform macular degeneration

o Histoplasmosis syndrome

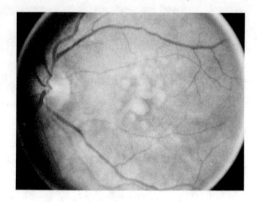

Fig. 6.18 Colloid drusen in the left eye of a 74-year-old white female. Visual acuity was 6/9 (20/30). The other eye had severe visual loss.

o Myopic degeneration

o Fundus flavimaculatus

o Central serous choroidopathy

References

Gass JDM: Pathogenesis of disciform detachment of the neuroepithelium: 3. Senile disciform macular degeneration. Am J Ophthalmol 63:617, 1967.

Gass JDM: Stereoscopic Atlas of Macular Diseases. St. Louis: Mosby, 1977.

Sarks SH: Aging and degeneration in the macular region: A clinicopathological study. Br J Ophthalmol 60:241, 1976.

c) GEOGRAPHIC (AREOLAR) ATROPHY (SORSBY'S CENTRAL AREOLAR CHOROIDAL SCLEROSIS) (Fig. 6.19; see also in color section)

There are several diseases that result in areolar retinal pigment epithelial and choroidal atrophy. The autosomal dominant type (Sorsby's central areolar choroidal sclerosis) described here can often be separated from similar-appearing atrophy in Stargardt's disease or juvenile macular dystrophy by age of onset. Serpiginous atrophy described in Chapter 7 has an age of onset and characteristic appearance by which it can be identified. Most confusing are the senile macular degeneration patients seen in a stage of areolar atrophy following serous effusion uncomplicated by subretinal neovascularization and hemorrhage. Central areolar dystrophy usually does not have a serous or hemorrhagic stage. It's included here because it's often considered a form of senile macular degeneration, even though fluorescein angiographic and histopathologic evidence suggest it starts as atrophy of the choriocapillaris vessels.

Ophthalmoscopic findings

o   Atrophy of central retinal pigment epithelium and choriocapillaris exposes larger choroidal vessels to view.

o   The borders are sharp and sometimes accentuated by fine black lines of relative hyperpigmentation. The retinal pigment epithelium may appear gray around margin of lesion.

o   Several smaller lesions may coalesce.

o   Fine black pigment dispersion is seen in the neurosensory retina over the lesion.

o   Subretinal pigment epithelium and subretinal blood may be present at the margin of lesion.

o   The neurosensory retina usually is not elevated or cystic, but often thin and atrophic; no shadow casting by vessels can be seen.

Symptoms & signs

o   Visual acuity loss may be profound — 6/120 (20/400) or worse.

o   Visual loss is often gradual and unassociated with metamorphopsia, sudden changes due to hemorrhage, or entopic phenomenon.

o   Visual loss in one eye may be worse than the other, but usually both are affected at the same time, unlike what happens with disciform degeneration.

o   There is a central scotoma on field testing.

Fig. 6.19 Areolar atrophy of the retinal pigment epithelium in the macula (arrows) in the acute stage (a, left) and four years later (b, right). Initial visual acuity of 6/120 (20/400) never improved. Similar difficulty was developing in the other eye. Also shown in color section.

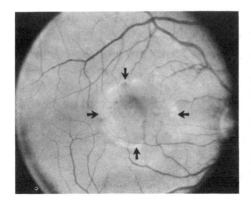 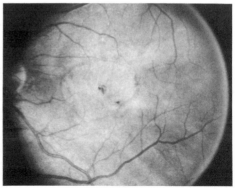

Other confirming findings

o Inheritance patterns are difficult to establish, but findings suggest that it is dominant.

o Affects males and females.

o Onset is after 40 years of age, perhaps even later than other forms of senile macular degeneration.

o Fluorescein angiography helps define the extent of the disease.

Main differential diagnosis

o Myopic degeneration

o Choroidal angiosclerosis (see Fig. 7.11).

o Serpiginous choroiditis

o Juvenile macular dystrophy

o Familial drusen

o Toxoplasmosis

References

Ashton N: Central areolar choroidal sclerosis: A histopathological study. Br J Ophthalmol 37:140, 1953.

Deutman AF: The Hereditary Dystrophies of the Posterior Pole of the Eye. Assen, The Netherlands: Van Gorcum, 1971, pp 409-425.

Gass JDM: Stereoscopic Atlas of Macular Diseases. St. Louis: Mosby, 1977, p 156.

Yannuzzi LA, Gitter KA, Schatz H: The Macula: A Comprehensive Text and Atlas. Baltimore: Williams & Wilkins, 1979, p 274.

d) DISCIFORM DEGENERATION (EXUDATION MACULOPATHY, KUHNT-JUNIUS DEGENERATION) (Figs. 6.20, 6.21; see 6.20b and 6.20d also in color section)

This form of senile macular degeneration may take several courses and, occasionally, different ones in opposite eyes of the same patient. Essential features include drusen of the retinal pigment epithelium, serous or hemorrhagic elevation of the retinal pigment epithelium, and neurosensory retina associated with subretinal neovascularization ending in a nonfunctional scar of the macula.

Ophthalmoscopic findings

o Drusen (see Figs. 6.17-6.18) are often subtle but almost invariably present in both eyes.

o Serous effusion of retinal pigment epithelium may be large, even extending into the periphery (usually inferiorly), or so small that it's difficult to detect. They are often more visible by proximal illumination and appear as a blurred spot that requires refocusing. Vessels and evenly spaced fine yellow dots may be seen on the retinal pigment epithelium.

o Hemorrhage under the retinal pigment epithelium is usually localized, but may be large and involve the whole posterior eye, bulging far forward and lifting the neurosensory retina. Blood under the retinal pigment epithelium has a slate-gray appearance, but is usually accompanied by red blood under the neurosensory retina at its margin.

o Subretinal neovascularization can be seen with the ophthalmoscope as a fine cartwheel of vessels with indistinct or scalloped edges or a gray-green circular or oval defect with a red-yellow center. Often there are hemorrhage at the borders and slight elevation and cystic change of the overlying neurosensory retina.

o Hemorrhage under the neurosensory retina does not hide retinal vessels and may lift the neurosensory retina so refocusing is needed. With changes in patient position, a fluid level does not form, as happens with preretinal blood. Yellow discoloration and indistinct margins occur with hemolysis.

o Elevated neurosensory retina is usually confined to the macula, but may be more extensive, occasionally extending to mid-periphery. The elevation may be subtle and overlie only areas of subretinal neovascularization or retinal pigment epithelial detachment. A cyst-like elevation may persist long after subretinal blood has been absorbed, leaving a yellow fibrous scar.

o Subretinal fibrosis is yellow to yellow-white, often distorts the retinal vessels, and may have retinal vessels disappearing into it to anastomose with the choroid or subretinal neovascularization. It may involve the whole macula.

o In some patients, hemorrhage may break through the retina into the vitreous.

o Rarely severe, sudden subretinal hemorrhage in macular degeneration may shallow the anterior chamber, precipitating acute glaucoma and corneal edema and preventing ophthalmoscopy.

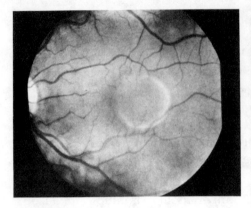

Fig. 6.20a

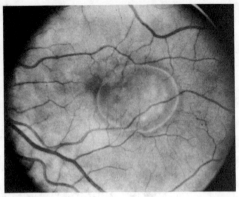

Fig. 6.20b

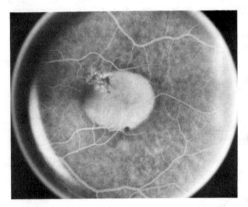

Fig. 6.20c

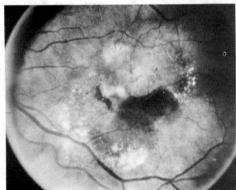

Fig. 6.20d

Fig. 6.20 Macular degeneration in a 48-year-old female, starting as a serous elevation of the retinal pigment (a) that gradually enlarged (b). The elevation filled with fluorescein (c). Three years later, subretinal hemorrhage occurred (d). Seven years after the onset, exudate surrounded the base of the elevated neurosensory retina (e). Visual acuity was 6/7.5 (20/25) at onset and 6/120 (20/400) seven years later. Fig. 6.20b and 6.20d also shown in color section.

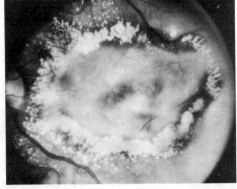

Fig. 6.20e

PHYSICIANS' GUIDE TO OCULOSYSTEMIC DISEASES

Symptoms & signs

o Decreasing vision may be gradual or precipitous. It's precipitous if serous or hemorrhagic retinal pigment epithelial or neurosensory retinal detachment occurs.

o Patient may discover poor vision only on chance covering of the better eye.

o Loss of vision in one eye may precede loss in second eye by many years.

o Serous retinal pigment epithelial detachment at the fovea may cause distortions (metamorphopsia), minification (micropsia), or enlargement (macropsia) of viewed objects. Vision may be improved with plus lenses to focus light on elevated, but still functional, retina.

o Hemorrhagic retinal pigment epithelial detachment involving the fovea interrupts function, and symptoms are severe loss of vision and a central scotoma.

o Color vision is diminished, if vision is severely affected.

o Light intensity may seem decreased to patient. Slow recovery after exposure to light, as in photo-stress test, may also be noted.

o In late stages, patients complain of central flashing lights, often colored or forming "pinwheels." These are different from peripheral field flashes that patients with a retinal tear or detachment experience.

o Decreased luminance perception curve is present.

Other confirming findings

o Inheritance is usually autosomal dominant with incomplete penetrance.

o The mean age of senile macular degeneration patients is 67 years.

o There is no sex predilection.

o Farsightedness (hyperopia) may predispose patient to disease. Farsightedness is 2.7 times more common in these patients.

o Blacks and Orientals rarely have the disease.

o Hypertension may be an aggravating factor. There are 6.1 times more patients with the disease who are hypertensive than patients who are normotensive.

o Fluorescein angiography helps define the extent of retinal pigment epithelium disturbance and identifies abnormal vascularization.

o Photo-stress testing, electroretinogram, and electro-oculogram aid physiologic identification of the disease.

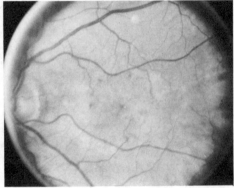
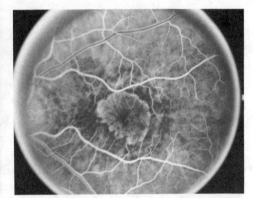
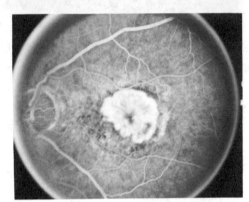

Fig. 6.21 Subretinal neovascularization in senile macular degeneration (a, above left). Fluorescein angiography defines the abnormal vessels that fill long after the choroid and perfuse slowly. There is a nine-second delay between 6.21b (above right) and 6.21c (right). The patient was a 75-year-old male with visual acuity of 6/60 (20/200) in this eye.

Main differential diagnosis

o   Choroidal angiosclerosis

o   Stargardt's disease

o   Myopic degeneration

o   Histoplasmosis syndrome

o   Familial drusen

o   Serpiginous choroiditis

o   Angioid streaks

o   Toxoplasmosis

o   Maculopathy secondary to retinal vascular disease

References

Braunstein RA, Gass JDM: Serous detachments of the retinal pigment epithelium in patients with senile macular disease. Am J Ophthalmol 88:652, 1979.

Delaney WV Jr, Oates RP: Senile macular degeneration and hypertension: A preliminary study. Ann Ophthalmol (accepted for publication).

Gass JDM: Pathogenesis of disciform detachment of the neuroepithelium: 3. Senile disciform macular degeneration. Am J Ophthalmol 63:617, 1967.

Gass JDM: Stereoscopic Atlas of Macular Diseases. St. Louis: Mosby, 1977.

Klien BA: Some aspects of classification and differential diagnosis of senile macular degeneration. Am J Ophthalmol 58:927, 1964.

Sarks SH: Aging and degeneration in the macular region: A clinicopathological study. Br J Ophthalmol 60:324, 1976.

Teeters VW, Bird AC: A clinical study of the vascularity of senile disciform macular degeneration. Am J Ophthalmol 75:53, 1973.

Yannuzzi LA, Gitter KA, Schatz H: The Macula: A Comprehensive Text and Atlas. Baltimore: Williams & Wilkins, 1979.

3. Onset usually in middle life (myopic macular degeneration, Foerster-Fuchs spot) (Figs. 6.22, 6.23; see 6.23a also in color section)

Simple and degenerative myopia are both undoubtedly inherited. Inheritance of the degenerative macular disease may be by a separate gene, but linked to myopia. Febrile illness in childhood, premature birth, and probably other environmental events are factors in causing myopia in the predisposed patient. The macular disease of myopia described here is only a small but symptomatic and very visible part of a disease that involves the retinal pigment epithelium, choroid, sclera, and vitreous.

Ophthalmoscopic findings

o Localized gray or black, slightly raised pigment spot in the fovea is rarely larger than ½ disc diameter in late stage.

o Often there are lacquer cracks, myopic conus, and posterior staphyloma with atrophy of the adjacent retinal pigment epithelium and choriocapillaris exposing blanched and thinned choroidal vessels. The sclera and choroid are obscured by the spot, even if visible in degenerative areas nearby.

o In the acute stage, a gray-green patch of subretinal neovascularization occurs at the margin of an atrophic area. The abnormal subretinal vessels may be visible.

o Subretinal hemorrhage occurs usually at the margin of subretinal neovascularization, and may cover it, hiding it from view.

o The overlying neurosensory retina may be thickened, elevated, or cystic.

o Usually, a Foerster-Fuchs spot occurs in only one eye — the more myopic.

Fig. 6.22 Focal pigmentation in the fovea in a highly myopic patient associated with a decrease in central vision. Visual acuity was counting fingers at 1 meter. Note the extensive atrophy of the retinal pigment epithelium and choroid as well.

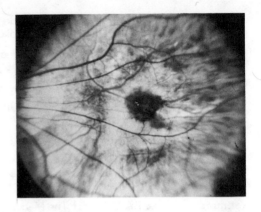

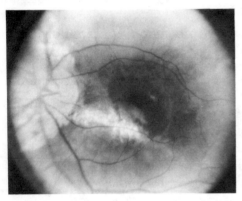

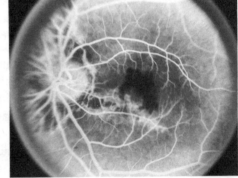

Fig. 6.23 Myopic degeneration with a lacquer crack and subretinal hemorrhage (a, above left). Fluorescein angiography shows the leak (arrow) in sequential photographs (b, above right, and c, right). Fig. 6.23a also shown in color section.

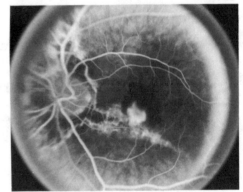

o   The disc may be pale, especially on temporal side (see Chapter 3: VIIIA).

o   Macular hole and retinal detachment are conditions associated with degenerative myopia, but are not associated with Foerster-Fuchs spot (see Chapter 5: IIA).

Symptoms & signs

o Decreased central vision may be sudden and associated with distortions, loss of color vision, micropsia, discoloration of vision — vision may be described as green — and after-image effect on exposure to light.

o Visual acuity may decrease to 6/60 (20/200) or less.

o Central scotoma is present.

o Color vision may be diminished in affected eye.

o Dark adaptation may be defective.

Other confirming findings

o Degenerative myopia accounts for 14 percent of blind patients under age 65.

o Most patients have more than 6 diopters of myopia.

o Inheritance is autosomal dominant with incomplete penetrance.

o History of prematurity or febrile illness in childhood can be elicited in some patients.

o Axial length of globe often greater than 26.76 mm on ultrasonography.

o Fluorescein angiography helps identify abnormal vessels.

o Electro-oculogram and electroretinogram are of minimal value.

Main differential diagnosis

o Senile macular degeneration

o Histoplasmosis syndrome

o Hereditary macular degeneration

o Choroideremia and gyrate atrophy

o Toxoplasmosis

o Angioid streaks

o Serpiginous uveitis

References

Gass JDM: Stereoscopic Atlas of Macular Diseases. St. Louis: Mosby, 1977, p 86.

Krill AE: Krill's Hereditary Retinal and Choroidal Diseases, vol 2. Hagerstown, Md: Harper & Row, 1977, p 911.

D. ACQUIRED MACULAR DISEASE

1. Drug-induced disease

There are a number of drugs known to cause maculopathy, and some result in loss of central vision. There may be others as yet undiscovered.

a) CHLOROQUINE (ARALEN) AND HYDROXYCHLOROQUINE (PLAQUE-NIL) (Fig. 6.24)

Ophthalmoscopic findings

o   Bull's-eye oval of pigment atrophy and clumping surround the foveola.

o   Findings are nearly always bilateral.

o   There may be extensive peripheral pigment atrophy in later stages.

o   Retina may be thinned, but vessels appear normal.

Symptoms & signs

o   Earliest symptoms may be blind spot near or in center of vision that gradually enlarges and reduces vision. Blindness may result from continued drug use.

o   Earliest sign may be a scotoma to recognition of a red test object in the central field.

o   Color vision becomes defective.

Other confirming findings

o   Most patients with maculopathy have received 100-300 grams total dose of 250 mg per day of chloroquine or 200 mg per day of hydroxychloroquine.

o   Drug has been used principally for treatment of lupus erythematosus and rheumatoid arthritis in this country, but also as an antimalarial elsewhere.

o   Pathology is due to toxicity from drug deposited in the retinal pigment epithelium and damage to ganglion cells rather than to idiosyncrasy. Disease may progress long after drug has been discontinued. Medications to increase excretion do not prevent further loss of vision.

Main differential diagnosis

o   Geographic (areolar) macular degeneration

o   Other senile macular degeneration

o   Histoplasmosis syndrome

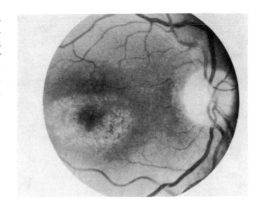

Fig. 6.24 Chloroquine bull's-eye maculopathy in a 51-year-old woman with disseminated lupus erythematosus. Visual acuity was 6/120 (20/400). From Wetterholm DH, Winter FC: Histopathology of chloroquine retinal toxicity. **Arch Ophthalmol 71**:82, 1964. Copyright © 1964, American Medical Association. Used with permission.

o   Stargardt's and other hereditary macular dystrophies

o   Ethambutol (Myambutol), chlorpromazine, indomethacin (Indocin)

o   Toxoplasmosis

o   Ring maculopathies of unknown cause

o   Cone-rod dystrophy of the macula

References

Brinkley JR, Dubois EL, Ryan SJ: Long-term course of chloroquine retinopathy after cessation of medication. Am J Ophthalmol 88:1, 1979.

Gass JDM: Stereoscopic Atlas of Macular Diseases. St. Louis: Mosby, 1977, p 204.

Ramsey MS, Fine BS: Chloroquine toxicity in the human eye: Histopathologic observation by electron microscopy. Am J Ophthalmol 73:229, 1972.

Weise EE, Yannuzzi LA: Ring maculopathies mimicking chloroquine retinopathy. Am J Ophthalmol 78:204, 1974.

b) THIORIDAZINE (MELLARIL), CHLORPROMAZINE, NP 207 (Fig. 6.25; see also in color section)

Ophthalmoscopic findings

o   Pigmentary mottling and subsequent clumping usually starts at the macula, but often involves the periphery with atrophy and pigment patches.

o   Pigment clumps are closer together at the macula than in the periphery; they may be evenly spaced in round or oval patches.

o   Pigment does not accumulate along blood vessels.

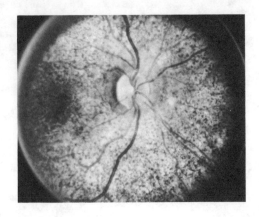

Fig. 6.25 Thioridazine damage to the retinal pigment epithelium in a young psychiatric patient. Courtesy of Paul Torrisi, M.D., Syracuse, New York. Also shown in color section.

Symptoms & signs

o   Decreased vision is associated with maculopathy and may be profound.

o   Central scotoma may be plotted.

Other confirming findings

o   Patients with a history of mental disorder receiving more than 1 gram of thioridazine or 2.5 grams of chlorpromazine over a year or more.

o   NP 207 was an experimental phenothiazine that is no longer used, principally because of the loss of vision it caused.

Main differential diagnosis

o   Geographic (areolar) macular degeneration

o   Senile macular degeneration

o   Histoplasmosis syndrome

o   Stargardt's and other hereditary macular dystrophies

o   Ethambutol (Myambutol), chlorpromazine, indomethacin (Indocin)

o   Toxoplasmosis

o   Ring maculopathies of unknown cause

o   Cone-rod dystrophy

o   Rubella retinitis

o   Luetic retinitis

References

Davidorf DF: Thioridazine pigmentary retinopathy. Arch Ophthalmol 90:251, 1973.

c) OTHER DRUGS

A number of drugs have been associated with retinal pigment epithelial abnormality. The strength of the evidence associating the drug with eye disease is variable. Some that are believed to be associated are listed here.

(1) Indomethacin (Indocin)
There are conflicting reports about pigmentary deposition in the macula associated with the use of this anti-inflammatory drug.

(2) Ethylhydrocupreine (Optoquine, Numoquin)
Although blindness from overdoses of this drug has been known for 100 years, the exact mechanism is still not understood. It binds to the retinal pigment epithelium just like chloroquine. Visual loss occurs within a few hours of ingestion. Retinal vascular narrowing and optic atrophy are followed by pigmentary deposition.

(3) Cephaloridine (Loridine)
Pigmentary retinopathy and loss of vision in a single case has raised the possibility of retinal toxicity.

(4) Sparsomycin
Pigmentary retinopathy has been reported to be associated with a central scotomata within two weeks of receiving this anticancer drug intravenously.

(5) Aminophenoxy alkanes
This group of drugs used as schistosomicidal medication may result in pigmentary retinopathy in about two months.

(6) Ethambutol (Myambutol)
A very subtle pigmentary disturbance, loss of vision, and inability to perceive red and green colors has been noted in patients on this antituberculosis drug.

(7) Iodates
These drugs are no longer used in the therapy of septicemia, because of their specific toxicity for the retinal pigment epithelium. They are now used only in research. Retinal edema, visual loss, and coarse pigmentary retinopathy may occur within a few days. Accidental ingestion may occur.

(8) Methoxyflurane (Penthrane)
Methoxyflurane undergoes degradation to oxalate in the liver. This anesthetic agent has resulted in myriads of oxalate crystals in the retinal pigment epithelium of one patient (see Fig. 6.40). Primary hyperoxaluria may cause similar findings.

(9) Tamoxifen (Nolvadex)
This drug is a chemotherapeutic agent used for treatment of breast carcinoma. Macular edema, refractile particles in the retinal pigment epithelium,

and whorl-like corneal opacities have been associated with decreased vision in patients receiving 60-100 mg/M^2 for over a year (see Fig. 5.51).

(10) Allopurinol

A drug used for the treatment of gout, allopurinol has been noted to cause depigmentation of the retinal pigment epithelium at the macula and occasionally subretinal hemorrhage resembling macular degeneration.

Ophthalmoscopic findings

o   The findings have been described briefly above with each drug; no consistent characteristic appearance for each drug has been seen.

Symptoms & signs

o   Visual loss,loss of color vision, and central scotoma are the major findings.

Other confirming findings

o   History of chemotherapy or accidental exposure to a specific drug can usually be elicited.

o   Fluorescein angiography defines retinal, choroidal, and optic disc vascular insufficiency.

o   Electroretinogram, electro-oculogram, and visually evoked potentials confirm the nature of functional loss.

o   Tissue or blood levels for the offending agent can be monitored in some of the drugs.

References

Ballingall DLK, Turpie AGG: Cephaloridine toxicity. Lancet 2:835, 1967.

Bullock JD, Albert DM: Flecked retina: Appearance secondary to oxalate crystals from methoxyflurane anesthesia. Arch Ophthalmol 93:26, 1975.

Carr RE, Siegel IM: Retinal function in patients treated with indomethacin. Am J Ophthalmol 75: 302, 1973.

Gilman AG, Goodman LS, Gilman A, eds: The Pharmacological Basis of Therapeutics. New York: MacMillan, 1980.

Grant WM: Toxicology of the Eye. Springfield, Ill: Thomas, 1962.

Hoddard HM: Nutritional therapy of metabolic eye disease. Metab Pediatr Ophthalmol 3:127, 1979.

Kaiser-Kupfer MI, Lippman ME: Tamoxifen retinopathy. Cancer Treat Rep 62:315, 1978.

Martino A, Lamberti O: Effects of a new synthetic antitubercular drug (ethambutol) on the visual apparatus. Arch Ottal 69:187, 1965. Asbtracted in Am J Ophthalmol 67:616, 1969.

McFarlane JR, Yanoff M, Scheie HG: Toxic retinopathy following sparsomycin therapy. Arch Ophthalmol 76:532, 1966.

2. Metals

Iron or copper foreign bodies in the eye undergo degradation, resulting in damage to the retinal pigment epithelium as well as the neurosensory retina.

a) SIDEROSIS (Fig. 6.26; see also Fig. 3.66)

Ophthalmoscopic findings

o   Fine pigmentation at fovea associated with loss of the normal foveal light reflection; more generalized pigment disturbance may resemble retinitis pigmentosa.

o   Generalized vascular narrowing and optic atrophy may be present in cases of longstanding intraocular iron foreign bodies.

o   The vitreous often has a yellow-brown color.

o   Foreign body may be visible.

Symptoms & signs

o   Decreased central vision and general constriction of field are variable.

o   The patient may complain of poor vision in bright light (hemeralopia).

o   There may be discoloration of iris — usually a golden brown — compared to other eye.

o   Pupil responses may be decreased, absent, or show escape (Marcus Gunn's pupil sign).

o   Chronic glaucoma may follow prolonged foreign-body retention, occasionally associated with pain.

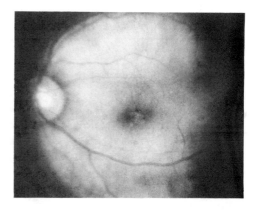

Fig. 6.26 Black pigmentation at the fovea and elsewhere from a longstanding intraocular iron foreign body.

Other confirming findings

o Usually, there's a history or physical evidence of a perforating injury.

o Roentgenogram, computerized axial tomography, and ultrasonic studies can demonstrate the foreign body; however, degradation of small foreign bodies may make them invisible on roentgenogram after one to two years.

o Analysis of aqueous or vitreous aspirate for iron.

o Electroretinogram shows specific changes in iron foreign bodies.

Main differential diagnosis

o Hemosiderosis

o Vogt-Koyanagi-Harada disease and other forms of uveitis

o Unilateral retinitis pigmentosa

o Choroideremia

o Gyrate atrophy

o Lipofuscinosis

o Thioridazine (Mellaril) toxicity

References

Cibis PA, Brown EB, Hong SM: Ocular effects of systemic siderosis. Am J Ophthalmol 44:158, 1957.

Cibis PA, Yamashita T, Rodriguez F: Clinical aspects of ocular siderosis and hemosiderosis. Arch Ophthalmol 62:46/180, 1959.

Zinn KM, Marmor MF, eds: The Retinal Pigment Epithelium. Cambridge, Mass: Harvard University Press, 1979, p 405.

b) CHALCOSIS (see Fig. 5.38)
Intercellular golden-yellow copper deposition may be reversible and consistent with good vision. It is uncertain if the copper is in the outer retinal layers or the retinal pigment epithelium.

3. Myopic degeneration (see IIIC, 3, above)

4. Histoplasmosis syndrome (Fig. 6.27)

This disease of unknown etiology was labeled the histoplasmosis syndrome, because it is endemic to areas where the fungus Histoplasma capsulatum is found in the soil. It's been reproduced in monkeys with some authenticity. The organism has rarely been found in the eye, however, even in patients

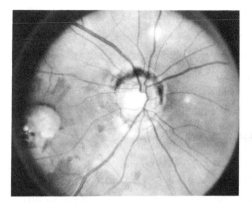

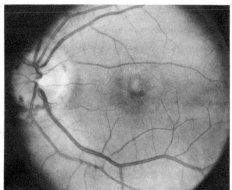

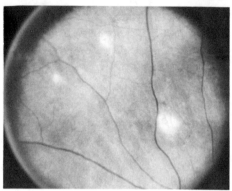

Fig. 6.27 Circumpapillary, peripheral, and macular scarring in a 53-year-old female with bilateral histoplasmosis syndrome (a, above left). Subretinal hemorrhage present in the macula. Gray-green circles with red center are characteristic of subretinal neovascularization (b, above right). Scattered punched-out peripheral chorioretinal lesions are a part of the typical histoplasmosis syndrome (c, right).

dying of systemic histoplasmosis. Even though, when it is found in the eye, the original lesions are in the choroid, it does not cause symptoms unless the retinal pigment epithelium is breached, particularly at the macula.

Ophthalmoscopic findings

Asymptomatic stage

o Pigment atrophy and hyperpigmentation around the disc in a band ¼ to ½ disc diameters wide, sometimes with pseudopodia extending further peripherally.

o Multiple yellow-white, punched-out defects in the retinal pigment epithelium and choroid, often with black pigment "signet-ring" border. Choroidal vessels may be exposed to view in lesions or may be completely absent, revealing the sclera. Lesions may be scattered from fovea to ora serrata. Clusters may be seen. The size varies from tiny, almost imperceptible defects to ½-disc-diameter scars. The lesions are unrelated to retinal or choroidal vessels. New lesions may appear, and old lesions may increase in size or pigmentation.

o The neurosensory retina appears uninvolved.

Symptomatic stage

o   The retinal pigment epithelium may be yellow and indistinct in localized area in or near the fovea. Lesions are usually ¼ to ½ disc diameter in size.

o   Highlights from edema of the neurosensory retina surround lesion.

o   Black pigment of old lesions nearby can be confused with the gray-green circular or oval doughnut of subretinal neovascularization.

o   There may be red subretinal blood at margins of retinal pigment epithelium detachment and gray-green neovascularization.

o   With proximal illumination, the retinal pigment epithelium around the lesion, compared to normal surrounding tissue, has a mottled golden glow.

o   Subretinal neovascularization may be seen in some patients as a cartwheel of fine red streaks on the retinal pigment epithelium.

o   Neurosensory retina over lesion may be multicystic. This is seen best with retroillumination (see Chapter 1).

o   The overlying vitreous remains clear, unlike with toxoplasmosis.

Advanced stage

o   Large subretinal hemorrhages with elevated, thinned neurosensory retina, and yellow exudates at the base. This finding may be replaced by the following.

o   Yellow-white elevated subretinal scar, heavy pigmentation,and, sometimes, anastomosis of retinal and choroidal vessels, resembling disciform macular degeneration.

Symptoms & signs

---

o   Sudden blurred or distorted vision may be central or paracentral.

o   Patients may describe objects as looking smaller than normal or say they have an after-image effect on exposure to light. Colors may be dull when viewed with affected eye.

o   Visual acuity varies with proximity to and destructiveness of a lesion near the fovea and may be as poor as counting fingers. In serous detachment of retinal pigment epithelium, vision may be improved by a 0.5 diopter plus lens over the patient's glasses.

o   Pupil reactions usually normal, unless the macula is destroyed.

o   A scotoma is present on field testing.

o   Exposure to the ophthalmoscope light reduces patient's visual acuity longer in the affected eye (photo-stress test).

o Twenty-five percent of patients with scars near the macula lose central vision in the second eye.

o It's rare for both eyes to have an acute lesion at same time, or for two active lesions to occur at same time in same eye.

Other confirming findings

o Histoplasmosis syndrome consists of bilateral circumpapillary and peripheral choroidal scars, associated with calcific scars of the lungs, spleen, and liver. Ninety percent of affected patients have a positive skin test to 1:1,000 histoplasmin.

o Patients are usually 20 to 45 years of age when symptoms occur and are otherwise in good health.

o Black and Oriental patients rarely have the syndrome.

o There is no strong evidence that the disease is hereditary.

o Fluorescein angiography helps define the ocular pathology.

Main differential diagnosis

o Myopic degeneration

o Senile macular degeneration

o Focal choroiditis

o Serpiginous choroiditis

o Toxoplasmosis

o Choroidal rupture with subretinal neovascularization

References

Davidorf FH, Anderson JD: Ocular lesions in the earth day histoplasmosis epidemic. Trans Am Acad Ophthalmol Otolaryngol 78:876, 1974.

Ganley JP: Epidemiologic characteristics of presumed ocular histoplasmosis. Acta Ophthalmol [Suppl] 119:1, 1973.

Gass JDM: Stereoscopic Atlas of Macular Diseases. St. Louis: Mosby, 1977, p 92.

Krill AE, Archer D: Choroidal neovascularization in multifocal (presumed histoplasmin) choroiditis. Arch Ophthalmol 84:595, 1970.

Meredith TA, Green WR, Key SN, et al: Ocular histoplasmosis: Clinicopathologic correlation of three cases. Surv Ophthalmol 22:189, 1977.

Smith RE, Ganley JP: Presumed ocular histoplasmosis: 1. Histoplasmin skin test sensitivity in cases identified during a community survey. Arch Ophthalmol 87:245, 1972.

5. Central serous choroidopathy (see Chapter 5: IIB, 2)

6. Angioid streaks (Fig. 6.28; see 6.28a also in color section)

These irregular dull red lines, sometimes radiating from the disc, taper and disappear in the periphery. They appear to be in the retinal pigment epithelium and histologically are associated with disruption of the elastic lamina of Bruch's membrane. Sometimes subtle, often damaging vision, they have been seen most with pseudoxanthoma elasticum (Grönblad-Strandberg syndrome), but may also occur in sickle cell disease, acromegaly, Paget's disease of bone, thrombocytopenic purpura, fibrodysplasia hyperelastica (Ehler-Danlos syndrome), occasionally with drusen of the disc and rarely with other conditions.

Ophthalmoscopic findings

o   Often radiating from disc, sometimes branching, these broad irregular dark red streaks may resemble choroidal vessels, but taper and disappear usually within 3 to 5 disc diameters of their origin.

o   May originate away from the disc, pass through the macula, or be concentric with disc.

o   Gray-green subretinal pigment epithelial neovascularization along streak may have red subretinal blood just ahead of it.

o   Atrophy of the retinal pigment epithelium and hyperpigmentation in longstanding disease follows the streaks initially, but may coalesce to form disciform macular scar. Retinal pigment epithelium disease is more widespread than just at the streaks.

o   Neurosensory retina is often cystic or mildly elevated over large streaks or subretinal hemorrhage.

Symptoms & signs

o   Blurred or distorted vision, either central or paracentral, is most frequent complaint.

o   Patient may describe decreased intensity of light in one eye, and colors may seem dull.

o   Visual acuity varies with proximity of disease to the fovea, but often is defective even without a streak in the fovea.

o   Pupil reaction normal initially, but becomes poorly responsive to light in late stages of the disease.

o   Scotomata are found on field testing.

o   Photo-stress test is positive.

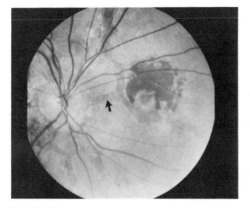

Fig. 6.28a

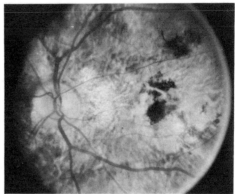

Fig. 6.28b

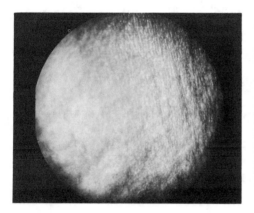

Fig. 6.28c

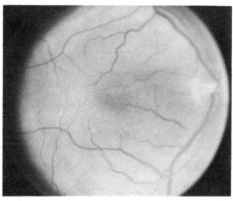

Fig. 6.28d

Fig. 6.28 Angioid streak (arrow) with sub-retinal hemorrhage in a 45-year-old male with pseudoxanthoma elasticum (a). Visual acuity of 6/30 (20/100) decreased to counting fingers in the next five years (b). The other eye was similar. Pseudoxanthoma elasticum of the skin (c). The neck and flexor surfaces are the most commonly affected. Subtle angioid streaks beneath the superior temporal vessels in a 45-year-old acromegalic (d). The first symptom of her pituitary tumor was blurred vision. Fluorescein angiography enhances the appearance (e). Fig. 6.28a also shown in color section.

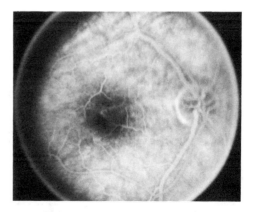

Fig. 6.28e

Other confirming findings

o   May occur in children, but most patients are between 30 and 60 years of age at diagnosis. History for the specific illnesses noted above under the heading Angioid streaks should be sought.

o   Most patients with pseudoxanthoma elasticum are unaware of their skin disease. Peau d'orange is most visible on the neck, axillae, and flexor surfaces of the elbows. Hyperextension of the joints may be known to the patient.

o   Increased hat size and other growth phenomenon later in life in patients with Paget's disease or acromegaly usually have to be elicited. Twenty percent of acromegalics have a family history of the disease.

o   Hypertension, sickle cell disease, and purpura are usually known to the patient.

o   Appropriate roentgenogram, laboratory, and skin biopsy evidence usually confirm the associated disease.

o   Fluorescein angiography is helpful in confirming the presence of questionable angioid streaks and the presence of subretinal neovascularization.

Main differential diagnosis

o   Myopic degeneration with lacquer cracks

o   Serpiginous uveitis

o   Histoplasmosis syndrome

o   Hypertension with Siegrist's pearls

o   Traumatic choroidal rupture

References

Gass JDM: Stereoscopic Atlas of Macular Diseases. St. Louis: Mosby, 1977, p 78.

Marmar MF: Inflammations and degenerations of the retinal pigment epithelium. In The Retinal Pigment Epithelium (Zinn KM, Marmor MF, eds). Cambridge, Mass: Harvard University Press, 1979, p 468.

7. Infection of the retinal pigment epithelium

a) RUBELLA RETINOPATHY (see IVB, 2, below)

b) ACUTE POSTERIOR MULTIFOCAL PLACOID PIGMENT EPITHELIO-PATHY (Fig. 6.29)
This acute disease of young, healthy patients is thought to be an infection, because it often follows a flu-like illness. No organism has been found.

Ophthalmoscopic findings

o   Multiple flat, gray, irregular ¼ to 1 disc diameter patches are seen in the retinal pigment epithelium.

o   Patches may coalesce, presenting an indistinct border and surface.

o   Neuosensory retina does not become elevated.

o   Macula and posterior retinal pigment epithelium around the disc are affected.

o   There may be sheathing of vessels, and sometimes they are slightly dilated and tortuous.

o   There may be cells in vitreous.

o   Papilledema occasionally accompanies disease.

o   Patches begin to fade from center within a few days.

o   Irregularly pigmented and depigmented retinal pigment epithelium is left at site of patches, and clumping and remodeling of pigment may go on for months after acute phase.

Symptoms & signs

o   Acute, rapid loss of vision one or both eyes may be to 6/60 (20/200) or less if fovea is involved.

o   Visual loss may be accompanied by symptoms of iritis, episcleritis, and papilledema.

o   Pupil response varies with degree of macular involvement, and there may be a Marcus Gunn's sign.

o   Scotoma on field testing may be permanent.

Fig. 6.29 Acute multifocal placoid epithelio-pathy in a 68-year-old man following an acute viral illness. Multiple subtle yellow patches in the retinal pigment epithelium are present nasal to the disc. Courtesy of Paul Torrisi, M.D., Syracuse, New York.

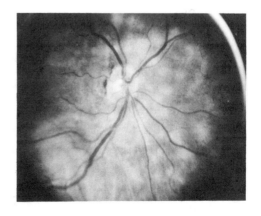

o Visual recovery is slow after exposure to light (photo-stress).

o Visual acuity usually improves to normal or near normal within six months.

Other confirming findings

o Average age of patients is 25.

o Affects both males and females.

o Diseases occasionally associated include erythema nodosum, regional enteritis, and hepatitis.

o Cerebral spinal fluid has pleocytosis, and increased protein may be present.

o Fluorescein angiography demonstrates the characteristic retinal pigment epithelial and choriocapillaris abnormalities.

o Electroretinogram and electro-oculogram define the electrical potential deficit.

Main differential diagnosis

o Serpiginous choroiditis

o Other acute choroiditis

o Histoplasmosis syndrome

o Regional choroidal atrophy

o Toxoplasmosis

o Cytomegalic inclusion virus disease

o Herpes simplex retinitis

References

Gass JDM: Stereoscopic Atlas of Macular Diseases. St. Louis: Mosby, 1977, p 212.

Yannuzzi LA, Gitter KA, Schatz H: The Macula: A Comprehensive Text and Atlas. Baltimore: Williams & Wilkins, 1979, p 247.

c) OPHTHALMOMYIASIS (see VIA, below)

d) DIFFUSE UNILATERAL NEURORETINITIS AND VITRITIS (WIPE-OUT SYNDROME) (see Chapter 5: VO)

E. SURGICAL EFFECTS

1. Pigment deposition (fall out) (Fig. 6.30)

Successfully treated retinal detachment patients may have deposition of pigment in the fovea. This occurs only when the macular retina was detached preoperatively. Cryotherapy may rupture cell walls and release pigment into the subretinal fluid. Visual acuity is not thought to be affected.

Ophthalmoscopic findings

o Black, scattered pigment particles resemble dispersed pepper.

o Usually at macula, but can be seen in other areas, including the disc or the margins of the detached retina. (This needs to be distinguished from demarcation lines indicating longstanding retinal detachment, since poor visual acuity is common when these pass through the fovea. See Fig. 6.46.)

Symptoms & signs

o Usually none related specifically to pigment. Recovering from retinal detachment of the macula, patients may describe improved field of vision, but a persistent shadow in the affected field after exposure to bright light; floaters — presumably the same ones as seen preoperatively now seen better with the retina reattached; and flickering or shimmering lights centrally located, compared to peripheral flashes seen preoperatively. They are unassociated with movement and may contain colors.

o A relative central scotoma is present.

Fig. 6.30 Pigment deposited at the fovea in a patient with successfully treated retinal detachment (a, left). Visual acuity was 6/6 (20/20). Similar deposition on the disc in another patient (b, right).

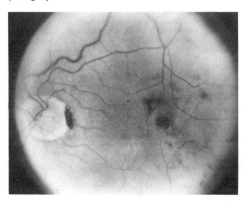 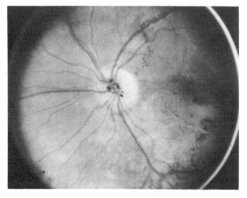

Other confirming findings

o History of retinal detachment surgery is easily elicited.

o Electroretinogram and electro-oculogram confirm retinal recovery.

o Fluorescein angiography aids definition of retinal pigment epithelium.

Main differential diagnosis

o Choroidal nevus

o Macular degeneration

o Myopic degeneration (Foerster-Fuchs spot)

o Demarcation lines due to retinal detachment, choroidal detachment, or retinoschisis

References

Hilton GF: Subretinal pigment migration: Effects of cryosurgical retinal detachment. Arch Ophthalmol 91:445, 1974.

Lincoff H, Kreissig I: Cryogenic and thermal effects on the retinal pigment epithelium. In The Retinal Pigment Epithelium (Zinn KM, Marmor MF, eds). Cambridge, Mass: Harvard University Press, 1979, p 314.

2. Photocoagulation (Fig. 6.31)

Light energy as a source of thermal cautery may be inadvertently or purposefully directed at the macula. The resulting scars are permanent and may be confused with scars from inflammatory or degenerative disease.

Ophthalmoscopic findings

o Localized circular lesion or lesions.

o Depending on photocoagulation used, spot size may vary from 1/30 to 1⅓ disc diameter in size.

o Fresh burns appear cloudy, with slightly indistinct margins. A very powerful burn may disperse pigment, cause a small gas bubble in adjacent tissue, and cause hemorrhage.

o Depending on energy used, spot may vary from just barely visible whitening of the retinal pigment epithelium to destruction of all layers, exposing the sclera. Therapeutic burns vary from faint to heavy whitening, according to purpose.

Fig. 6.31 Intentional laser burns near fovea (a, left) and an accidental burn in a laser research engineer (b, right). See also Fig. 4.78.

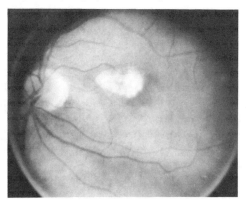 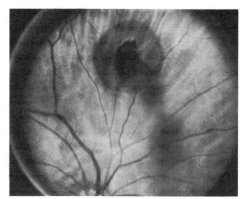

- o Late burns may remain white — from the exposed sclera — or have varying degrees of pigmentation.
- o Retinochoroidal vascular anastomosis may traverse a scar, or subretinal neovascularization may be present.

Symptoms & signs

- o Photocoagulation of the fovea results in immediate loss of visual acuity and distortion of images. Visual loss is usually permanent, unless part of the fovea has been spared.
- o Extensive treatment, as in diabetic retinopathy, may reduce patient's field of vision and dark adaptation.

Other confirming findings

- o History of photocoagulation treatment or accidental laser or xenon light is usually known, except in infants (see F1, below).
- o The discrete, uniform size and grouping of lesions usually confirm the man-made scars.

Main differential diagnosis

- o Histoplasmosis syndrome
- o Myopic degeneration
- o Retrolental fibroplasia
- o Paving stone degeneration

o   Regional choroidal atrophy

o   Radiation trauma

References

L'Esperance FA Jr: Ocular Photocoagulation: A Stereoscopic Atlas. St. Louis: Mosby, 1975.

3. Cryocoagulation (see Fig 4.34)

Thermal cautery by cold application is widely used in ocular surgery.

Ophthalmoscopic findings

o   Most scars are from the mid-periphery to the ora serrata, since the freezing is applied to the scleral surface and the back of the eye is difficult to reach.

o   Size of scars is larger than photocoagulation, usually 2 to 3 disc diameters. They often coalesce.

o   Immediate evidence of treatment is only a faint whitening of the neurosensory retina and the retinal pigment epithelium.

o   Late effects are retinal pigment epithelial atrophy, pigment dispersion, and exposure of the choroidal vessels or sclera. Pigment clumping is common.

o   The borders are sharp.

Symptoms & signs

o   There are no late symptoms, unless the macula or optic nerve has been damaged by treatment or the disease process. In that instance, visual acuity may be counting fingers or less.

o   Symptoms and signs are of the disease for which treatment was used.

Other confirming findings

o   History of treatment is known, except in infants.

o   Discrete, uniform size and grouping of lesions is confirmatory.

Main differential diagnosis

o   Histoplasmosis syndrome

o   Myopic degeneration

o   Retrolental fibroplasia

o   Paving stone degeneration

o   Regional choroidal atrophy

References

Lincoff H, Kreissig I: Cryogenic and thermal effects on the retinal pigment epithelium. In The Retinal Pigment Epithelium (Zinn KM, Marmor MF, eds). Cambridge, Mass: Harvard University Press, 1979, p 314.

F. RADIATION TRAUMA

Accidental irradiation may occur from the sun, other bright light sources, ultrasonic devices, or electricity. Photochemical and thermal changes in tissue proteins result.

1. Solar, welder's arc, accidental laser burn retinopathy (see Figs. 5.30, 6.31)

This rare injury results from both thermal and photochemical damage to the retinal pigment epithelium and overlying retina.

Ophthalmoscopic findings

---

o   Yellow-white spot at or near the foveola has a faint gray halo in acute phase. Severe burns may cause hemorrhage.

o   Central reddish partial thickness hole or cyst in the neurosensory retina appears within 15 days. It's permanent, if exposure is severe.

o   Hyperpigmentation may occur at the impact site.

Symptoms & signs

---

o   Patients usually note loss of vision and a central scotoma immediately after exposure.

o   They may describe a constant effect resembling the after-image of a flashbulb. Symptoms include yellow-red discoloration of vision, distortions, and sometimes headache.

o   Visual acuity reduction is variable, but usually 6/18 (20/60) or better.

o   Central scotoma is difficult to plot because of its small size. The Amsler grid works best.

o   Color vision is usually not affected.

Other confirming findings

o Macular burns are dependent on the wavelengths involved, distance from the source, intensity of the light, pupil size at the time of exposure, the duration of the flash, light transmission of the ocular media, pigment at the macula, the heat-dissipating effect of ocular blood flow, and other factors. The burns are due to visible and infrared light.

o Sungazing — during an eclipse, especially through a telescope, or at the normal sun under the influence of intoxicants or during a psychiatric disorder — is the usual cause of solar burn.

o Electric arcs, either in welding or by accidental exposure, are rare causes of maculopathy, since they infrequently exceed 156,000 erg-secs/CM^2 at 40 cm distance (noon sunlight at sea level is about 1,000,000 erg-secs/CM^2).

o Lightning, aside from its electrical effects, and atomic blast may cause maculopathy.

o Ruby, argon-helium, yag-yttrium, and neodymium lasers produce wavelengths of light that can photocoagulate the retina. Carbon dioxide lasers do not, although they may cause perforation of the cornea.

o Prolonged exposure to the light of the indirect ophthalmoscope or operating microscope and to intraocular fiberoptic light has been shown to cause microscopic retinal damage.

o Fluorescein angiography helps define the extent of pathology.

Main differential diagnosis

o Focal choroiditis

o Histoplasmosis syndrome

o Toxoplasmosis

o Hereditary maculopathies

o Electric shock maculopathy

o Photocoagulation treatment

References

Duke-Elder S: System of Ophthalmology, vol 14. St. Louis: Mosby, 1972, p 893.

Ewald RA, Ritchey CL: Sun Gazing as the cause of foveomacular retinitis. Am J Ophthalmol 70:491, 1970.

Friedman E, Kuwabara T: The retinal pigment epithelium: 4. The damaging effects of radiant energy. Arch Ophthalmol 80:265, 1968.

Gass JDM: Stereoscopic Atlas of Macular Diseases. St. Louis: Mosby, 1977, p 322.

Naidoff MA, Sliney DH: Retinal injury from a welding arc. Am J Ophthalmol 77:663, 1974.

2. Electric shock

Patients surviving severe electric shock may have macular injury.

Ophthalmoscopic findings

o   There is gray-white edema of the neurosensory retina in the macula immediately after injury.

o   Splinter hemorrhages may be seen.

o   Within 10 days, edema subsides and mottled pigmentation and depigmentation of the foveal retinal pigment epithelium is evident.

o   Optic disc may become pale at same time.

o   Ophthalmoscopy may be hindered by an electric cataract.

Symptoms & signs

o   Patient has immediate loss of vision following injury that varies from a slight reduction to no light perception.

o   One or both eyes may be involved, depending on the electrical current traverse.

o   Initial good vision may diminish as cataracts progress (see Chapter 2: VIA). Macular and optic nerve damage appears to be instantaneous.

Other confirming findings

o   The history and other findings of electric shock are confirmatory.

Main differential diagnosis

o   Focal choroiditis

o   Hereditary maculopathies

o   Toxoplasmosis

References

Freeman HM, ed: Ocular Trauma. New York: Appleton-Century-Crofts, 1979, p 313.

IV. SCATTERED BLACK PARTICLES

Multiple black, flake-like deposits in the retinal pigment epithelium first described in 1828 were thought to be due to inflammation, and the term retinitis pigmentosa was chosen by Donders. The majority of patients don't have an inflammatory disease but a family inheritance. There are patients, however, with black deposit disease who have undergone deprivation of vitamin A, infection, trauma, radiation, or drug toxicity.

A. RETINITIS PIGMENTOSA (ROD-CONE DYSTROPHY, PRIMARY HEREDITARY PIGMENTARY RETINOPATHY, LEBER'S CONGENITAL AMAUROSIS, RETINITIS PIGMENTOSA SINE PIGMENTO, RETINITIS PUNCTATA ALBESCENS) (Fig. 6.32; see 6.32b also in color section)

Classic rod-cone dystrophy is hereditary nightblindness with onset before age 30, showing scattered peripheral retinal pigment epithelium disturbance. It's been associated and confused with many conditions that are detailed below. Credit should be given to Krill and Deutman (see references to their works below) for organizing our thinking about the tapetoretinal degenerations.

Ophthalmoscopic findings

o   Bilateral spidery or bone corpuscular black pigment, usually within 5 disc diameters of the disc, is often along veins. With age, pigment approaches the disc and macula and also the ora serrata. Large clumps may occur.

o   Atrophy of the retinal pigment epithelium around black particles exposes the choroid to view, although it may be seen through a glistening, sometimes crystalline, depigmented retinal pigment epithelium.

o   Disc is pale with sharp margins.

o   Both arteries and veins are narrow at the disc and become more narrowed peripherally. They may be of normal caliber in young patients.

o   White defects may predominate (retinitis punctata albescens), but eventually pigment deposits occur.

Fig. 6.32 Retinitis pigmentosa with pallor of disc, circumpapillary chorioretinal atrophy, and attenuated retinal vessels (a), associated with typical spider pigmentation in the periphery (b). Note pigment clumping along the veins. Advanced pigment changes in a 93-year-old male with nightblindness for life, but no family history of the disease (c). Visual acuity was 6/15 (20/50). Retinitis punctata albescens with myriads of yellow dots in the peripheral pigment epithelium (d). Fig. 6.32b also shown in color section.

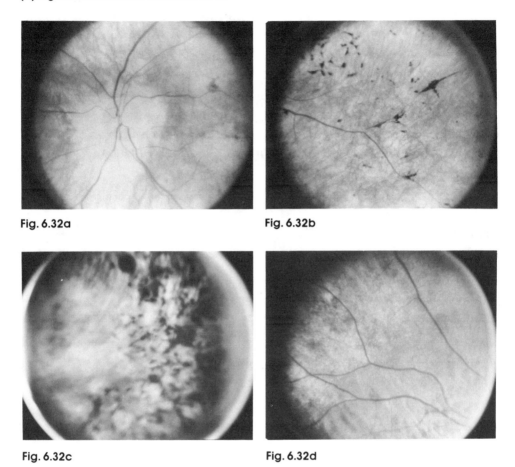

Fig. 6.32a   Fig. 6.32b

Fig. 6.32c   Fig. 6.32d

o In early disease, vessel, disc, and pigment findings may be present without typical spider pigmentations (retinitis pigmentosa sine pigmento).

o The ophthalmoscopic findings have in some patients been seen in only one eye. These patients never developed functional visual loss in the other eye.

o Partial ocular (usually inferior) bilateral pigment clumping and atrophy associated with some functional deficit has led to the conclusion that sector retinitis pigmentosa occurs.

- Rarely, ophthalmoscopic findings are confined to the macular area (pericentral retinitis pigmentosa), but most of these patients prove to have cone-rod dystrophy.
- Cystoid macular edema may occur early in the disease.
- Myopia, drusen of disc, cataracts, and hamartomas of the retinal pigment epithelium at the disc or nearby retina may be associated.
- Microphthalmos, keratoconus, and external third nerve palsy have been described in retinitis pigmentosa patients.

Symptoms & signs

- Daylight visual acuity is normal early in the disease, but eventual blindness is common in the majority of patients, except those with late autosomal recessive form.
- Reading vision decreases suddenly in those who develop cystoid macular edema.
- Inability to adapt to dim light.
- Color vision for blue is defective in advanced disease.
- Annular scotoma on field testing early in disease is usually between 30 and 50 degrees from fixation.

Symptoms & signs by inheritance form

Early autosomal recessive (Leber's amaurosis congenita)
- Blindness, often in first year of life.
- Ophthalmoscopic appearance usually normal.
- Very limited field.
- Severe nightblindness.

Early autosomal recessive (most common form)
- Visual loss and nightblindness in first few years of life.
- Rapid progression.
- Ocular complications — macular degeneration and cataracts.

Late autosomal recessive (after age 30)
- Mild visual impairment.
- Good central vision.
- Slow progression.

Autosomal dominant

o   Mild initially.

o   Slow progression.

o   Eventual severe functional loss.

Sex-linked

o   Female carriers show peripheral retinal pigment epithelial atrophy.

o   Usually slow progression.

Other confirming findings

o   There are three main modes of inheritance: autosomal recessive —
    about 41 percent of retinitis pigmentosa patients; autosomal dominant —
    about 39 percent of retinitis pigmentosa patients; and sex-linked —
    17 percent of retinitis pigmentosa patients.

o   Dark adaptation, inverted profile — sensitivity to dim light appears
    greatest at the macula instead of 15 to 20° from fixation as is the case in
    normal patients.

o   Electroretinogram — depressed or absent response in the dark-adapted
    eye in most patients. This usually precedes ophthalmoscopic findings.

o   Electro-oculogram is abnormal in most patients.

o   Table 6.3 lists diseases sometimes accompanied by atypical pigmentary
    retinal dystrophy, often described as retinitis pigmentosa.

Main differential diagnosis

o   Congenital rubella and acquired rubeola retinopathy

o   Phenothiazine, chloroquine (Aralen), indomethacin (Indocin) toxicity

o   Syphilis

o   Radiation retinopathy

o   Smallpox

o   Cytomegalic inclusion virus retinopathy

o   Herpes simplex retinopathy

o   Trauma

o   Pigmentation following retinal reattachment

o   Pigmentation following spontaneous collapse of retinoschisis

Table 6.3

DISEASES SOMETIMES ASSOCIATED WITH
RETINITIS PIGMENTOSA-LIKE FINDINGS

Bone disease
   Marfan's syndrome
   Osteogenesis imperfecta
   Osteoporosis
   Paget's disease of bone
Dresbach's elliptocytosis
Familial myoclonic epilepsy
Generalized muscular dystrophy
Hallervorden-Spatz syndrome
Hearing loss
   Alstrom's syndrome — obesity, diabetes mellitus, deafness,
     and pigmentary retinopathy
   Cockayne's syndrome — labyrinthine deafness, progeria, oligophrenia,
     childhood dwarfism
   Hallgren's syndrome — congenital deafness, vestibulocerebellar ataxia,
     mental disturbance
   Usher's syndrome — congenital labyrinthine deafness and pigmentary
     retinopathy
Hooft's hypolipidemia syndrome
Idiopathic intracerebral vascular calcification
Klinefelter's syndrome
Laurence-Moon-Biedl syndrome
Lipid storage disease
   Batten-Mayou disease
   Ceroid lipoid fuscinosis
   Vogt-Spielmeyer disease
Marinesco-Sjörgren syndrome
Mucopolysaccharidosis
Mytonic dystrophy
Pelizaeus-Merzbacher disease
Pipecolic acidemia
Porphyria cutanea tarda
Progressive external ophthalmoplegia
   Bassen-Kornzweig syndrome of spinocerebellar degeneration,
     acanthocytosis, abetalipoproteinemia, and celiac disease
     may affect vitamin A absorption

Table 6.3

DISEASES SOMETIMES ASSOCIATED WITH
RETINITIS PIGMENTOSA-LIKE FINDINGS

Progressive external ophthalmoplegia (continued)
  Kearns-Sayre syndrome — in addition to ophthalmoplegia, these patients have
    pigmentary retinopathy and heart block. The syndrome also includes
    short stature, kyphoscoliosis, pes cavus, hirsutism, sexual immaturity, weakness
    of bulbar and limb girdle muscles, ataxia, sensory losses,
    reflex abnormalities, deafness, increased spinal fluid protein, and
    electroencephalogram abnormalities. Onset before age 20. Early death
    from Stokes-Adams episodes are common. Diagnosis can be confirmed
    when, by muscle biopsy, tissues show characteristic "ragged-red"
    fibers on trichrome stain.
  Refsum's syndrome — cerebellar ataxia, nystagmus, pes cavus, inner ear
    deafness, increased cerebral spinal fluid protein, ichthyosis,
    epiphysial dysplasia, abnormal cardiac conduction, and high levels
    of phytanic acid; condition in some patients is reversible by diet with
    preservation of vision
Progressive hypertrophic neuritis (Dejerine-Sottas disease)
Progressive muscular atrophy
Renal disease
  Cystinosis (Fanconi's syndrome)
  Cystinuria
  Familial juvenile nephrophthisis (Fanconi's nephrophthisis)
  Oxalosis
  Renoretinal dysplasia
Rud's syndrome
Sjörgren-Larsson syndrome
Skin disease
  Psoriasis
  Werner's syndrome
Spinopontocerebellar degeneration
Other conditions
  Coats's disease
  Exudative vasculopathy
  Foveal cysts or areolar atrophy
  Fuchs's heterochromic cyclitis
  Myopia (75% of patients, in contrast to 12% in normal population)
  Vitreous degeneration

Adapted from Krill AE: Krill's Hereditary Retinal and Choroidal Diseases, vol 2. Hagerstown, Md:
Harper & Row, 1977. Used with permission.

References

Deutman AF: The Hereditary Dystrophies of the Posterior Pole of the Eye. Assen, The Netherlands: Van Gorcum, 1971.

Fishman GA: Retinitis pigmentosa: Genetic percentages. Arch Ophthalmol 96:822, 1978.

Gass JDM: Stereoscopic Atlas of Macular Diseases. St. Louis: Mosby, 1977.

Hansen E, Bachen NI, Flage T: Refsum's disease: Eye manifestations in a patient treated with low phytol and low phytanic acid diet. Acta Ophthalmol 57:899, 1979.

Krill AE: Krill's Hereditary Retinal and Choroidal Diseases, vol 2. Hagerstown, Md: Harper & Row, 1977.

Leveille AS, Newell FW: Autosomal dominant Kearns-Sayre syndrome. Ophthalmology 87:99, 1980.

Merin S, Auerbach E: Retinitis pigmentosa. Surv Ophthalmol 20:303, 1976.

B. INFECTIONS OF THE RETINAL PIGMENT EPITHELIUM (PSEUDORETINITIS PIGMENTOSA)

1. Syphilis (lues) (Fig. 6.33; see 6.33a also in color section)

The primary ocular syphilitic lesion is usually in the choroid. It's discussed here, because secondary involvement of the retinal pigment epithelium provides an ophthalmoscopic appearance that resembles retinitis pigmentosa and some viral retinopathies.

Ophthalmoscopic findings

o   Diffuse atrophy of retinal pigment epithelium and "salt and pepper" appearance.

o   Pigment clumps often larger and less spider-like than in retinitis pigmentosa.

o   Pigment clumps are diffuse and more likely to be along arterioles than in retinitis pigmentosa.

o   In young patients, vessel attenuation and optic atrophy may be less marked in syphilis than in retinitis pigmentosa.

o   Circumpapillary scarring and disturbance of the retinal pigment epithelium.

o   Far peripheral pigment changes are more advanced in syphilis.

o   Patches of chorioretinal atrophy are common.

Symptoms & signs

o Visual acuity may be good, if early treatment limited optic atrophy and macular involvement.

o Nightblindness occurs in extensive peripheral disease.

o Constricted fields or sector defects are usual.

o Argyll Robertson pupil is often present.

o Residuum of interstitial keratitis may be seen.

Other confirming findings

o Historical or physical findings known to be associated with syphilis, such as chancre, aortitis, optic neuritis, central nervous system disease.

o Laboratory and radiological evidence of disease, such as VDRL and fluorescent treponemal antibody absorption, are not conclusive evidence that the pigmentary retinopathy is luetic.

o Electroretinogram and electro-oculogram help define the functional loss and separate the disease from retinitis pigmentosa.

Main differential diagnosis

o Retinitis pigmentosa

o Rubella retinopathy

o Other viral retinopathies

Fig. 6.33 Congenital syphilitic retinitis resembling retinitis pigmentosa (a, left). Note optic atrophy, vessel attenuation, and retinal pigment epithelial atrophy except at the macula (b, right). Fig. 6.33a also shown in color section.

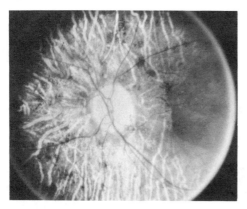 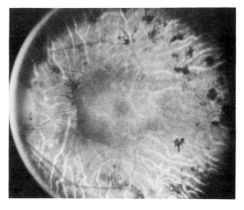

o   Thioridazine (Mellaril), phenothiazine, and chloroquine (Aralen) retinopathy

o   Paravenous atrophy

o   Diffuse choroiditis

o   Histoplasmosis syndrome

References

Elder-Duke S, Dobree S: System of Ophthalmology, vol 10. St. Louis: Mosby, 1967, p 252.

Marmor MF: Inflammations and degenerations of the retinal pigment epithelium. The Retinal Pigment Epithelium (Zinn KM, Marmor MF, eds). Cambridge, Mass: Harvard University Press, 1979, p 460.

2. Rubella (Fig. 6.34)

Congenital rubella syndrome results in a diffuse pigmentary retinopathy in a large percentage of afflicted infants—50 percent according to some authors.

Ophthalmoscopic findings

o   Fine, diffuse pigment stippling is present at birth or develops in first years of life.

o   Pigment changes may involve or come close to the fovea, but are usually more in mid-periphery.

o   No specific accumulation of pigment occurs along veins.

o   Pigment does not take spider or bone-corpuscular shape.

Fig. 6.34 Rubella retinopathy in a 46-year-old female (a, left). Visual acuity was 6/12 (20/40). The macula may also be involved apparently without severe visual loss (b, right). Fig. 6.34b courtesy of William Havener, M.D., Ohio State University.

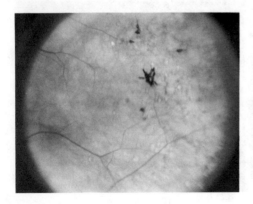
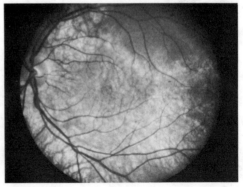

o Optic disc is normal.

o Blood vessels are normal caliber.

o The disease is nearly always bilateral and frequently is an accidental finding on routine ophthalmoscopy.

o Rarely, subretinal neovascularization and hemorrhage have been reported.

Symptoms & signs

o Visual acuity is usually normal or near normal.

o Pupil reactions are normal.

o There is no field loss.

o Cataracts and glaucoma result in severe visual deficit. Cardiac abnormalities and deafness are present in the full syndrome.

Other confirming findings

o Cataract and glaucoma associated with gestational rubella characteristically occur with disease contracted in the first trimester. Retinopathy has been found after exposure at different periods — usually second or third trimester — throughout pregnancy.

o Serologic testing and tissue culture from lens material identify the virus.

o Electroretinogram, electro-oculogram help define retinal function.

o Fluorescein angiography confirms blood-flow patterns.

Main differential diagnosis

o Retinitis pigmentosa

o Other viral retinopathies

o Thioridazine (Mellaril), phenothiazine, and chloroquine (Aralen) retinopathy

o Syphilis

o Radiation retinopathy

References

Gass JDM: Stereoscopic Atlas of Macular Diseases. St. Louis: Mosby, 1977, p 210.

Krill AE: The retinal disease of rubella. Arch Ophthalmol 77:445, 1967.

Marmor MF: Inflammations and degenerations of the retinal pigment epithelium. The Retinal Pigment Epithelium (Zinn KM, Marmor MF, eds). Cambridge, Mass: Harvard University Press, 1979, p 460.

3. Measles (rubeola) and subacute sclerosing panencephalitis
(Fig. 6.35)

Retinopathy is a rare but distinct complication of measles.

Ophthalmoscopic findings

o Retinal artery occlusions with edema, hemorrhage, and exudate occur in acute phase.

o Pale disc, attenuated vessels, and diffuse pigmentary changes, including bone spicules, are seen within a few weeks.

o In subacute sclerosing panencephalitis, focal area of retinal edema may leave larger pigment scars as they subside.

Symptoms & signs

o Visual acuity starts to deteriorate in the second week of measles infection. May progress to severe loss of visual acuity in both eyes long after acute phase is over.

o In subacute sclerosing panencephalitis, the post-measles period is followed by an insidious onset of mental deterioration along with edema of the retina. The disease progresses to seizures, cortical blindness, and death in one to two years.

o Congenital pigmentary retinopathy due to measles has been reported.

Fig. 6.35 Acute retinitis in a 12-year-old boy with subacute sclerosing panencephalitis (a, left). Visual acuity was limited to hand movement. The other eye was similar. During the month after the photograph, he became lethargic, mute, and blind. Irregular pigmentary disturbance of the macula and mild papilledema in an eight-year-old boy who became lethargic, incontinent, and comatose (b, right). He died three weeks after the photograph. Fig. 6.35a from Landers MB, Klintworth GK: Subacute sclerosing panencephalitis (SSPE): A clinicopathologic study of the retinal lesions. **Arch Ophthalmol** 86:156, 1971. Copyright © 1971, American Medical Association. Used with permission. Fig. 6.35b from Font RL, Jenis EH, Tuck KD: Measles maculopathy associated with subacute sclerosing panencephalitis. **Arch Pathol** 96:168, 1973. Copyright © 1973, American Medical Association. Used with permission.

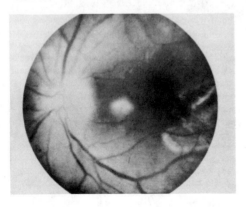 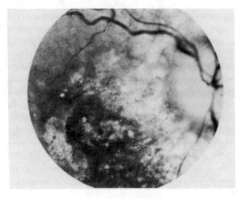

Other confirming findings

o   History and physical evidence of measles.

o   Measles antibody titer elevated and increasing in cerebral spinal fluid.

o   Viral inclusions in nuclei of cells of central nervous system and retina.

Main differential diagnosis

o   Cytomegalic inclusion virus or herpes simplex retinitis

o   Bacteremia

o   Coccidioidomycosis

o   Other viral retinopathies

o   Rocky Mountain spotted fever

References

Gass JDM: Stereoscopic Atlas of Macular Diseases. St. Louis: Mosby, 1977, p 302.

Marmor MF: Inflammations and degenerations of the retinal pigment epithelium. The Retinal Pigment Epithelium (Zinn KM, Marmor MF, eds). Cambridge, Mass: Harvard University Press, 1979, p 461.

4. Other infections

Pseudoretinitis pigmentosa syndromes have been reported in mumps, influenza, varicella, poliomyelitis, herpes zoster, herpes simplex, infectious hepatitis, diphtheria, typhoid fever, cytomegalic inclusion disease, Behcet's disease, Vogt-Koyanagi-Harada disease, and periarteritis nodosa. Some infections (such as myiasis) cause streaks and lines.

References

Duke-Elder S, Dobree JH: System of Ophthalmology, vol 10. St. Louis: Mosby, 1967, pp 264, 530.

Gass JDM: Stereoscopic Atlas of Macular Diseases. St. Louis: Mosby, 1977, p 302.

Marmor MF: Inflammations and degenerations of the retinal pigment epithelium. The Retinal Pigment Epithelium (Zinn KM, Marmor MF, eds). Cambridge, Mass: Harvard University Press, 1979, p 462.

Yannuzzi LA, Gitter KA, Schatz H: The Macula: A Comprehensive Text and Atlas. Baltimore: Williams & Wilkins, 1979, p 247.

C. RADIATION RETINOPATHY (see IIIF, above)

D. DRUG TOXICITY (see IIID, 1, above)

E. FOLLOWING SUCCESSFUL RETINAL REATTACHMENT, CHOROIDAL EFFUSION, OR COLLAPSE OF RETINOSCHISIS (Fig. 6.36)

The function of the retinal pigment epithelium is undoubtedly altered by these three conditions. Evidence may be apparent only later, when restoration of the anatomy is achieved.

Ophthalmoscopic findings

o Irregular black pigment clumping is localized to area of previous retinal detachment, choroidal effusion, or retinoschisis.

o Pigment is best seen in proximal illumination.

o Loss of pigment between clumps exposes choroidal vessels to view and contrasts with retinal pigment epithelium at unaffected areas.

o Choroidal elevation and scarring from diathermy or cryocoagulation may be found at site of treatment for retinal breaks.

Symptoms & signs

o Visual acuity varies, depending on whether macula was involved in the original disease.

o Field loss corresponds to affected area in retinoschisis and may persist for some time after successful retinal detachment repair. Usually, field is relatively normal with uveal effusion.

o Pupil response when light is directed at affected field may be less than when light is directed at unaffected area.

Other confirming findings

o History of retinal or choroidal disease and treatment.

o Physical evidence of surgical treatment for retinal detachment, retinoschisis, or choroidal effusion.

o Retinal degeneration, retinal breaks, or retinoschisis may be found in the other eye.

o Electroretinogram and electro-oculogram are abnormal.

o Fluorescein angiography aids definition of retinal vascular disease.

Main differential diagnosis

o Coloboma of the choroid

o Regional choroidal atrophy

Fig. 6.36 Scattered fine black flecks after retinal reattachment. The pigmentation was confined to the area where the retina had been detached.

Fig. 6.37 Photocoagulation for diabetic retinopathy leaves pigmented scars about two weeks later.

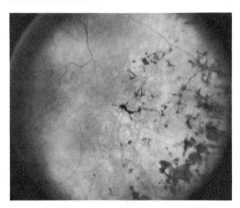
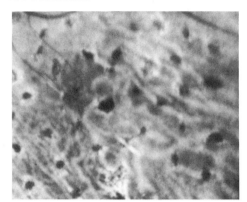

- o Retinitis pigmentosa
- o Histoplasmosis syndrome
- o Photocoagulation treatment or cryotherapy
- o Retrolental fibroplasia
- o Subretinal hemorrhage
- o Radiation retinopathy
- o Rubella retinopathy
- o Metastatic tumor of choroid
- o Syphilis
- o Thioridazine (mellaril) toxicity

References

Hollenberg MJ, Ghosh M: Epithelial changes after retinal detachment: The fine structure of retinal pigment epithelium following retinal detachment. Ann Ophthalmol 2:264, 1970.

F. FOLLOWING PHOTOCOAGULATION (Fig. 6.37)

Photocoagulation has been described in IIIE, 2, above. Multiple peripheral photocoagulation scars are commonly seen now in patients suffering diabetic retinopathy or intravitreal bleeding from various vascular abnormalities. The evenly spaced scars may be very faint.

V. SCATTERED WHITE FLECKS

Some diseases give such an unusual appearance through the ophthalmoscope that they are rarely forgotten. The abnormalities described here constitute such a group. It's often difficult to determine the tissue location of the tiny scattered white flecks. Some diseases in this group have already been described, but are noted here again to aid in differential diagnosis.

A. FUNDUS ALBIPUNCTATUS (STATIONARY OR NONPROGRESSIVE, RETINITIS PUNCTATA ALBESCENS, ALBIPUNCTATE DYSTROPHY)
(Fig. 6.38; see also in color section)

Fundus albipunctatus is a term for nonprogressive disease. Progressive retinitis punctata albescens is thought to be a form of retinitis pigmentosa with delayed pigmentation.

Ophthalmoscopic findings

o   Fine, yellow-white dots seen at retinal pigment epithelial level.

o   Often evenly spaced, but sometimes coalescent.

o   Macula is usually spared.

o   Greatest concentration in mid-periphery, sometimes a radial arrangement.

o   Two eyes are similar.

o   No pigment is associated with the dots.

o   Disc and blood vessels normal.

o   Deposits do not change in size or number in most patients.

Symptoms & signs

o   Congenital nightblindness is the only symptom. Since the disease is nonprogressive, many patients are unaware of it.

o   Visual acuity may be normal.

o   Fields are full.

o   Dark adaptation is variable.

Other confirming findings

o   The disease has an autosomal recessive inheritance often with consanguinity in the history.

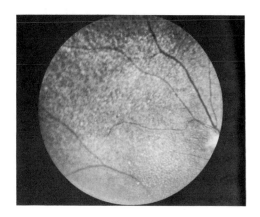

Fig. 6.38 Fundus albipunctatus, a non-progressive hereditary form of nightblindness in a nine-and-one-half-year-old female. Also shown in color section.

o Crystalline corneal dystrophy, cataracts, spherophakia and lenticonus are sometimes associated with it.

o Alport's syndrome (deafness, cataracts, and hereditary nephropathy) is associated in some patients. Retinitis pigmentosa and fundus albipunctatus have been present in same pedigree occasionally.

o Fluorescein angiography aids localization of the dots.

o Electroretinographic and electro-oculographic studies confirm rod malfunction.

Main differential diagnosis

o Familial drusen

o Fundus flavimaculatus

o Progressive retinitis punctata albescens

o Vitamin A deficiency with nightblindness

o Talc embolization in drug abuse

o Oxalosis

o Tamoxifen (Nolvadex) therapy

References

Krill AE: Krill's Hereditary Retinal and Choroidal Diseases, vol 2. Hagerstown, Md: Harper & Row, 1977, p 739.

B. FUNDUS FLAVIMACULATUS (see IIIC, 1a, above)

C. FAMILIAL DRUSEN (see IIIC, 2a, above)

D. FLECK RETINA OF KANDORI

Ophthalmologists consider this rare disease a distinct entity.

Ophthalmoscopic findings

o Yellow, irregular deposits occur in the retinal pigment epithelium.

o Located between macula and equator.

o Size of deposits varies from diameter of small retinal vessel to 1.5 disc diameter.

o Defects are surrounded by brown discoloration of retinal pigment epithelium.

Symptoms & signs

o Nightblindness is present from birth.

o Normal vision and fields are found.

o Dark adaptation is mildly affected.

Other confirming findings

o Rare disease.

o Autosomal recessive with consanguinity.

o Electroretinogram is abnormal.

o Fluorescein angiography helps localize the retinal pigment epithelial disease.

Main differential diagnosis

o Familial drusen

o Fundus flavimaculatus

o Histoplasmosis syndrome

o Gyrate atrophy of choroid

o Fundus albipunctatus

References

Krill AE: Krill's Hereditary Retinal and Choroidal Diseases, vol 2. Hagerstown, Md: Harper & Row, 1977, p 817.

Fig. 6.39 Yellowish deposits in the macula with fine crystalline deposits in a 31-month-old black boy with mental and motor retardation, ichthyosis, generalized weakness, and spasticity. Note the narrowing of the arterioles. From Gilbert WR Jr, Smith JL, Nyhan WL: The Sjögren-Larrson syndrome. **Arch Ophthalmol** 80:308, 1968. Copyright © 1968, American Medical Association. Used with permission.

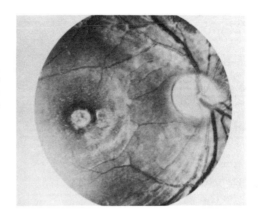

E. SJÖGREN-LARSSON SYNDROME (Fig. 6.39)

This rare pigment epithelial disease has been defined by careful study.

Ophthalmoscopic findings

o Glistening white-yellow flecks are seen especially at the macula.

o There may be pigmentary irregularity.

o Arterioles may be slightly narrowed.

o Ophthalmoscopic findings occur in 25 percent of patients with disease.

Symptoms & signs

o Visual acuity is defective.

Other confirming findings

o Autosomal recessive inheritance.

o Congenital low-grade stationary mental deficiency.

o Congenital ichthyosis.

o Symmetrical spastic paresis, especially of legs.

o Convulsions.

o Defective sweating.

o Hypertelorism.

o Dental and osseous dysplasia.

o Limited life expectancy.

Main differential diagnosis

o Cystinosis

o Oxalosis

o Familial drusen

o Retinitis punctata albescens

o Gyrate atrophy of choroid

References

Gass JDM: Stereoscopic Atlas of Macular Diseases. St. Louis: Mosby, 1977, p 200.

F. OXALOSIS AND OTHER CRYSTALLINE DEPOSITS (Fig. 6.40)

Primary hyperoxaluria and oxaluria due to ethylene glycol (antifreeze) ingestion or methoxyflurane (Penthrane) anesthesia hypersensitivity have resulted in fine crystalline deposits histologically confirmed within the retinal pigment epithelium.

Ophthalmoscopic findings

o Multiple glistening fine white flecks.

o Macula involved, as well as periphery.

o Blood vessels normal.

Symptoms & signs

o Visual acuity is usually normal, but may be affected if gyrate atrophy is present.

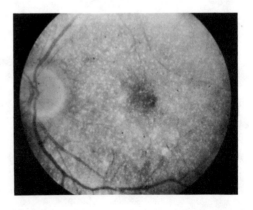

Fig. 6.40 Retinal oxalosis in a 63-year-old man who developed renal failure following methoxyflurane anesthesia. From Bullock JD, Albert DM: Flecked retina: Appearance secondary to oxalate crystals from methoxyflurane anesthesia. Arch Ophthalmol 93:26, 1975. Copyright © 1975, American Medical Association. Used with permission.

Other confirming findings

o Primary hyperoxaluria is a rare disease associated with ethylene glycol poisoning or recent anesthesia associated with renal failure, and family history of gyrate atrophy of the choroid or atypical pigmentary retinal dystrophy.

o Fluorescein angiography confirms retinal pigment epithelial disease.

o Electroretinogram and electro-oculogram are confirmatory.

Main differential diagnosis

o Talc emboli in drug abuse

o Tamoxifen (Nolvadex) therapy

o Retinitis punctata albescens

o Familial drusen

o Photocoagulation scars

References

Bullock JD, Albert DM: Flecked retina: Appearance secondary to oxalate crystals from methoxyflurane anesthesia. Arch Ophthalmol 93:26, 1975.

Gottlieb RP, Ritter JA: Flecked retina: An association with primary hyperoxaluria. J Pediatr 90:939, 1977.

Zinn KM, Marmor MF: Toxicology of the human retinal pigment epithelium. The Retinal Pigment Epithelium (Zinn KM, Marmor MF, eds). Cambridge, Mass: Harvard University Press, 1979, p 406.

G. VITAMIN A DEFICIENCY (Fig. 6.41)

This nutritional defect may be due to deprivation, poor gastrointestinal absorption, or liver malfunction.

Ophthalmoscopic findings

o Tiny, dull white deposits in mid-periphery.

o Macula is not usually affected.

o Blood vessels are normal.

Symptoms & signs

o Reversible nightblindness, poor dark adaptation is present.

o Visual acuity is good.

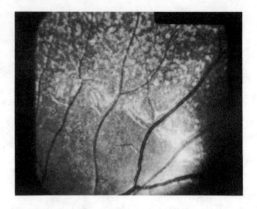

Fig. 6.41 Vitamin A deficiency in a 25-year-old female with photophobia and corneal xerosis. The retinal lesions cleared with one and one-half months of vitamin A replacement. From Sommer A, Tjakrasudjatma S, Djunaedi E, et al: Vitamin A-responsive pan-ocular xerophthalmia in a healthy adult. **Arch Ophthalmol** 96:1630, 1978. Copyright © 1978, American Medical Association. Used with permission.

o   Dryness of eyes and skin (xerosis).

o   Bitot's spots can be seen on the conjunctiva.

Other confirming findings

o   History of deficiency of diet, poor gastrointestinal absorption, or liver malfunction.

o   Serum vitamin A level is below normal.

o   Electroretinogram abnormalities are present.

Main differential diagnosis

o   Other forms of nightblindness

o   Fundus albipunctatus

o   Tamoxifen (Nolvadex) ingestion

o   Talc emboli

o   Familial drusen

References

Fuchs A: White spots of the fundus combined with nightblindness and xerosis (Uyemura's syndrome). Am J Ophthalmol 48:101, 1959.

VI. WRINKLES AND STREAKS

Linear retinal pigment epithelial abnormalities are often confusing when seen with the ophthalmoscope, since only a small part is seen at one time. You have to make a mental mosaic of the actual appearance. Note that the photographic field of the illustrations is several times larger than the ophthalmoscope's view. There are many causes for the lines. Some of the more common are illustrated and discussed.

A. MYIASIS (OPHTHALMOMYIASIS) (Fig. 6.42)

Larval parasites in the eye may arrive there through the blood stream or by burrowing through the ocular coats after hatching on the conjunctiva.

Ophthalmoscopic findings

o   Criss-crossing white or partially pigmented lines may involve a part or nearly the whole interior of the eye.

o   Usually the disease is unilateral.

o   Focal areas of hyperpigmentation may follow localized hemorrhage.

o   Larvae may be seen in motion, and the motion may increase under the ophthalmoscope's light.

o   Larvae are white or semitransparent, may have visible stoma, scolex, and alimentary canal. They vary from ½ to 1½ disc diameters in length and may be identified within the eye if characteristic findings can be seen. They may be seen in the anterior chamber, on or in the disc and subretinal space, or in the vitreous. Reports of the disappearance of motile larvae and the absence of inflammatory reaction suggests they may leave the eye.

o   Severe inflammatory cellular reaction may be present in the vitreous, retina, and choroid.

Symptoms & signs

o   Visual acuity may be nearly normal, even with considerable "tracking" through the macula — a common area of track confluence. Profound visual loss may follow subretinal hemorrhage or the inflammatory response to death of the larvae.

o   Some patients have described intense itching and a crawling sensation in the affected eye.

o   Some patients may describe a floating spot, which is due to the larva in the vitreous.

o   Most patients have no complaints or describe only decreased vision.

Other confirming findings

o   History reveals that the patient lives in an area where there are botflies (order Diptera) that use sheep, cattle, deer, or horses for their larval host. Ticks, mosquitos, the patient's hands, or the adult fly may carry the eggs

Fig. 6.42 Tracks criss-crossing the retinal pigment epithelium (a, left) due to migration of an intraocular larva (b, right). Fig. 6.42a from Gass JDM, Lewis RA: Subretinal tracks in ophthalmomyiasis. **Arch Ophthalmol** 94:1500, 1976. Copyright © 1976, American Medical Association. Used with permission. Fig. 6.42b from Fitzgerald CR, Rubin ML: Intraocular parasite destroyed by photocoagulation. **Arch Ophthalmol** 91:162, 1974. Copyright © 1974, American Medical Association. Used with permission.

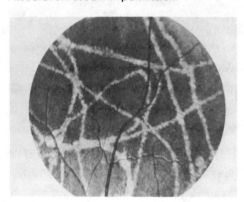 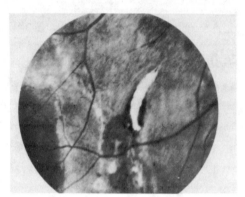

to the conjunctiva. Toxocara canis and trematodes may migrate in the subretinal space but do not produce lines.

o   When surgical removal of the organism is required because of inflammation, laboratory identification is often possible.

o   Fluorescein angiography presents a characteristic picture.

o   Photocoagulation may be used as a diagnostic and therapeutic tool. It stops migration of the larvae by killing them.

o   Clinic appearance of multiple tracks is pathognomonic. Indirect ophthalmoscopy gives a better overall view.

Main differential diagnosis

o   Demarcation lines of retinal detachment, retinoschisis, or choroidal detachment

o   Serpiginous uveitis

o   Chorioretinal folds

References

Gass JDM: Stereoscopic Atlas of Macular Diseases. St. Louis: Mosby, 1977, p 222.

Santos R, Dalma A, Ortiz E, et al: Management of subretinal and vitreous cysticercosis: Role of photocoagulation and surgery. Ophthalmology 86:1501, 1979.

Slusher, MM, Holland WD, Weaver RG, et al: Ophthalmomyiasis interna posterior. Arch Ophthalmol 97:885, 1979.

B. CHORIORETINAL AND CHOROIDAL FOLDS
(Figs. 6.43, 6.44; see 6.43a also in color section)

The choroid, Bruch's membrane, and retinal pigment epithelium are involved in histologic studies of eyes with folds. Ophthalmoscopically, the appearance is wrinkling of the retinal pigment epithelium. Tissue displacement by choroidal, scleral, or orbital swelling or tumor and low pressure (hypotonia) may also cause folding.

Ophthalmoscopic findings

o Alternate dark and yellow streaks are seen.

o These streaks may be nearly parallel lines, circular (like ripples in a pond), or irregular.

o Larger folds are readily seen, short ones may be difficult to see.

o Folds may be present anywhere that scleral edema, choroidal congestion, or orbital mass occurs. Spontaneous choroidal folds in acquired hyperopia are usually in or near the macula.

o Folds associated with acquired hyperopia are fine, whereas retrobulbar masses cause large folds.

o Retinal blood vessels are uninvolved, unless hypotony is present, and then the veins appear large, tortuous, and overfilled.

o Subretinal neovascularization with or without subretinal hemorrhage occurs rarely.

Symptoms & signs

o Blurred vision — usually unilateral — is the most common complaint.

o Worsening of distance or reading vision occurs in farsighted patients.

o Sudden improvement in distance vision or deterioration of reading vision in a previously myopic patient may indicate that the back of the eye is being pushed in. Distance visual acuity is improved in nearsighted and farsighted by weaker minus or stronger plus lens (or by a pinhole).

o The visual loss can usually be corrected by lenses.

o Proptosis, conjunctival edema, redness, pain, restriction of ocular movement, and diplopia are indications of an orbital tumor.

Fig. 6.43 Chorioretinal folds in a 64-year-old hyperopic male (a, left). The patient complained of blurred vision, although he could read 6/6 (20/20). The other eye was normal. Fluorescein accentuates the appearance (b, right). Fig. 6.43a also shown in color section.

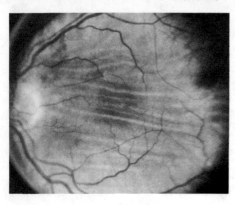

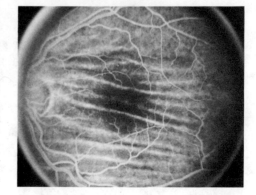

Fig. 6.44 Chorioretinal folds in a 60-year-old female with thyroid exophthalmos.

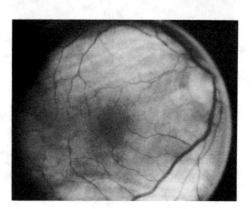

Other confirming findings

o   Most patients with spontaneous idiopathic acquired or congenital folds are healthy, young farsighted adults, and only one eye is affected.

o   Family history of farsightedness and good vision.

o   History of recent ocular surgery—particularly for glaucoma, cataract, retinal detachment, or ocular trauma—or of hyperthyroidism or thyroidectomy.

o   External ocular evidence of inflammation, trauma, orbital or choroidal tumors, proptosis and impaired muscle function.

o   Low intraocular pressure (hypotony) is confirmed by tonometry.

o   Fluorescein angiography confirms vascular insufficiency and choroidal tumors.

o Radiographic studies (including computerized axial tomography) of eye, orbit, and skull aid diagnosis.

o Laboratory evaluation of thyroid function may be indicated.

Main differential diagnosis

o Papilledema

o Choroidal tumor, primary or metastatic

o Orbital tumor

o Thyroid exophthalmos

o Scleral buckling for retinal detachment

o Surface wrinkling retinopathy

o Retinal detachment

o Senile macular degeneration

References

Fastenberg DM, Fetkenhour CL, Choromokos E, et al: Choroidal vascular changes in toxemia of pregnancy. Am J Ophthalmol 89:362, 1980.

Friberg TR, Grove AS: Subretinal neovascularization and choroidal folds. Ann Ophthalmol 12:245, 1980.

Gass JDM: Stereoscopic Atlas of Macular Diseases. St. Louis: Mosby, 1977, p 147.

Kalina RE, Mills RP: Acquired hyperopia with choroidal folds. Ophthalmology 87:44, 1980.

C. DEMARCATION LINES
(Figs. 6.45-6.47; see 6.46a also in color section)

Pigmented, partially pigmented, or depigmented lines mark the border of retinal or choroidal elevations on the retinal pigment epithelium. These lines take four to six months to form and usually persist permanently after the elevation has subsided or been corrected surgically. Retinal detachments account for most demarcation lines. Because the elevations that cause these "high water marks" usually originate peripherally, the lines often present a convex contour in the posterior eye.

Ophthalmoscopic findings

o Disease-caused lines are usually curvilinear, but when two meet they may appear angulated.

o May be multiple, often concentric, forming expanding partial rings.

o Lines may be black, yellow, or mottled.

Fig. 6.45 Demarcation line at the margin of a longstanding retinal detachment.

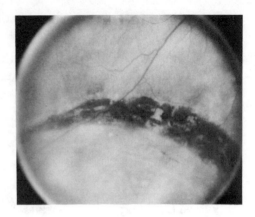

Fig. 6.46 Multiple demarcation lines. After successful retinal reattachment, these lines are more easily seen. Each line probably indicates a four- to six-month period while the retinal detachment did not advance (a, left). They can be subtle (b, right). Fig. 6.46a also shown in color section.

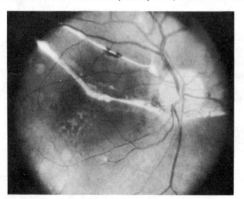
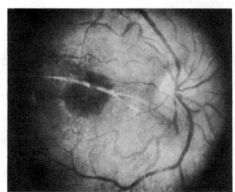

Fig. 6.47 Band of pigment disturbance in an 18-year-old female underlying an encircling silicone band placed on the scleral surface for retinal detachment.

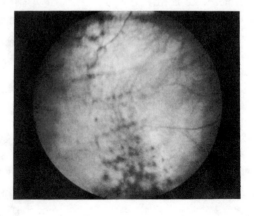

- There may be as many lines as there are borders to the elevation. They may be multilobulated or scalloped.
- Lines of pigment disturbance outline the area of former elevation after it has subsided.
- Pigment lines caused by surgical indentation of the globe correspond to the surgical site.

Symptoms & signs

- Demarcation lines are a finding in the disease process, and the symptoms and signs are those of retinal and choroidal elevations.
- Visual acuity following successful retinal reattachment is often poor, if a demarcation line goes through the fovea.
- Patients with demarcation lines through the fovea may describe a split image or double vision with one eye (monocular diplopia). This usually lasts only a few months.

Other confirming findings

- History of known predisposing causes of retinal detachment, retinoschisis, or choroidal elevation.
- History of lung, breast, or other neoplasms known to metastasize to choroid.
- Retinal detachment or retinoschisis surgery.
- Ocular radiation by external portal or direct application to the sclera.
- Family history of retinal detachment, high myopia, aphakia, trauma, retinoschisis, or other cause of retinal or choroidal elevations.
- Indirect ophthalmoscopy provides a larger binocular field to show the extent of lines.

Main differential diagnosis

- Old chorioretinitis scars, including histoplasmosis syndrome and trauma
- Photocoagulation, diathermy, or cryotherapy scars
- Choroidal rupture
- Angioid streaks
- Lattice degeneration
- Retinal folds associated with chlorthalidone or originating from some unknown cause

References

Norton EWD: Differential diagnosis of retinal detachment. In Symposium on Retina and Retinal Surgery, pp 52-65. Transactions of the New Orleans Academy of Ophthalmology. St. Louis: Mosby, 1969.

Tolentino FI, Schepens CL, Freeman HM: Vitreoretinal Disorders. Philadelphia: Saunders, 1976.

D. ACQUIRED FOLDS OF UNKNOWN CAUSE OR DRUG-RELATED
(Fig. 6.48)

Rare and unusual folds or wrinkles in the retina or retinal pigment epithelium have been reported without known cause or apparently due to drug hypersensitivity.

Fig. 6.48 Fine retinal folds in a 22-year-old female who bilaterally developed acute myopia on chlorthalidone 5 mg qid for two weeks following delivery of an infant (a, left). Visual acuity corrected to 6/7.5 (20/25) OD and 6/6 (20/20) OS. Medication was discontinued, visual acuity returned to 6/4.5 (20/15) OU without correction within 24 hours. The retinal folds disappeared. Intraocular pressure was normal before and after cessation of the medication. Retinal folds of unknown cause in a 20-year-old male with bilateral visual acuity of 6/200 (20/666) in both eyes (b, right). Neurological examination and electroretinogram were normal. Visual evoked responses were subnormal. From Gass, J. Donald M.: Stereoscopic atlas of macular diseases, ed. 2, St. Louis, 1977, The C. V. Mosby Co. Used with permission.

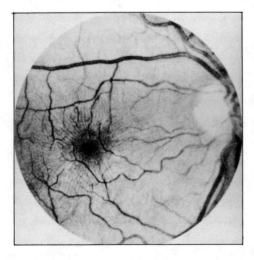 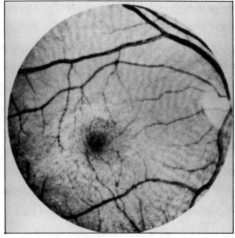

Ophthalmoscopic findings

o   Fine radiating or pond-ripple folds.

o   Blood vessels of retina undisturbed.

o   May be exaggerated retinal highlights.

Symptoms & signs

o   May be profound decrease in visual acuity.

o   Loss of visual acuity may be correctable with lenses, if caused by induced myopia.

o   Visual loss may be reversible by discontinuing drug.

o   Intraocular pressure is normal.

Other confirming findings

o   History of drug use, recent surgery, trauma, or anesthesia in some patients.

o   Laboratory studies of specific drug levels.

o   Electroretinogram, electro-oculogram, visually evoked potentials detail retinal function.

o   Fluorescein angiography defines vascular permeability.

Main differential diagnosis

o   Papilledema

o   Hypotonia

o   Chorioretinal folds associated with hyperopia

o   Choroidal or orbital tumor

References

Gass JDM: Stereoscopic Atlas of Macular Diseases. St. Louis: Mosby, 1977, p 153.

E. PAPILLEDEMA

Concentric rings of tissue displacement may be seen around the disc in papilledema. These rings may involve the retinal pigment epithelium and neurosensory retina. They are frequently seen best as the papilledema is subsiding (see Chapter 3: VII7, C).

Fig. 6.49 Dark line traversed the circumference of eye at the vortex vein ampullae (arrows) in a patient with normal vision and no history of ocular disease.

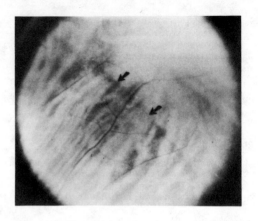

F. VARIATIONS OF NORMAL PIGMENTATION
(Fig. 6.49; see also Figs. 6.2, 7.5b)

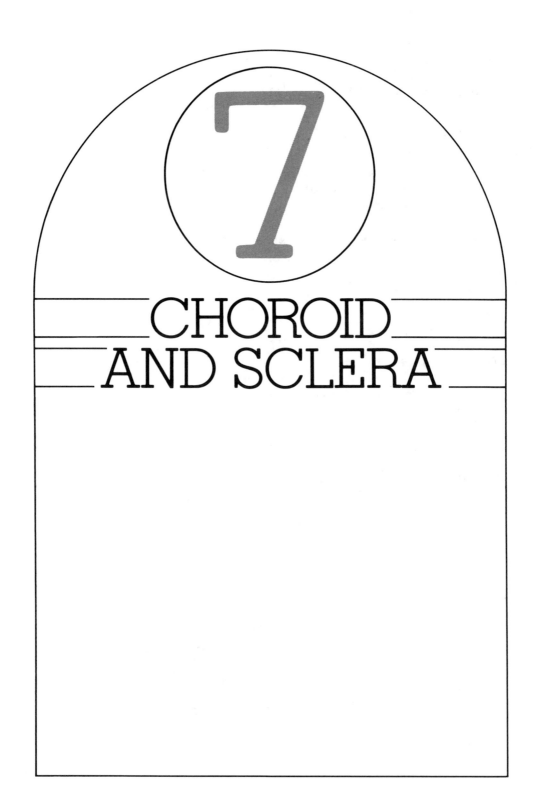

7

CHOROID AND SCLERA

The neurosensory retina and retinal pigment epithelium sometimes distract us from the choroid. But we must always keep it in mind in order to make a proper interpretation of any pathology we may observe.

I. NORMAL ANATOMY

Derived from embryonic mesoderm, the pigment cells of the choroid differ from those of the ectodermal retinal pigment epithelium both histologically and ophthalmoscopically. Choroidal melanin granules are yellow-brown, in contrast with the black melanin of the retinal pigment epithelium, and they are of a finer grain. Pigmentation of the choroid is greatest near the sclera, diminishing in the inner layers so that the choriocapillaris is essentially devoid of pigment cells (see Fig. 1.5).

In detailed studies in rhesus monkeys and in man, Hayreh has found that two or three branches of the ophthalmic artery divide and penetrate the posterior sclera to enter the choroid. Usually, these arteries are medial and lateral to the optic nerve, but in 20 percent of eyes they are superior and inferior. Despite the marked vascularity of the choroid there is little functional anastomosis between areas supplied by specific vessels. Hayreh has described a common pattern to the vascular zones (Fig. 7.1).

Receiving over three-fourths of all blood flow to the eye, the choroid contains very large vessels (see Figs. 1.5, 1.7). Flattened laminae with considerable pigment are interposed between the largest vessels (Haller's layer) and the sclera. Medium-sized vessels (Sattler's layer) in the mid-choroid give way to fine, uniform vessels called the choriocapillaris directly beneath Bruch's membrane and the retinal pigment epithelium. This layer of vessels, critical to nourishment of the outer retina, ends anteriorly with the

Fig. 7.1 Diagrammatic representation of the zones of choroidal arterial perfusion. From Hayreh SS: Segmental nature of the choroidal vasculature. **Br J Ophthalmol** 59:631, 1975. Used with permission.

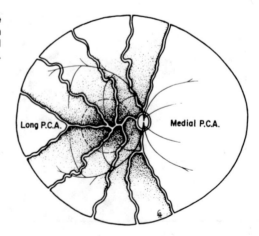

retina at the ora serrata, while the other layers continue forward. Choroidal arterioles supply part of the optic nerve.

In the posterior eye around the disc, the choriocapillaris consists of a polygonal mosaic with a central, nonanastomosing arteriole for each one-quarter disc diameter lobule (Fig. 7.2). Venous drainage from the periphery of each lobule joins that from others to empty into the vortex vein for that quadrant. Vortex veins (Fig. 7.3; see 7.3a also in color section) drain a quadrant from the front to the back of the eye and receive blood from the iris, ciliary body, and choroid. Variation in the number of vortex veins is common. These vessels exit from the eye, after an approximately 1.25 mm intrascleral course, 19-23 mm from the limbus. This puts their visible internal

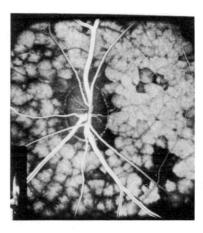

Fig. 7.2 Fluorescein angiogram of the choroid in monkey, showing various units of the choriocapillaris mosaic. Note presence of some nonperfused (black) units. From Hayreh SS: Segmental nature of the choroidal vasculature. **Br J Ophthalmol** 59:631, 1975. Used with permission.

Fig. 7.3 Rendering of a normal fundus, showing details of choroidal pattern (a, left). Fundus with the principal structures labeled (b, right). From Rutnin U: Fundus appearance in normal eyes: 1. The choroid. **Am J Ophthalmol** 64:821, 1967. Fig. 7.3a by William Stenstrom. Fig. 7.3b by David Tilden. Used with permission. Fig. 7.3a also shown in color section.

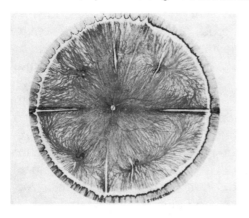
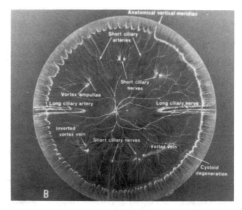

Fig. 7.4 Vortex vein ampulla (arrow) and feeding choroidal veins in a lightly pigmented patient.

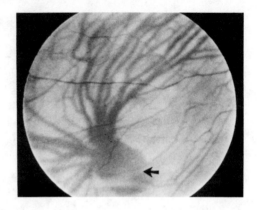

Fig. 7.5 Scleral foramina for the short posterior ciliary arteries (arrows) exposed to view by myopic degeneration (a, left). Long posterior ciliary nerve (arrow) and artery (curved arrow) are easily identified because of the pigmentation along their margins (b, right).

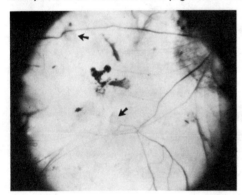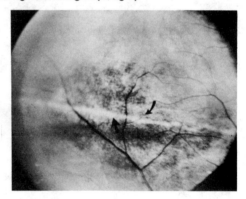

location in the mid-peripheral fundus, providing an excellent ophthalmoscopic landmark (Fig. 7.4).

The choroid is traversed by branches of the ophthalmic (first) division of the fifth cranial nerve. The long and short ciliary nerves (Fig. 7.3, 7.5b) arise directly from the nasociliary nerve or pass to the globe via the ciliary ganglion. Together these nerves provide all sensation of the eyeball. Sympathetic fibers from the ciliary ganglion seem to affect only the central retinal and not choroidal arteries.

Bruch's membrane (lamina vitrea) derives its name from its smooth, glass-like microscopic appearance. A noncellular structure, it's a product of adjoining retinal pigment epithelium and choriocapillaris cells. It figures significantly in the all-important exchange between the neurosensory retina and choriocapillaris.

The high oxygen content of choroidal venous blood suggests a very inefficient system, requiring a volume of choroidal blood flow in excess of tissue oxygen demands. This apparent inefficiency may be explained by the heat-dissipating effect of rapid blood flow. Temperature measurements in monkeys give evidence that the choroid also acts as a cooling device to counteract the heat generated when light energy is absorbed at the retinal pigment epithelium.

The sclera is relatively avascular in its inner layers and presents a bone-white appearance when exposed to ophthalmoscopic view (see Fig. 1.10). In some patients, the scleral foramina for the short ciliary arteries are visible (Fig. 7.5a). Only the absence or thinning of the overlying choroid, retinal pigment epithelium, and neurosensory retina allows a view of the sclera.

References

Hayreh SS: Segmental nature of the choroidal vasculature. Br J Ophthalmol 59:631, 1975.

Hayreh SS, Baines JAB, McLeod D: Occlusion of the posterior ciliary artery. Br J Ophthalmol 56:719, 1972.

Parver LM, Auker C, Carpenter DO: Choroidal blood flow as a heat dissipating mechanism in the macula. Am J Ophthalmol 89:641, 1980.

Ring HG, Fujino T: Observations on the anatomy and pathology of the choroidal vasculature. Arch Ophthalmol 78:431, 1967.

Rutnin U: Fundus appearance in normal eyes: 1. The choroid. Am J Ophthalmol 64:821, 1967.

Wolff E: The Anatomy of the Eye and Orbit. New York: McGraw-Hill, 1955.

II. MISSING CHOROID

Patchy exposure of the sclera from absence of the choroid is a nonspecific finding. Even a good family and personal history, observation in various stages of disease, characteristic location and associated pathology, such as myopia, do not always allow confirmation of the etiology.

A. LARGE DEFECTS

1. Coloboma (Fig. 7.6; see also Figs. 2.27, 3.19)
Failure of the fetal fissure to close in the fourth to fifth week of gestation (7-14 mm stage) results in a choroidal and retinal defect. Such defects may be small and multiple or very large.

Ophthalmoscopic findings

o   Typically involves only the inferior eye at the site of the fetal fissure. Atypical colobomata occur in any quadrant.

o   Central part of defect exposes the mostly white sclera, sometimes with a bluish cast. Often the defect is depressed, which requires refocusing the ophthalmoscope.

Fig. 7.6 Large coloboma involving the disc and macula in a 47-year-old male with poor vision from birth (a, left). Minimal congenital coloboma along the embryonic fetal fissure (b, right).

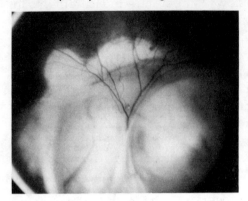 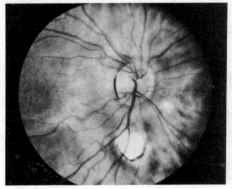

o Edges of a coloboma are sharp, often with dark line of increased pigmentation.

o Retinal blood vessels often dip into a coloboma or appear to arise from it.

o Choroidal blood vessels in a coloboma are tortuous and broad.

o Defect may extend the whole length of the eye from the disc anteriorly to iris and lens. It also may be limited to the disc or the peripheral location.

o Typical colobomata occur in both eyes in 60 percent of afflicted patients.

Symptoms & signs

o Nonprogressive defect.

o Visual acuity is normal, unless the coloboma involves optic disc or macula.

o An absolute field defect corresponds to the coloboma.

o Retinal detachment may develop from holes along margin of the coloboma.

o Dislocation or subluxation of lens may occur (see Chapter 2: VIC).

o Glaucoma may occur if an iris coloboma is present.

Other confirming findings

o Findings are present from birth in both typical and atypical forms.

o The typical form has dominant inheritance with incomplete penetrance — 20-30 percent.

o Iris and lens coloboma are often present.

- o Fluorescein angiography aids in defining vascular and neurosensory retina abnormalities.
- o Electro-oculogram and electroretinogram determine electrophysiology of the neurosensory retina and retinal pigment epithelium.

Main differential diagnosis

- o Congenital toxoplasmosis
- o Retinoblastoma
- o Retrolental fibroplasia
- o Glaucomatous cupping of optic disc
- o Falciform retinal fold
- o Retinal dysplasia
- o Myelinated nerve fibers

References

Duke-Elder S: System of Ophthalmology, vol 3, part 2. St. Louis: Mosby, 1964, p 456.

Mann I: Developmental Abnormalities of the Eye. Philadelphia: Lippincott, 1957.

2. Gyrate atrophy (Fig. 7.7)

This hereditary disease causes large areas of choroidal destruction, exposing the sclera to view. Although it probably begins in the retinal pigment epithelium, the extensive choroidal involvement dominates the appearance.

Ophthalmoscopic findings

- o Starts in mid-periphery, usually within 3-4 disc diameters from disc.
- o Lesions have sharply defined margins.
- o Lesions often a disc diameter in size, but variable.
- o Defects coalesce, giving a scalloped border.
- o Retinal pigment epithelium, choriocapillaris, and even large choroidal vessels disappear and may be in different stages of atrophy in individual lesions; pigment often is chocolate. The vitreous is clear.
- o The disease spreads peripherally and centrally at variable rate, eventually reaching the macula in most patients.
- o Retinal blood vessels narrow in advanced stages.
- o A bilateral disease.

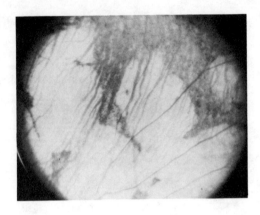

Fig. 7.7 Gyrate atrophy of the choroid that started in the mid-periphery and gradually extended toward the macula.

Symptoms & signs

o   Nightblindness is usually noted before age 20.

o   Unless cataracts occur — in 30-50 percent of patients — visual acuity is often normal until the macula becomes involved late in the disease.

o   Eighty to 90 percent of patients are myopic to some degree.

o   Visual field is restricted peripherally, or ring scotoma may be present.

o   Pupil reactions are normal, except in very late stages.

Other confirming findings

o   Autosomal recessive, consanguinity is common.

o   Early mild defect in dark adaptation becomes progressively worse with disease.

o   Electroretinogram and electro-oculogram are normal early, but deteriorate with disease.

o   Fluorescein angiography shows that choriocapillaris perfuses in diseased areas only at low intraocular pressure, suggesting resistance to blood flow. There's a simultaneous deficiency of flow in whole choroid, in contrast to choroideremia.

o   Plasma ornithine levels are usually elevated, and the enzyme ornithine aminotransferase may be deficient. Relatives may also be deficient.

Main differential diagnosis

o   Choroideremia

o   Myopic degeneration

o   Regional choroidal atrophy

- Serpiginous choroidal atrophy
- Choroidal vascular occlusion
- Retinitis pigmentosa
- Histoplasmosis syndrome

References

Berson EL, Schmidt SY, Shih VE: Ocular and biochemical abnormalities in gyrate atrophy of the choroid and retina. Ophthalmology 85:1018, 1978.

Kaiser-Kupfer MI, Valle D, Del Valle LA: A specific enzyme defect in gyrate atrophy. Am J Ophthalmol 85:200, 1978.

Krill AE: Krill's Hereditary Retinal and Choroidal Diseases, vol 2. Hagerstown, Md: Harper & Row, 1977, p 1002.

Simell O, Takki K: Raised plasma-ornithine and gyrate atrophy of the choroid and retina. Lancet 1:1031, 1973.

Takki K: Gyrate atrophy of the choroid and retina associated with hyperornithinaemia. Br J Ophthalmol 58:3, 1974.

Weleber RG, Kennaway NG, Buist NR: Vitamin B_6 in management of gyrate atrophy of choroid and retina. Lancet 2:1213, 1978.

3. Choroideremia (Fig. 7.8; see 7.8a and 7.8d also in color section)

Inheritance of choroideremia is now well established, but whether the disease is manifest at birth has not been determined. Like gyrate atrophy, it probably originates with retinal pigment epithelium, but it's included here because the extensive choroidal disease dominates the picture.

Ophthalmoscopic findings

- Starts with fine pigment stippling and atrophy (pepper-and-salt appearance).
- Often begins around the disc and equator at the same time.
- Large choroidal vessels become exposed and disappear first in the periphery. A similar process starts at the disc, spreading outward but sparing the macula. Some clumps of pigment may be seen.
- Optic disc may become pale and retinal vessels narrowed.

Symptoms & signs

- Nightblindness may be noted at five to 10 years of age.
- Visual acuity is usually good until 40 years of age.
- General constriction of field.

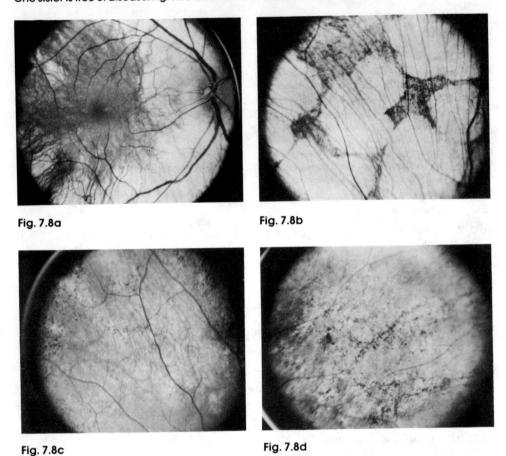

Fig. 7.8 Choroideremia, an X-linked disease in a 16-year-old boy with 6/4.5 (20/15) vision (a and b). His mother (c) and sister (d) both show the fine peripheral pigmentation of the carrier state. One sister is free of disease. Fig. 7.8a and 7.8d also shown in color section.

Fig. 7.8a

Fig. 7.8b

Fig. 7.8c

Fig. 7.8d

o Pupil reactions are normal, until visual acuity is affected.

o Myopia in affected males is more prevalent than hyperopia.

Other confirming findings

o Inheritance is felt to be linked to the X chromosome, although some females have the disease.

o Earliest known manifestation occurred in a patient age 12 months.

o Fluorescein angiography shows a diffuse and widespread hyperfluorescence of the retinal pigment epithelium and more visible choroidal vessels than expected.

o Electroretinogram may be normal early in the disease.

o Dark adaptation is usually poor, even when the patient first comes in.

Main differential diagnosis

o Gyrate atrophy

o Retinitis pigmentosa

o Myopic degeneration

o Regional choroidal atrophy

o Serpiginous choroidal atrophy

o Histoplasmosis syndrome

o Choroidal vascular occlusion

References

Gass JDM: Stereoscopic Atlas of Macular Diseases. St. Louis: Mosby, 1977, p 158.

Krill AE: Krill's Hereditary Retinal and Choroidal Diseases, vol 2. Hagerstown, Md: Harper & Row, 1977, p 1013.

4. Myopic degeneration (Fig. 7.9; see 7.9a and 7.9b also in color section; see also Fig. 6.23)

Simple myopia (shortsightedness) is distinguished from secondary myopia associated with increased refractive power of the lens and degenerative myopia. In degenerative myopia, an increase in axial length of the eye is associated with changes in the sclera, choroid, and retina. One important complication of progressive myopia, the Foerster-Fuchs spot, has been described in Chapter 6: IIIC, 3. The more generalized choroidal and scleral abnormalities are described here.

Ophthalmoscopic findings

o At least a minus 6.00 lens is needed to view the disc. The ophthalmoscopic view is often better if observed with patient's glasses in place.

o Disc is often gray and misshapen, with vessels entering at unusual angles.

o Retinal pigment epithelial atrophy around the disc may be a simple myopic crescent (see Fig. 3.4), usually, but not always, on the temporal side. The atrophy may be much more extensive and involve the whole posterior eye.

o Temporal retinal vessels are usually straight.

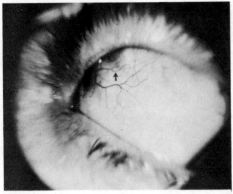

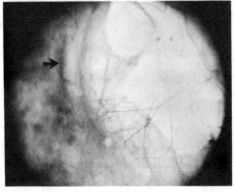

Fig. 7.9 Myopic degeneration with a bulge, or staphyloma (arrow), in the sclera (a, above left). The margin of staphyloma (arrows) could be focused with a −6.00 lens (b, above right), while the disc could be focused only with a −10.00 lens. Note the ripple in the pigment (arrow) at the margin of the staphyloma (c, right). Fig. 7.9a and 7.9b also shown in color section.

o   Retinal pigment epithelial atrophy peripherally may be mild or extensive, exposing choroidal vessels and sclera to view. Hyperpigmentation at the margins of atrophic areas is uncommon.

o   White lines of atrophy (lacquer cracks) may radiate from the disc or involve the fovea and result in subretinal hemorrhage (see Fig. 6.23).

o   Paving stone and lattice degeneration (see Figs. 5.52, 5.57) may involve the periphery. Atrophic round or oval retinal holes may occur.

o   Weiss ring may be seen over the disc, if vitreous degeneration and separation have occurred.

o   May be unilateral, but more often bilateral.

Symptoms & signs

o   Poor distance visual acuity without corrective lenses requires the patient to squint (stenopeic slit) to increase depth of focus and to hold objects close.

o Onset is often before age five, with rapid increases in myopia associated with skeletal growth. Progression may continue into patient's fourth decade or even longer, but usually maximum myopia is achieved before age 30.

o Corrected visual acuity may vary from 6/6 (20/20) to counting fingers, depending on macular function. Decreased visual acuity may occur suddenly from Foerster-Fuchs spot or retinal detachment. It may be poor from infancy, due to amblyopia in patients with only one myopic eye or to associated optic atrophy.

o Floaters may be described by patients with vitreous degeneration.

o Visual fields are often unreliable, even with patient's glasses in place. Reliable fields to define scotomas corresponding to patient's chorioretinal atrophy are achieved with contact lenses.

o Color vision, especially blue-yellow, is often defective in severe degeneration.

o Difficulty with seeing in the dark and poor dark adaptation are common symptoms.

o Myopic eyes may be more susceptible to increased intraocular pressure (glaucoma), and pressure readings with Schiøtz tonometers may be unreliable.

Other confirming findings

o Degenerative myopia probably occurs in about 5 percent of world population. In the United Kingdom, it accounts for 14 percent of newly registered blind.

o Autosomal dominant and sex-linked inheritance is reported, but the majority of pedigrees appear to be autosomal recessive. There may be an association of myopia to retrolental fibroplasia and febrile illnesses in childhood.

o Inheritance of myopia in association with gyrate atrophy, retinitis pigmentosa, albinism, microphthalmos, and other diseases is well known.

o About one-third of all retinal detachment patients are myopic. The prevalence increases directly with the degree of myopia.

o Among glaucoma patients, those with myopia may be more susceptible to loss of visual field at lower intraocular pressures than those who are nonmyopic.

o Cataracts may be more common in myopic patients.

Main differential diagnosis

o   Gyrate atrophy

o   Regional choroidal atrophy

o   Serpiginous choroidal atrophy

o   Histoplasmosis syndrome

o   Retinitis pigmentosa

o   Choroideremia

o   Angioid streaks

References

Gass JDM: Stereoscopic Atlas of Macular Diseases: St. Louis: Mosby, 1977, p 86.

Krill AE: Krill's Hereditary Retinal and Choroidal Diseases, vol 2. Hagerstown, Md: Harper & Row, 1977, p 911.

B. SMALL DEFECTS

Localized small patches of atrophy are the result of various choroidal injuries. Traumatic and vascular causes are often explainable, but many inflammatory causes cannot be diagnosed. For example, the histoplasmosis syndrome is a choroiditis resulting in many small punched-out choroidal defects. Despite the name, the etiology of this disease still cannot be attributed to the organism Histoplasma capsulatum, because it has rarely been found in the eye, even at autopsies of patients with the systemic disease.

1. Histoplasmosis syndrome (see Chapter 6: IIID, 4)

2. Toxoplasmosis (see Chapter 5:VA)

3. Choroiditis and chorioretinitis (see VG, below)

4. Trauma (see VF, below)

III. FLUSHED CHOROID

Slow blood flow through large, dilated choroidal vessels or increased hemoglobin content of the blood give the choroid a redder than normal appearance.

A. DIFFUSE HEMANGIOMA OF THE CHOROID (TOMATO CATSUP FUNDUS) (Fig. 7.10; see 7.10a also in color section)

The diffuse, flat choroidal hemangioma (tomato catsup) is most common in patients with Sturge-Weber syndrome (encephalotrigeminal angiomatosis).

Ophthalmoscopic findings

o   Diffuse bright red color of most of the interior of the eye, compared with other eye, which is usually normal.

o   Retinal vessels may be tortuous, dilated, or sheathed or have aneurysms.

o   Optic disc often cupped from glaucoma.

o   Drusen or focal atrophy or hypertrophy of the retinal pigment epithelium may be present.

o   View of choroid may be impaired by intravitreal blood, dislocated lens, corneal edema, or iris synechiae.

o   Unilateral.

o   There may be shallow elevation of choroid and retina.

Symptoms & signs

o   Port wine stain (nevus flammeus) on the affected side of the face may be large or easily overlooked. Often, there are associated dilated conjunctival or episcleral vessels, an orbital hemangioma with proptosis, and, in some patients, an oculocutaneous melanosis.

Fig. 7.10 Diffuse choroidal hemangioma in a five-year-old female gave a red tomato catsup appearance appreciated only by contrasting it with the other eye or observing the margin of the hemangioma (a, left). Facial hemangioma in a patient with Sturge-Weber disease (b, right). The facial lesions may also be very small. Fig. 7.10a also shown in color section.

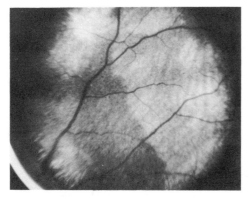
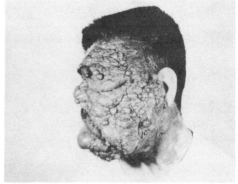

- o Globe on affected side, as well as surrounding soft tissue and bone, may be larger than other eye.
- o Iris is darker on affected side, and occasionally there is a coloboma.
- o Pupils are unequal; on affected side, the pupil may be small or large.
- o Vision is usually poor from birth in the affected eye, but may become worse from strabismus (amblyopia), dislocated lens, glaucoma, corneal opacity, or anisometropia (greater myopia in affected eye, leading to amblyopia).
- o Nystagmus (rotary type) may be present.
- o Ocular muscle palsy with double vision may result from sixth cranial nerve injury.
- o Glaucoma occurs in 68 percent of affected eyes, sometimes with pain.
- o Intravitreal hemorrhage from retinal vascular anomalies may result in sudden loss of vision.
- o Facial paralysis of supranuclear type occurs.

Other confirming findings

- o No hereditary pattern emerges.
- o Mental retardation is common — one of every 1,000 admissions to hospitals for the retarded; most patients with full syndrome die before age 30.
- o Epilepsy (contralateral side) occurs in two-thirds of patients.
- o Cerebral calcifications and cortical atrophy can be seen on computerized axial tomography.
- o Fluorescein angiography yields a characteristic picture.
- o Ultrasonography can help define both ocular and orbital disease.

Main differential diagnosis

- o Preretinal and intravitreal hemorrhage from any cause
- o Brunescent (brown) nuclear cataract, which often gives the retina and choroid a reddish hue (see Fig. 2.48)
- o Neurofibromatosis
- o Incontinentia pigmenti
- o Klippel-Trenaunay-Weber syndrome (nevus varicosus osteohypertrophicus)
- o Louis-Bar syndrome (ataxia-telangiectasia)

References

Krill AE: Krill's Hereditary Retinal and Choroidal Diseases, vol 2. Hagerstown, Md: Harper & Row, 1977, p 1275.

Susac JO, Smith JL, Scelfo RJ: The "tomato-catsup" fundus in Sturge-Weber syndrome. Arch Ophthalmol 92:69, 1974.

Walsh FB, Hoyt WF: Clinical Neuro-Ophthalmology, vol 3. Baltimore: Williams & Wilkins, 1969, pp 1976-1985.

B. LOCALIZED (CAVERNOUS) HEMANGIOMA (see VIIB, below)

C. POLYCYTHEMIA (see Chapter 4: IXE)

D. CARBON MONOXIDE POISONING (see Chapter 4: IXF)

IV. PALE CHOROID

Anemia from blood loss, iron deficiency, hemolysis, and bone marrow malfunction are severe when noticeable in the choroid. Of course, the choroid is not the only affected tissue, but it's a readily visible one. Choroidal pallor, by displacement of the red blood cells by white blood cells or fat, also occurs. Thickening of vascular walls may hide blood from view as well.

A. LIPEMIA RETINALIS (see Chapter 4: IXB)

B. LEUKEMIA (see Chapter 4: IXC)

C. ANEMIA (see Chapter 4: IXA)

D. MYOPIC DEGENERATION (see II4, above)

E. ALBINISM (see Chapter 6: IIA)

F. CHOROIDAL ANGIOSCLEROSIS
(Fig. 7.11; see also in color section)

Opacification and thickening of vessel walls can hide the red color of blood in the choroid, even when hemoglobin content is normal. It's doubtful that perfusion is normal under these circumstances. Large or small pale areas may be seen (see VE, below).

Ophthalmoscopic findings

o Choroidal vessels are readily seen and appear yellow-white.

o Whole choroid or only localized areas may be involved.

o Retinal pigment epithelium may be missing in patches, and there may be areas of pigment clumping.

o Small localized patches of atrophy over a yellow-white choroidal vessel were described by Elschnig (see references); sometimes several occur in a row (Siegrist's pearls).

o Retinal vessels usually also show evidence of arteriosclerotic and hypertensive disease.

Symptoms & signs

o Vision may be surprisingly good, despite apparent lack of blood in choroidal vessels.

o Amaurosis fugax (fleeting loss of vision) may bring the patient for examination.

o Pupil response to light varies with vision, ischemic iris atrophy, or rubeosis iridis.

o Field loss corresponds to areas of defective choroidal perfusion or optic nerve damage.

o Tonography shows difference between the two eyes in intraocular pressure and pulse pressure.

Other confirming findings

o History of giant cell arteritis or of arteriosclerotic, hypertensive, or other vascular occlusive disease needs review.

o Physical evidence of defective blood flow to the head, including, among other signs, loss of hair, diminished pulse, cool skin, loss of sweating, carotid murmurs, hearing loss.

o Plethysmography helps define ocular blood flow.

o Angiography confirms insufficiency of blood flow to the head.

o Fluorescein angiography defines specific ocular blood-flow problems.

o Radionuclear brain or carotid scan aid blood-flow definition.

Main differential diagnosis

o Regional and diffuse choroidal atrophies

o Choroideremia

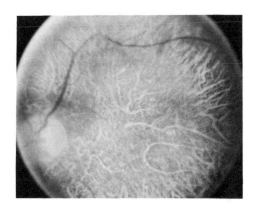

Fig. 7.11 Choroidal angiosclerosis in a 71-year-old man with carotid and coronary artery disease. Visual acuity was reduced to counting fingers at 1 meter. Also shown in color section.

o Gyrate atrophy

o Retinitis pigmentosa

o Myopic degeneration

References

Archer D, Krill AE, Newell FW: Fluorescein studies of choroidal sclerosis. Am J Ophthalmol 71:266, 1971.

de Venecia GT, Wallow I, Houser D, et al: The eye in accelerated hypertension: 1. Elschnig's spots in nonhuman primates. Arch Ophthalmol 98:913, 1980.

Krill AE: Krill's Hereditary Retinal and Choroidal Diseases, vol 2. Hagerstown, Md: Harper & Row, 1977, p 979.

Wise GN, Dollery CT, Henkind P: The Retinal Circulation. New York: Harper & Row, 1971, p 320.

G. OSSEOUS CHORISTOMA OF CHOROID (see VID, 2, below)

H. METASTATIC TUMOR OF CHOROID (see VIC, below)

I. AMELANOTIC MELANOMA (see VIA, below)

V. LOCALIZED PIGMENT DISTURBANCE IN THE CHOROID

Choroidal melanocytes are concentrated near the sclera, deep in the choroid and out of the ophthalmoscopist's view. Unlike the retinal pigment epithelium, the melanocytes of the choroid don't become hyperpigmented with healing. Once injured, depigmentation usually follows. Much of what is thought to be hyperpigmentation of the choroid is attempted repair by melanocytes of the retinal pigment epithelium.

A. MELANOSIS OCULI AND NEVUS OF OTA (MELANOSIS BULBI, OCULAR MELANOCYTOSIS)

(Fig. 7.12; see also in color section)

Increased pigmentation of the uvea throughout the eye is called melanosis oculi or bulbi. When the skin around the eye is also pigmented, as occurs more commonly in black or Oriental patients, the term nevus of Ota is used. Melanosis oculi should not be confused with ocular albinism and Waardenburg's syndrome (see Chapter 6: IIA), in which the eye without pigment is the diseased one.

Ophthalmoscopic findings

o All structures appear normal, except for generalized darker choroidal colors on affected side, in contrast with other eye.

o Usual segmental variations of choroidal color may be seen.

o It is unilateral.

Symptoms & signs

o Scleral pigmentation is a common sign and is best seen by raising upper lid.

o In nevus of Ota, skin of lids and around the orbit gives a mask-like appearance on the affected side. Skin may appear blue or gray. Most patients are black or Oriental.

o Vision is usually normal, unless melanoma occurs.

o Pupil reactions are normal.

o Dark adaptation and color vision normal.

Other confirming findings

o Melanosis oculi is uncommon, but not rare. The incidence is unknown. There is no confirmed inheritance pattern.

o Melanosis oculi may slightly increase the patient's chance of a malignant melanoma.

o Serial photography helps in keeping track of suspicious lesions.

o Fluorescein angiography may help differentiate a change.

o Ultrasonography is especially helpful in defining elevation.

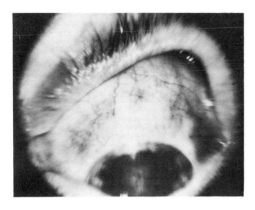

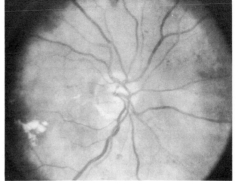

Fig. 7.12 Melanosis oculi involving the sclera (a, above left). Contrast the color of the choroid in the unaffected right eye (b, above right) with the left eye (c, right). The patient also has diabetic retinopathy. Also shown in color section.

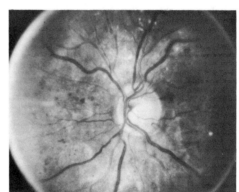

Main differential diagnosis

o Ocular albinism and Waardenburg's syndrome

o Heterochromia iridis (Fuchs's heterochromia)

o Precancerous conjunctival melanosis

o Carotid artery disease with ocular ischemia, central retinal artery occlusion, iris atrophy

o Malignant melanoma

o Pseudometastatic disease

References

Blodi FC: Ocular melanocytosis and melanoma. Am J Ophthalmol 80:389, 1975.

Mohandessan M, Fetkenhour C, O'Grady R: Malignant melanoma of choroid in a case of nevus of Ota. Ann Ophthalmol 11:189, 1979.

Yanoff M, Fine BS: Ocular Pathology: A Text and Atlas. Hagerstown, Md: Harper & Row, 1975.

B. CHOROIDAL NEVI (Fig. 7.13; see also in color section)

By definition, nevi are benign tissues composed of normal or atypical melanocytes. They probably are cell rests and may grow in response to unknown factors, since they are rarely present at birth. Malignant melanomas have in some patients started in nevi followed for years as benign.

Ophthalmoscopic findings

o   Can be located anywhere in choroid, but 80 percent are temporal to the disc and one-third are within 2 disc diameters of the macula.

o   May be multiple and bilateral.

o   Usually, they are ½ to 2 disc diameters in size.

o   May be slightly elevated, but are usually flat.

o   Margins often irregular, without a halo of depigmentation as seen in retinal pigment hyperplasia (see Fig. 6.11).

o   Color varies from subtle gray to near black and is usually uniform, unless drusen occurs. Hypopigmented nevi also occur. Orange pigment (lipofuscin) suggests malignant melanoma (see VIA, below).

o   Disruption of retinal pigment epithelium with drusen-like defects may be present over nevi.

o   Subretinal neovascularization and serous elevation of retinal pigment epithelium and neurosensory retina may occur; latter may extend considerable distance from the nevus.

Symptoms & signs

o   Visual acuity is usually normal, unless serous retinal pigment epithelial or neurosensory retina detachment secondary to nevus involves the fovea.

o   Pupil reactions are normal.

o   Scotomata corresponding to nevi can be found in some patients on careful testing.

o   Most nevi of choroid are found on routine examination. Observation at regular intervals is necessary to rule out malignant melanoma.

Other confirming findings

o   Incidence in children is about 0.40 percent, adults 30 percent, bilaterality 3.5 percent, multiple nevi 7 percent.

o   About 55 percent of patients with choroidal nevi have iris nevi also.

Fig. 7.13 Nevus of the choroid. Note the difference in color between 7.13a (left) and 7.13b (right) aside from the multiple drusen. Subtle nevi are easily overlooked when the pigmentation is light. Also shown in color section.

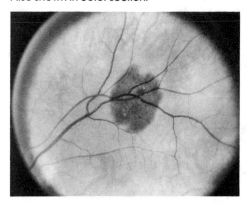 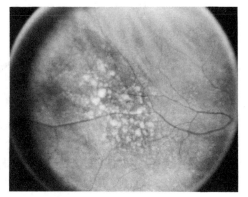

o Serial photography and close observation allow early detection of change.

o Fluorescein angiography helps determine activity and confirm diagnosis.

o Multiple pigmented nevi or pigmented melanocytomas have been seen in patients with undifferentiated lung cancer. The ocular disease is benign, but occurs coincidentally with disease elsewhere. A remote malignancy should be considered when multiple nevi are seen.

Main differential diagnosis

o Malignant melanoma

o Metastatic tumor

o Choroidal effusion (detachment)

o Retinal pigment epithelial hyperplasia (bear track)

o Chorioretinal scarring (multiple causes)

o Normal pigmentation variations (see Figs. 6.3, 6.4)

o Pseudometastatic disease

References

Ferry AP: Lesions mistaken for malignant melanoma of the posterior uvea. Arch Ophthalmol 72:463, 1964.

Gass JDM: Problems in the differential diagnosis of choroidal nevi and malignant melanoma. Am J Ophthalmol 83:299, 1977.

Gass JDM: Stereoscopic Atlas of Macular Diseases. St. Louis: Mosby, 1977, p 134.

CHOROID AND SCLERA

MacIlwaine WA, Anderson B Jr, Klintworth GK: Enlargement of a histologically documented choroidal nevus. Am J Ophthalmol 87:480, 1979.

Ryll DL, Campbell RJ, Robertson DM, et al: Pseudometastatic lesions of the choroid. Ophthalmology 87:1181, 1980.

Yannuzzi LA, Gitter KA, Schatz H: The Macula: A Comprehensive Text and Atlas. Baltimore: Williams & Wilkins, 1979, p 302.

C. MALIGNANT MELANOMA (see VIA, below)

D. METASTATIC TUMOR OF CHOROID (see VIC, below)

E. VASCULAR OCCLUSIVE DISEASE (Fig. 7.14; see 7.14a also in color section)

Localized choroidal infarction from arteriosclerosis, hypertension, giant cell arteritis, and other causes often go unrecognized, if the macula or optic nerve are uninvolved. As indicators of arteriosclerosis and hypertension, choroidal vascular abnormalities may exceed retinal vascular disease in importance. (See also IVF, above, and Chapter 3: VIIB, 4b).

Ophthalmoscopic findings

o Depigmentation or pigment clumping in the retinal pigment epithelium is seen over occluded vessels.

o Choroidal vessels are exposed to view by atrophy of retinal pigment epithelium.

o Color of choroid is variable, depending on the area supplied by the occluded vessel. Defects may be large (5-10 disc diameters), small (Elschnig's spot), or in a line of atrophy along vessels (Siegrist's pearls).

o Sclera may be exposed to view.

o In acute phases, gray clouding of the choroid with slight elevation is present in the involved area.

Symptoms & signs

o Vision is often good, unless macula or optic nerve are involved.

o Pupil responses are normal, except in large infarctions involving the macula or optic nerve.

o Field loss corresponds to damaged choroid.

o Amaurosis fugax is uncommon in embolic disease of choroid, probably because the large vessels pass the embolus to periphery.

Fig. 7.14 Choroidal infarction in a 68-year-old hypertensive female (a, left). Area of choroidal atrophy developed along with a central retinal artery occlusion. Note proliferation by the retinal pigment epithelium and the white sclera showing in the center. Local spots of pigmentation over white choroidal vessels (Elschnig's spots) sometimes form a line (Siegrist's pearls) (b, right). Fig. 7.14a also shown in color section.

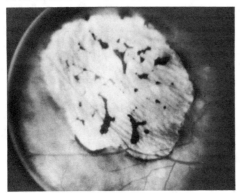 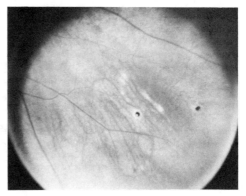

Other confirming findings

o History of giant cell arteritis or of arteriosclerotic, hypertensive, or other vascular occlusive disease needs review.

o Physical evidence of defective blood flow to the head, including, among other signs, loss of hair, diminished pulse, cool skin, loss of sweating, carotid murmurs, hearing loss.

o Plethysmography helps define ocular blood flow.

o Angiography confirms insufficiency of blood flow to the head.

o Fluorescein angiography defines specifc ocular blood-flow problems.

o Radionuclear brain or carotid scan aid blood-flow definition.

Main differential diagnosis

o Regional and diffuse choroidal atrophies

o Choroideremia

o Gyrate atrophy

o Retinitis pigmentosa

o Myopic degeneration

References

Archer D, Krill AE, Newell FW: Fluorescein studies of choroidal sclerosis. Am J Ophthalmol 71:266, 1971.

de Venecia G, Wallow I, Houser D, et al: The eye in accelerated hypertension: 1. Elschnig's spots in nonhuman primates. Arch Ophthalmol 98:913, 1980.

Krill AE: Krill's Hereditary Retinal and Choroidal Diseases, vol 2. Hagerstown, Md: Harper & Row, 1977, p 979.

Wise GN, Dollery CT, Henkind P: The Retinal Circulation. New York: Harper & Row, 1971, p 320.

F. TRAUMA (Figs. 7.15, 7.16; see 7.15b also in color section)

Contusion injuries may fracture Bruch's membrane and rupture choroidal blood vessels, even though the globe is not penetrated. If the injury comes from a large object, like a fist, the rupture commonly is in the posterior eye, often near the disc. Ruptures may occur at the impact site of smaller objects, like BB pellets.

Ophthalmoscopic findings

o   Yellow-white curved line or lines are concentric with the disc.

o   Retinal pigment may outline and accentuate the yellow-white split; usually this takes a few weeks.

o   Lines may be of various lengths and sometimes star-shaped at impact sites.

o   Subretinal pigment epithelial, subretinal, intraretinal, and intravitreal hemorrhage may all be present in the acute stage. Intraretinal hemorrhage may obscure the choroidal rupture initially.

o   Late subretinal neovascularization may occur with new subretinal hemorrhage.

Symptoms & signs

o   Vision varies from normal to hand motion, depending on whether the choroidal rupture damaged the fovea, papillomacular retinal fibers, or the disc or caused severe intravitreal hemorrhage.

o   Pupil is often fixed and dilated from traumatic mydriasis and iris injury; fixed pupil can also result from severe visual loss, due to optic nerve injury.

o   Poor vision may occur suddenly, months after injury, in some patients who develop subretinal neovascularization through a defect in Bruch's membrane.

o   Pain and photophobia right after injury are common, due to traumatic iritis.

Fig. 7.15 Choroidal rupture from blunt injury (a, left). Curvilinear orientation around the disc is common. Visual acuity was 6/90 (20/300). If the fovea is injured, visual recovery is poor (b, right). Acuity was counting fingers at 1 meter. Fig. 7.15b also shown in color section.

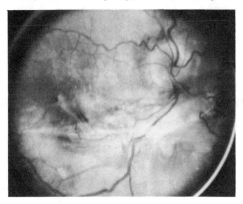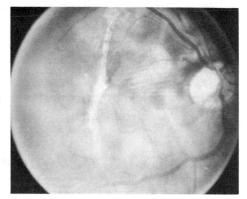

Fig. 7.16 Shotgun pellet injury of the right eye (a) seen 23 days (b), 53 days (c), and one year later (d). The white material under the hemorrhage at the second visit was not exposed sclera but hemolyzed blood.

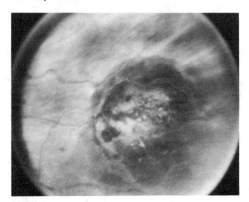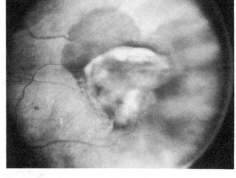

Fig. 7.16a

Fig. 7.16b

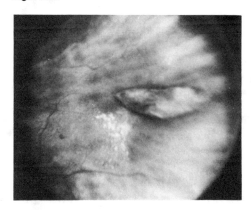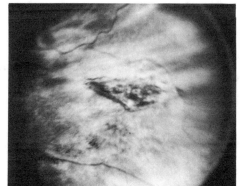

Fig. 7.16c

Fig. 7.16d

o   Glaucoma from contusion angle deformity may occur initially or after a delay of years. Follow-up is needed.

o   Retinal disinsertion and detachment from severe blunt trauma must always be kept in mind (see Chapter 5: IIIB, 4).

Other confirming findings

o   History of trauma is usually elicited easily, except in the battered-child syndrome. Old injuries that cause new disorders, such as subretinal neovascularization, may have been forgotten by the patient.

o   Gonioscopic evidence of contusion angle deformity may be found.

o   Fluorescein angiography demonstrates subretinal neovascularization.

o   Ultrasonography may be helpful, if intravitreal blood obscures the choroid.

Main differential diagnosis

o   Intraocular foreign body

o   Acute focal choroiditis

o   Histoplasmosis syndrome

o   Serpiginous choroiditis

o   Senile macular degeneration

o   Myopic degeneration (Foerster-Fuchs spot)

o   Rhegmatogenous retinal detachment

References

Freeman HM, ed: Ocular Trauma. New York: Appleton-Century-Crofts, 1979.

Gass JDM: Stereoscopic Atlas of Macular Diseases. St. Louis: Mosby, 1977, p 126.

G. INFLAMMATION (CHOROIDITIS, CHORIORETINITIS, POSTERIOR UVEITIS)

There are many known causes of choroidal inflammation (see Table 7.1). Some authors include diseases that histologic studies show originate in the retina, such as toxoplasmosis. Choroidal inflammation cannot be isolated from disease of the retinal pigment epithelium, neurosensory retina, or vitreous, and disease starting in the choroid often has its greatest clinical effect when these other tissues become involved. For example, in the histoplasmosis syndrome, patients are usually unaware of choroidal lesions until the macular retinal pigment epithelium and neurosensory retina are injured.

Not all diseases causing redness, pain, and swelling are due to inflammation. Retinoblastoma in children, melanomas, metastatic tumors, and vascular disease in adults may be mistaken as inflammatory disease.

In some cases of choroiditis, the cause is known or can be strongly presumed; others present with characteristic findings that label them, but the etiology remains obscure. With still others, the cause continues to escape every investigative effort. This last group is probably the largest.

The list of causes of uveitis in Table 7.1 will undoubtedly be expanded in time. Selected examples are discussed here.

1. Disseminated Choroiditis

a) HISTOPLASMOSIS SYNDROME (see Chapter 6: IIID, 4)

b) MILIARY TUBERCULOSIS (Fig. 7.17; see 7.17b also in color section)
Tuberculosis may be seen in the iris, ciliary body, and choroid. Miliary tuberculosis of the choroid is occasionally found in patients known to have the disease but are refractory to treatment or have failed to take it.

Ophthalmoscopic findings

o Gray-white nodules of various sizes and indistinct margins.

o Rarely a localized, elevated, single tumor-like tuberculoma.

o Size of nodules may vary from pinpoint to larger than a disc diameter.

o Confluence may occur, and nodules may enlarge within a week.

o Posterior choroid around disc is the most common site.

o Margins become more distinct with healing, and color becomes white or yellow.

o Pigmented scar is the residue of healing.

Symptoms & signs

o Patients with miliary tuberculosis are usually seriously ill, while those with solitary tuberculomas are in apparent good health.

o Blurred and distorted vision may be noted in one or both eyes.

o Visual acuity is reduced if the fovea is involved or there is vitreous cellular reaction.

o Scotomata can be plotted.

o Pupil responses depend on severity of choroidal and optic nerve disease.

o Symptoms and signs of iritis occur with iris nodules.

Table 7.1

CAUSES OF UVEITIS

Infectious uveitis

A. Bacterial uveitis

Cocci: staphylococci, streptococci, pneumococci, gonococci, meningococci, Neisseria catarrhalis

Gram negatives: Pseudomonas, diplobacillus, subtilis, coliform, Proteus, Shigella, Salmonella typhi (agent of typhoid fever), Yersinia pestis (agent of plague), Brucella

Clostridium sp: gas gangrene

Actinomycosis (nocardiosis) listeriosis

Mycobacterium sp: tuberculosis, leprosy

Spirochetes: syphilis, yaws, relapsing fever, leptospirosis

Pleuropneumonia-like organism

B. Rickettsial uveitis

Epidemic typhus	Boutonneuse fever
Scrub typhus	Q fever
Murine typhus	Neorickettsiae

C. Viral uveitis

PLT viruses: psittacosis, lymphogranuloma venereum, trachoma

Herpes simplex

Exanthematous viruses: measles, varicella (chicken pox), herpes zoster

Pox viruses: variola (smallpox), vaccinia

Myxoviruses: mumps, influenza

Arbor viruses: dengue, sandfly fever, Rift Valley fever

Other: cytomegalic inclusion disease, epidemic kerato-conjunctivitis, foot and mouth disease, infectious hepatitis, verrucae (warts)

Presumed viral etiology: Behcet's disease, Vogt-Koyanagi-Harada disease, infectious mononucleosis

D. Mycotic uveitis

Sporotrichosis	Candidiasis (moniliasis)
Blastomycosis	Cryptococcosis (torulosis)
Aspergillosis	Mucormycosis
Coccidioidomycosis	Histoplasmosis

E. Parasitic infection

Protozoa: toxoplasmosis, malaria, amebiasis, giardiasis, leishmaniasis, trypanosomiasis

Nemathelminthes: onchocerciasis, wuchereriasis, and loiasis, angiostrongyliasis, gnathostomiasis, ascariasis, toxocariasis, oxyuriasis (enterobiasis), ankylostomiasis, trichinosis

Platyhelminthes: schistosomiasis (bilharziasis), echinococcosis (hydatid disease), cysticercosis, coenurosis (gid)

Arthropoda: endocular myiasis, Apterygota, porocephaliasis

Table 7.1 (continued)

CAUSES OF UVEITIS

Hypersensitivity uveitis

A. Foreign agents

Serum sickness

Angioneurotic edema

Atopic uveitis

B. Autoimmune disease

Lens-induced uveitis

Pigment-induced uveitis

Toxic and irritative uveitis

Phthisis bulbi

Retinal detachment

Hemolysis (ghost cell) of intraocular blood

Necrotic neoplasm

Chemical irritants and drugs

Trauma (contusion)

Noninfective systemic disease

A. Sarcoidosis

B. Collagen disease

Rheumatoid arthritis, Still's disease

Rheumatic fever

Necrotizing angiitis (polyarteritis nodosa)

Disseminated lupus erythematosus

Scleroderma

Polychondritis

C. Central nervous system disease

Disseminated sclerosis (multiple sclerosis)

Diffuse leucoencephalopathy

D. Skin disease

Pyogenic dermatoses

Pemphigus

Rosacea

Nodular nonsuppurative panniculitis

Erythema

Psoriasis

Lichen planus

Xeroderma pigmentosum

Uveitis of unknown cause

A. Sympathetic ophthalmia

B. Heterochromic cyclitis

Adapted from Duke-Elder S, Perkins ES: System of Ophthalmology, vol 9. St. Louis: Mosby, 1966. Used with permission.

Fig. 7.17 Choroidal lesion in a patient with miliary tuberculosis (a, left). Raised choroidal lesion with surrounding serous elevation of the retina, intraretinal exudation, and macular star in a patient with positive sputum and other findings of tuberculosis (b, right). Fig. 7.17a courtesy of William Havener, M.D., Ohio State University. Fig. 7.17b from Cangemi FE, Friedman AH, Josephberg R: Tuberculoma of the choroid. **Ophthalmology** 87:252, 1980. Used with permission. Fig. 7.17b also shown in color section.

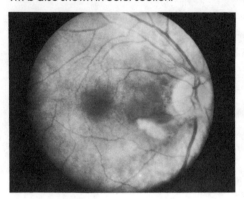 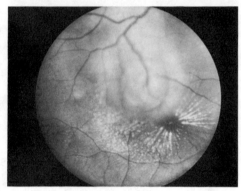

Table 7.2

DIAGNOSTIC TESTING IN CHOROIDAL INFLAMMATION

Possible cause	Some tests of value
Cytomegalic inclusion virus	Acute and convalescent sera for complement fixation Urine cytology
Filariasis (onchocerciasis)	Skin biopsy
Herpes simplex	Acute and convalescent sera for complement fixation
Herpes zoster	Vesicle cytology
Infectious mononucleosis	Heterophile or mono spot test
Intraocular foreign body	Radiologic, ultrasonic examination
Leptospirosis	Latex agglutination Acute and convalescent sera for complement fixation Anterior chamber tap
Moniliasis	Vitreous biopsy
Parasites	Stool specimen Proctoscopy with biopsy

Other confirming findings

o Acute miliary tuberculosis patients usually have active acute chest disease, while isolated tuberculoma patients are usually healthy and well nourished, but with a history of healed tuberculosis elsewhere in the body.

o May occur at any age, but most are young adults. No sex predilection.

o Sputum and node and other tissue analysis is indicated, including spinal fluid and node biopsy.

o Radiologic and radionuclear studies are indicated.

o Fluorescein angiography may aid ophthalmoscopic diagnosis.

o See Table 7.1 and Table 7.2.

Table 7.2

DIAGNOSTIC TESTING IN CHOROIDAL INFLAMMATION

Possible cause	Some tests of value
Rheumatoid collagen disease	Antinuclear antibody titer Rheumatoid factor Lupus erythematosus preparations VDRL
Sarcoidosis	Serum angiotensin-converting enzyme Gallium scan (chest) Chest and hand X-rays Conjunctival biopsy
Streptococcus	ASO titer AH titer
Syphilis	FTA-absorption VDRL
Toxocara canis or catis	ELISA test
Toxoplasmosis	Indirect hemagglutination Sabin-Feldman dye test ELISA test for toxoplasmosis
Tuberculosis	Skin test, PPD (intermediate) Chest X-ray, sputum, urine, Node biopsy, bone marrow

Main differential diagnosis

o Septic — both bacterial and fungal — embolization from such causes as drug abuse and prolonged intravenous therapy.

o Histoplasmosis syndrome

o Acute multifocal placoid epitheliopathy

o Vogt-Koyanagi-Harada disease

o Sympathetic ophthalmia

o Cytomegalic inclusion virus

o Herpes simplex retinitis

References

Cangemi FE, Friedman AH, Josephberg R: Tuberculoma of the choroid. Ophthalmology 87:252, 1980.

Duke-Elder S, Perkins ES: System of Ophthalmology, vol 9. St. Louis: Mosby, 1966, pp 246-285.

c) SARCOIDOSIS (see Chapter 5: VN)

d) VOGT-KOYANAGI-HARADA DISEASE (see Chapter 6: IIC)

e) SYMPATHETIC OPHTHALMIA (Fig. 7.18)

The incidence of sympathetic ophthalmia has been reported at 0.1-0.2 percent of injured eyes. While the incidence is low, the significance is great, since both eyes are threatened with blindness. No cases of sympathetic ophthalmia have been reported without severe disease or penetrating injury to the exciting eye. The penetration may have been surgical incision.

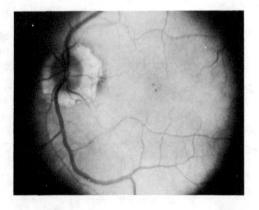

Fig. 7.18 Sympathetic ophthalmia in a 73-year-old patient following complicated cataract surgery. Note the circumpapillary choroidal atrophy, fine pigment in the fovea, poor foveal definition, and narrowed arteries. The other eye was similar. Visual acuity was 6/18 (20/60) OD, 6/9 (20/30) OS five years later.

Ophthalmoscopic findings

o Media may be turbid, due to cells and protein in aqueous and vitreous, although some patients have clear media and most of disease — at least in the early stages — is in posterior choroid.

o Gray, scattered, coalescent nodules with indistinct margins may be slightly elevated.

o Greatest concentration of nodules is near the disc, but may extend anteriorly to equator or beyond.

o Serous retinal detachment with shifting subretinal fluid sometimes develops, as in Vogt-Koyanagi-Harada disease.

o Optic disc may be swollen.

o As nodules subside with treatment, areas of pigment atrophy remain.

Symptoms & signs

o Vision of the injured exciting eye is usually impaired and becomes worse with onset of the disease.

o Transient obscure vision in normal eye, especially for reading, is often a first sign of involvement.

o Light sensitivity and tearing in the uninjured eye follow.

o Redness, miosis, and circumcorneal flush resembling acute iritis occur.

o Multiple scotomata or altitudinal field loss can be found.

Other confirming findings

o History of penetrating injury, surgery, severe ocular disease, or removal of the other eye is available in every patient.

o Onset of inflammation in the normal eye has been reported from five days to 12 years after injury to other eye.

o The disease can occur at any age. It's less common in black patients.

o Males suffer more injuries and, therefore, have a higher incidence of disease. Sympathetic ophthalmia after surgery has equal frequency in males and females. Trauma causes about 54 percent, surgery 40 percent, perforating corneal ulcers 6 percent.

o Fluorescein angiography helps define macular involvement.

o Histologic evaluation of blind exciting eye is used to confirm the diagnosis.

o See Table 7.1 and Table 7.2.

Main differential diagnosis

o   Vogt-Koyanagi-Harada disease

o   Choroidal effusion

o   Hypotony

o   Acute multifocal placoid epitheliopathy

o   Behcet's disease

o   Miliary tuberculosis

o   Multifocal choroiditis

References

Gass JDM: Stereoscopic Atlas of Macular Diseases. St. Louis: Mosby, 1977, p 120.

Lewis ML, Gass JDM, Spencer WH: Sympathetic uveitis after trauma and vitrectomy. Arch Ophthalmol 96:263, 1978.

Lubin JR, Albert DM, Weinstein M: Sixty-five years of sympathetic ophthalmia: A clinico-pathologic review of 105 cases (1913-1978). Ophthalmology 87:109, 1980.

Marak GE Jr: Recent advances in sympathetic ophthalmia. Surv Ophthalmol 24:141, 1979.

f)   BEHCET'S DISEASE (see Chapter 4: VD)

g) ACUTE MULTIFOCAL PLACOID EPITHELIOPATHY
(see Chapter 6: IIID, 7b)

h) RETICULUM CELL SARCOMA (see Chapter 8)

i) WHIPPLE'S DISEASE (INTESTINAL LIPODYSTROPHY)
(see Figs. 7.19, 7.20)

This uncommon systemic disease may have both ocular and central nervous system involvement. The cause is unknown.

Ophthalmoscopic findings

o   Many gray indistinct choroiditis lesions.

o   Rarely larger than 1 disc diameter.

o   Small hemorrhages often near active lesions.

o   May be several at the same time.

o   Vitreous is hazy from cells and protein.

o   Both eyes usually involved, but not always simultaneously.

o   Lesions may heal without scarring.

o   Blood vessel attenuation and optic disc pallor may develop.

Symptoms & signs

o   Visual loss may be mild to severe.

o   Double vision, nystagmus, broad gait, and ophthalmoplegia occur.

o   Iritis and keratitis cause ocular pain when present.

Other confirming findings

o   Males over age 35 most commonly affected.

o   Nondeforming polyarticular arthritis.

o   Intermittent low-grade fever.

o   Cough, hearing loss, lymphadenopathy.

o   Pericardial, pleural, or peritoneal effusion, endocarditis.

o   Gastrointestinal bleeding, abdominal pain.

o   Anemia and hypoproteinemia.

o   Weakness and weight loss.

o   See Table 7.1 and Table 7.2.

Fig. 7.19 Multiple foci of choroiditis, sometimes called birdshot choroiditis, in a 22-year-old female. The other eye was similar.

Fig. 7.20 Cryptococcal chorioretinitis in a 41-year-old male. Note the creamy subretinal lesion with intraretinal hemorrhage, dependent exudates, and retinal detachment. Courtesy of Jerry Shields, M.D., and James Augsburger, M.D., Philadephia.

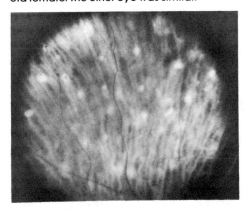

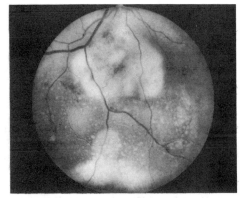

Main differential diagnosis

o   Vogt-Koyanagi-Harada disease

o   Behcet's disease

o   Sympathetic ophthalmia

o   Leukemia

o   Sarcoidosis

References

Knox DL, Bayless TM, Yardley JH, et al: Whipple's disease presenting with ocular inflammation and minimal intestinal symptoms. Johns Hopkins Med J 123:175, 1968.

Walsh FB, Hoyt WF: Clinical Neuro-Ophthalmology, vol 2. Baltimore: Williams & Wilkins,
1969, p 1196.

j) BIRDSHOT RETINOCHOROIDOPATHY (Fig. 7.19)

Ophthalmoscopic findings

o   Many depigmented areas from disc to equator.

o   Both eyes affected.

o   Sheathing of veins, especially in the temporal retina.

o   Vitreous hazy with cells and protein.

o   Cystoid edema of macula common.

Symptoms & signs

o   Chronic, recurrent course with complaints of decreasing vision.

o   Visual acuity varies from normal to 6/60 (20/200).

o   Patient may note loss of dark adaptation and color vision.

Other confirming findings

o   Male and females usually over age 40.

o   Patients are generally in good health.

o   Electroretinogram, electro-oculogram, and dark adaptation usually
    abnormal.

o   Fluorescein angiography confirms macular edema, decompensated
    disc vessels, and window defects in the retinal pigment epithelium.

o   See Table 7.1 and Table 7.2.

Main differential diagnosis

o   Histoplasmosis syndrome

o   Vogt-Koyanagi-Harada disease

o   Sympathetic ophthalmia

o   Reticulum cell sarcoma

o   Acute multifocal placoid epitheliopathy

References

Kaplan HJ, Aaberg TM: Birdshot retinochoroidopathy. Am J Ophthalmol 90:773, 1980.

Ryan SJ, Maumonee AE: Birdshot retinochoroidopathy. Am J Ophthalmol 89:31, 1980.

k) CRYPTOCOCCOSIS (TORULOSIS) (Fig. 7.20)

Infection of the eye by Cryptococcus neoformans involves the choroid in most of the afflicted patients. Both healthy and immunosuppressed patients have had the disease.

Ophthalmoscopic findings

o   Yellow or white patch in the choroid.

o   May be single or multiple.

o   Margins are indistinct.

o   Dilated or telangiectatic retinal vessels over lesions.

o   Vitreous is usually clear.

o   May be bilateral.

o   Papilledema or optic atrophy may be present in severe central nervous system disease.

Symptoms & signs

o   Visual acuity varies from normal to no light perception, depending on the location of the lesions and the extent of retinal or optic disc disease.

o   Pupil reactions vary with the extent of retinal, optic nerve, or central nervous system injury.

o   Visual field loss corresponds to location of the lesions, involvement of the optic nerve tract, or radiations.

o   Double vision from muscle paresis occurs.

Other confirming findings

o   History of immunosuppressive therapy, debilitation from malignant lymphoma, systemic lupus erythematosus, or severe meningoencephalitis in many patients. Less common are antecedent history of subclinical pneumonitis or corneal transplantation.

o   Lethargy, weakness, speech impairment, ataxia, and other neurologic signs are common.

o   Computed axial tomography confirms central nervous system disease, often including obstructive hydrocephalus.

o   Cerebrospinal fluid analysis, culture, and India ink preparations.

o   Fluorescein angiography confirms telangiectasis, and late staining suggests infectious disease.

o   Biopsy of the vitreous or removal of a blind eye may aid diagnosis when severe ocular involvement is present and diagnosis is difficult.

Main differential diagnosis

o   Cytomegalovirus retinitis

o   Herpes simplex retinitis

o   Histoplasmosis choroiditis

o   Candidiasis

o   Coccidioidal endophthalmitis

o   Toxoplasmosis

References

Avendano J, Tanishima T, Kuwabara T: Ocular cryptococcosis. Am J Ophthalmol 86:110, 1978.

Francois J, Rysselaere M: Oculomycoses. Springfield, Ill: Thomas, 1972, pp 316-326.

Shields JA, Wright DM, Augsburger JJ, et al: Cryptococcal chorioretinitis. Am J Ophthalmol 89:210, 1980.

1) COCCIDIOIDOMYCOSIS (VALLEY FEVER, SAN JOAQUIN VALLEY FEVER) (Fig. 7.21)

The choroid and retina have been involved in disseminated Coccidiodes immitis infection. Less than one in 200 males infected has disseminated disease, but, when it occurs, any organ system may be included. Anterior uveal tissue is the second most common intraocular site. External conjunctivitis, keratitis, and episcleritis are seen in the initial acute pulmonary disease.

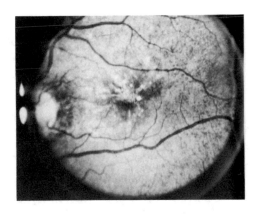

Fig. 7.21 Coccidioidomycosis choroiditis in a patient from the San Joaquin Valley. Courtesy of David Stevens, M.D., San Jose, California.

Ophthalmoscopic findings

o   White plaque-like lesions in the choroid. Some have hazy borders and others are more discrete.

o   Diffuse dissemination of lesions may be present in preterminal patients.

o   Large juxtapapillary lesions may be associated with edema, hemorrhage, and exudate.

o   Lesions may also originate in the retina.

o   Angioid streaks may radiate from the disc.

o   Peau d'orange appearance of the fundus is said to be characteristic.

o   Neovascularization may occur on the disc.

Symptoms & signs

o   May be no ocular symptoms unless macula or disc is involved.

o   Pupil reactions usually are normal.

o   Scotoma corresponds to large choroidal lesions or disc involvement.

o   Granulomas of eyelids, phlyctenular keratoconjunctivitis, or episcleritis may yield the organism.

Other confirming findings

o   This disease is endemic in the hot, dry San Joaquin Valley of California, particularly after dust storms that disseminate the mycelial form of the organism.

- o History of upper respiratory infection or pneumonitis with associated fever, malaise, cough, and chest pain, usually three weeks after exposure.
- o Erythema nodosum or multiforme occurs three days to three weeks after onset of symptoms.
- o Chest roentgenogram reveals pneumonitis, granulomata, nodules, or thin-walled cavities.
- o Central nervous system disease may result in bahavioral changes, meningeal signs, muscle paresis.
- o Complement fixation antibody tests on serum and cerebrospinal fluid aid diagnosis.
- o Cerebrospinal fluid and lid granulomas may reveal the organism on culture.

Main differential diagnosis

- o Histoplasmosis choroiditis
- o Candidiasis
- o Cryptococcosis
- o Cytomegalovirus retinitis
- o Toxoplasmosis
- o Herpes simplex retinitis

References

Blumenkranz MS, Stevens DA: Endogenous coccidioidal endophthalmitis. Ophthalmology 87:974, 1980.

Zakka KA, Foos RY, Brown WJ: Intraocular coccidioidomycosis. Surv Ophthalmol 22:313, 1978.

2. Localized choroiditis (Figs. 7.22, 7.23; see also in color section)

Some patients have a localized sudden inflammatory choroidal lesion that heals spontaneously, leaving a scar, and never have another episode.

Ophthalmoscopic findings

- o Single lesion near fovea often initiates examination.
- o Usually less than 1 disc diameter size.
- o Usually unilateral.

o Gray or yellow lesions are slightly elevated with indistinct margins.

o May be patch or halo of subretinal blood.

o Retinal vessels pass over lesions without much apparent involvement; later, they may enter scar.

o Neurosensory retina may be microcystic over lesion.

o Margins become sharp; patchy black pigmentation occurs during healing. In some patients, a punched-out defect without pigment is left, exposing the sclera.

Symptoms & signs

o Vision varies with proximity of lesion to fovea. Lesion in fovea may reduce visual acuity to counting fingers. Juxtapapillary lesions interrupting nerve fiber layer from the fovea or damaging optic nerve conduction may do the same.

o Distortion or micropsia (decreased size of image) may be chief complaint in lesions near, but not in, fovea; vision otherwise may be normal.

o Scotoma corresponds to lesions and any nerve fiber layer disruption (sector defect).

o Pupil reactions are usually normal, unless a large lesion has destroyed the macula or injured the optic nerve or anterior uveitis is also present.

o Pain or photophobia are usually not present.

o Patient finds light is dim and color weak in affected eye.

Fig. 7.22 Acute localized choroiditis with subretinal hemorrhage in a 20-year-old female. The etiology was never found. Visual acuity was 6/30 (20/100). Also shown in color section.

Fig. 7.23 One of several similar choroidal infiltrates in both eyes of a 39-year-old diabetic with pneumococcal bacteremia. Retinal detachment in the left eye required surgery. Also shown in color section.

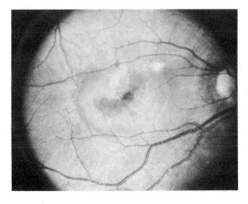 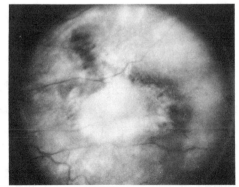

Other confirming findings

o No hereditary pattern.

o Patients are usually in the second to fourth decade of life and in previous good general health.

o May be history of recent injection, as with drug abuse and dental work.

o Physical, laboratory, and radiologic evidence of an infectious focus elsewhere in the body should be sought as indicated by history and physical examination.

o Fluorescein angiography helps define activity, location, and damaging effects of the disease.

o See Table 7.1 and Table 7.2.

Main differential diagnosis

o Atypical histoplasmosis syndrome

o Embolic infectious disease

o Macular degenerative disease, senile or juvenile

o Toxoplasmic retinochoroiditis

o Toxocara canis

o Behcet's disease

o Vogt-Koyanagi-Harada disease

o Tuberculosis

o Leprosy

o Syphilis

References

Campinchi R, ed: Uveitis: Immunologic and Allergic Phenomena. Springfield, Ill: Thomas, 1973.

Schlaegel TF Jr: Ocular toxoplasmosis and pars planitis. New York: Grune & Stratton, 1978.

3. Finger-like expanding (serpiginous, geographic, or helicoid) choroiditis (Fig. 7.24; see 7.24a also in color section)

This disease starts at the disc and extends peripherally, leaving behind areas of destruction of the choriocapillaris and retinal pigment epithelium. The term serpiginous describes the progressive twisting course of the disease.

Fig. 7.24 Serpiginous (geographic) choroiditis (a, left) in a 15-year-old white female is more readily apparent on fluorescein angiography (b, right). Both eyes were affected by progressive choroiditis starting at the disc and extending peripherally in all directions. Maculae became involved; visual acuity reduced to 6/60 (20/200) in both eyes. Fig. 7.24a also shown in color section.

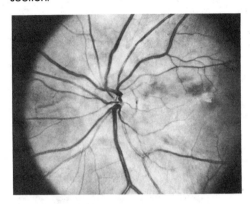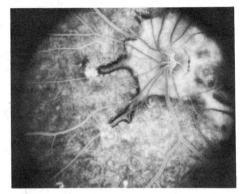

Ophthalmoscopic findings

o   Nearly always bilateral, often at same time.

o   Starts at the disc and extends peripherally.

o   Atrophy and pigment clumping at the disc give way to fingers with indistinct margins. In some patients, there is visible subretinal neovascularization or subretinal blood. A trench of atrophy may be left by advancement of the finger-like projections.

o   Neurosensory retina often is gray at ends of fingers and becomes thin and microcystic later. It's often elevated over lesions.

o   Margins of lesions may be hyperpigmented, like a black line drawn around the edges.

o   Skip areas ahead of finger-like projections may be seen .

o   Fingers rarely extend more than 8-10 disc diameters from disc.

o   Macula is often involved, but occasionally may be circumvented by the lesion.

o   Disc becomes pale and retinal vessels narrowed in longstanding, extensive disease.

o   Vitreous cellular reaction is common over lesions.

Symptoms & signs

o   Blurred or distorted vision is the chief complaint. The patient may be unaware of disease in other eye.

o   Visual acuity usually 6/12 (20/40) or less.

o Scotomata coincide with the disease and may become absolute — the patient is unable to see any test object.

o Light may seem dim, and color perception is diminished.

o Photophobia and pain usually are not present.

Other confirming findings

o Patients are young or middle-aged.

o No hereditary pattern is known.

o Progresses and extends over a period of months or years, often by recurrent episodes.

o Fluorescein angiography helps define the margin and subretinal neovascularization.

o Table 7.2 is a brief diagnosis guide for some of the common causes of ocular inflammation. Specific tests initiated by reason of clinical suspicion are of more value than all-inclusive battery of examinations.

Main differential diagnosis

o Acute multifocal placoid epitheliopathy

o Histoplasmosis syndrome

o Regional choroidal atrophy

o Gyrate atrophy

o Choroideremia

References

Baarsma GS, Deutman AF: Serpiginous (geographic) choroiditis. Doc Ophthalmol 40:269, 1976.

Gass JDM: Stereoscopic Atlas of Macular Diseases. St. Louis: Mosby, 1977, p 112.

Weiss H, Annesley WH, Shields JA, et al: The clinical course of serpiginous choroidopathy. Am J Ophthalmol 87:133, 1979.

H. PIGMENT LINES (see Chapter 6: VI)

VI. ELEVATED CHOROID

Elevation of choroid toward the center of the eye necessarily pushes the retina and retinal pigment epithelium ahead of it and displaces fluid from the vitreous. Such choroidal swelling may originate in the choroid itself, the suprachoroidal space (between choroid and sclera), the sclera, or the orbit.

Unless accompanied by retinal detachment, choroidal elevations usually present to the viewer a smooth contour that is fixed rather than undulating with eye movement.

The magnitude of elevation varies from very subtle and indiscernible without binocular viewing to extreme and visible in the pupil with the help of a hand-held light.

Tumors, both primary and metastatic, are a grave concern when an elevated lesion appears in the choroid. Decisions about choroidal elevations center about whether they are neoplasms, originate in or outside the eye, and are malignant or benign. Common examples are described here.

A. CHOROIDAL MELANOMA (MALIGNANT MELANOMA OF THE CHOROID, CHOROIDAL MELANOSARCOMA) (Figs. 7.25-7.29; see 7.26-7.29 also in color section)

The worldwide age-adjusted incidence of choroidal melanoma ranges from two of every 100,000 in Asian countries to 10 per 100,000 in Scandinavia. In the U.S.A., an age-adjusted incidence of seven per 100,000 in whites and 0.7 per 100,000 in blacks has been reported. Age adjustment of the figures is necessary, because the average age at diagnosis is 56 years. There are indications that the incidence may be increased by chemical exposure.

Ophthalmoscopic findings

o   Slightly more melanomas arise posterior to the equator than anterior.

o   Size varies from less than one disc diameter to tumor large enough to fill the eye.

o   Flat, laterally extending melanomas may circle the globe, extend anteriorly to block Schlemm's canal and cause glaucoma. Others break through Bruch's membrane in a collar-button shape into the subretinal or intravitreal space. Refocusing the ophthalmoscope is often required to see the apex of the tumor.

o   The majority are mottled gray with pigment clumping, drusen, or orange lipofuscin pigment on the surface. Some contain very little pigment. A dark red reflection in the quadrant of a melanoma may be all the detail possible in highly elevated tumors.

o   Large choroidal blood vessels within the tumor substance, called sinusoids, appear as large red ribbons. They may blanche and flush with gentle pressure on the eye.

o   Intravitreal hemorrhage may obscure or completely hide a tumor from view. Mild subretinal hemorrhage is common in rapidly growing tumors, and occasionally severe hemorrhage causes acute glaucoma by flattening the anterior chamber.

Fig. 7.26 Mildly elevated choroidal melanoma in a 60-year-old man that enlarged to involve the macula over a four-year observation period. Note the mottled pigment in the tumor. Histologic diagnosis was malignant melanoma of choroid, mixed-cell type, predominantly spindle B. Compare with Fig. 7.13. Also shown in color section.

Fig. 7.25 Presumed small choroidal melanoma in a 41-year-old female. A detachment of the neurosensory retina was present. Note the pigmentation in the slightly elevated tumor. Compare with Fig. 7.13.

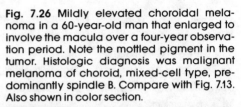

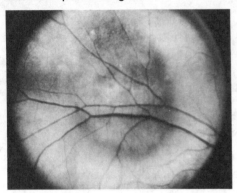

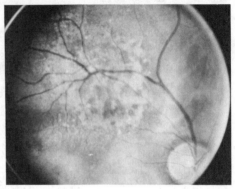

Fig. 7.27 Choroidal melanoma covered with orange pigment and subretinal blood. The highly elevated anterior part is out of focus. Also shown in color section.

Fig. 7.28 Choroidal melanoma obliterating the disc. The color of the tumor is similar to the surrounding normal choroid. Also shown in color section.

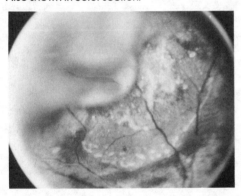

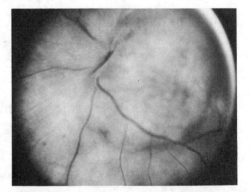

Fig. 7.29 Choroidal melanoma with very little pigment. Note the large choroidal vessels (sinusoids). Also shown in color section.

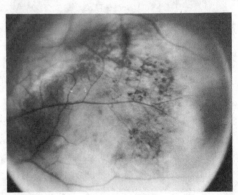

PHYSICIANS' GUIDE TO OCULOSYSTEMIC DISEASES

o Retinal detachment is common and not limited to the immediate tumor area. Shifting subretinal fluid remote from the tumor may cause the retina to undulate with eye movement. Careful notation of surrounding landmarks and comparision with disc size (see Fig. 1.36) help determine growth on repeat examination.

o Cystic macular edema may occur, even though the tumor is remote from the macula.

o Bilateral choroidal melanomata are rare.

Symptoms & signs

o Visual acuity is often reduced severely, but may be totally unaffected even by large tumors, if tumor, cystic edema, retinal detachment, or subretinal hemorrhage does not involve the macula. Intravitreal hemorrhage and, occasionally, corneal edema from acute glaucoma may reduce vision.

o Most melanomas are painless, but acute inflammatory signs — pain, redness, swelling — suggesting infection may follow hemorrhage or necrosis within a tumor. Acute glaucoma associated with pain is also an occasional presenting sign.

o Patient may notice a loss of visual field, often gradually progressive, for some months. This may be due to retinal detachment or the tumor itself. A scotoma on field testing corresponds with the tumor or retinal detachment.

o Floaters from vitreous separation or intravitreal cells may prompt examination.

o Pupil reactions may be normal in small tumors or totally absent in severe optic nerve and macular involvement.

o Spread of choroidal melanomas prior to their discovery or clinically detectable growth has been reported and must be considered in patients who present with liver, lung, or other melanotic metastasis.

Other confirming findings

o Ocular melanoma does not have the dominant inheritance patterns of skin melanoma. The incidence of ocular melanoma is probably slightly greater in patients with melanosis oculi and nevus of Ota.

o Indirect ophthalmoscopy is invaluable in choroidal tumor diagnosis.

o Transillumination of choroid is sometimes helpful.

o Serial stereoscopic photography and fluorescein angiography are essential, especially in small suspicious tumors.

o Ultrasonography to verify growth, particularly elevation, is useful, if the view of tumor is obscured by intravitreal blood or retinal detachment. Some indication of tissue consistency within the tumor can also be obtained, and tissue diagnosis may be possible.

o Computerized axial tomography can demonstrate tumor location, size, and orbital extension.

o Radioactive phosphorous study of posterior masses requires surgical placement of the probe directly over the tumor.

o Skin test hypersensitivity and serum tumor-associated antibodies under study have not yet reached a level of high reliability.

Main differential diagnosis

o Choroidal effusion (detachment)

o Kuhnt-Junius disciform macular degeneration

o Choroidal nevi

o Melanosis oculi

o Melanocytoma

o Metastatic tumors

o Other choroidal tumors (hemangioma, choristoma, neurofibroma, and others)

o Scleral buckle for retinal detachment

o Congenital hyperplasia of the retinal pigment epithelium

References

Albert DM, Puliafito CA, Fulton AB, et al: Increased incidence of choroidal malignant melanoma occurring in a single population of chemical workers. Am J Ophthalmol 89:323, 1980.

Anderson DE: Clinical characteristics of the genetic variety of cutaneous melanoma in man. Cancer 28:721, 1971.

Bloome MA, Ruiz RS: Massive spontaneous subretinal hemorrhage. Am J Ophthalmol 86:630, 1978.

Brownstein S, Sheikh KM, Lewis MG: Tumor-associated antibodies in the serum of patients with uveal melanoma. Can J Ophthalmol 11:147, 1976.

Canny CLB, Shields JA, Kay ML: Clinically stationary choroidal melanoma with extraocular extension. Arch Ophthalmol 96:436, 1978.

Char DH, Hollinshead A, Cogan DG, et al: Cutaneous delayed hypersensitivity reactions to soluble melanoma antigen in patients with ocular malignant melanoma. N Engl J Med 291:274, 1974.

Gass JDM: Observation of suspected choroidal and ciliary body melanomas for evidence of growth prior to enucleation. Ophthalmology 87:523, 1980.

Gass JDM: Problems in the differential diagnosis of choroidal nevi and malignant melanomas. Am J Ophthalmol 83:299, 1977.

Gass JDM: Stereoscopic Atlas of Macular Diseases. St. Louis: Mosby, 1977, p 136.

Gundersen T, Smith TR, Zakov N, et al: Choroidal melanocytic tumor observed for 41 years before enucleation. Arch Ophthalmol 96:2089, 1978.

Kline LB, Bright M, Brownstein S: Uveal melanoma presenting as post-traumatic choroidal hemorrhage and panophthalmitis. Can J Ophthalmol 12:226, 1977.

McLean IW, Foster WD, Zimmerman LE: Prognostic factors in small malignant melanomas of choroid and ciliary body. Arch Ophthalmol 95:48, 1977.

Shields JA, Augsburger JJ, Brown GC, et al: The differential diagnosis of posterior uveal melanoma. Ophthalmology 87:518, 1980.

Shields JA, McDonald PR: Improvements in the diagnosis of posterior uveal melanomas. Arch Ophthalmol 91:259, 1974.

Thomas JV, Green WR, Maumenee AE: Small choroidal melanomas: A long-term follow-up study. Arch Ophthalmol 97:861, 1979.

B. LOCALIZED (CAVERNOUS) HEMANGIOMA (Fig. 7.30; see also in color section)

Unlike diffuse choroidal hemangiomas (see Fig. 7.10) localized hemangiomas are rarely associated with the Sturge-Weber syndrome and therefore create a problem in differential diagnosis.

Ophthalmoscopic findings

o   Nearly all localized hemangiomas occur near the disc and are round or oval.

o   Choroidal elevation may be subtle, rarely high.

o   Retinal elevation occurs and may be shallow, resembling central serous retinopathy, or very high, obscuring a view of tumor.

o   Color is red, orange-red, or, in some patients, white-red with indistinct margins.

o   Transilluminates easily.

o   Size is usually larger than ophthalmoscope field (2-10 disc diameters), requiring careful comparison of the tumor with surrounding areas to see contrast in color and elevation (indirect ophthalmoscopy with larger field of view makes this much easier).

o   Pigment clumping and yellow exudates may occur on surface or around the base of the tumor. The neurosensory retina often develops microcystic changes over tumor.

Fig. 7.30 Localized choroidal hemangioma (arrows). The red color of the choroid blanched and flushed with slight digital pressure on the eye (a, left). Compare with Fig. 7.10a. On fluorescein angiography the tumor vessels fill with the choroid (b, right). Fig. 7.30a also shown in color section.

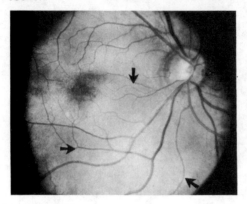 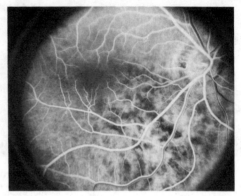

Symptoms & signs

o Usually asymptomatic, unless macula is involved by tumor or serous elevation of the neurosensory retina.

o Visual acuity is normal, unless macula is involved, in which case it may decrease to less than 6/120 (20/400).

o Pupil reactions are normal, unless the central vision is severely impaired.

o Scotoma corresponds to tumor or nerve fiber sector interrupted by it.

Other confirming findings

o These tumors are hamartomas with no hereditary pattern.

o They are more common in white than black patients.

o Males and females are equally affected.

o They are rarely seen before the third decade of life and usually are asymptomatic until fourth or fifth decade.

o Indirect ophthalmoscopy provides a binocular, large field view.

o Transillumination shows the lack of pigment proliferation.

o Fluorescein angiography usually confirms the vascular nature of the tumor.

o Ultrasonography measures elevation and the fluid (blood) spaces in the tumor.

o Radioactive phosphorous (^{32}P) uptake is usually low.

Main differential diagnosis

o Malignant melanoma

o Metastatic tumors

o Other choroidal tumors, such as neurofibroma

o Kuhnt-Junius disciform macular degeneration

o Vitelliform macular degeneration

o Rhegmatogenous retinal detachment

o Central serous retinopathy

References

Gass JDM: Stereoscopic Atlas of Macular Diseases. St. Louis: Mosby, 1977, p 130.

Yannuzzi LA, Gitter KA, Schatz H: The Macula: A Comprehensive Text and Atlas. Baltimore: Williams & Wilkins, 1979, p 316.

C. METASTATIC TUMORS
(Figs. 7.31, 7.32; see 7.31 also in color section)

The most common malignant tumor of the eye is probably metastatic carcinoma. In nearly half the patients with eye or orbital metastatic tumor, the eye is the first indication of metastatic disease. The most common sites of the primary tumor are the breast in females and the lung in males. In the next largest group, the primary site cannot be determined with certainty.

Ophthalmoscopic findings

o Tumors involve posterior eye alone in nearly 50 percent of patients and bilaterally in 5 percent. There's no predilection for right or left eye.

o Slightly elevated white-yellow or yellow lesions in choroid may be of various sizes, usually from ¼ disc diameter to 8 disc diameters.

o Retinal detachment may occur over tumors and extend into the periphery. The retinal detachment may be subtle or highly elevated. Retinal elevation posterior to the equator that fails to reach the ora serrata suggests tumor, rather than rhegmatogenous retinal detachment.

o Mottling or salt-and-pepper disturbance of the retinal pigment epithelium over the tumors is common. This is most noticeable in regression or following treatment.

o Hazy vitreous and aqueous may make ophthalmoscopy difficult in some patients.

Fig. 7.31 Metastatic carcinoma in a white female with primary breast tumor. Note the flat pale elevation of the choroid (a, left) that is even more subtle at another site (b, right). Also shown in color section.

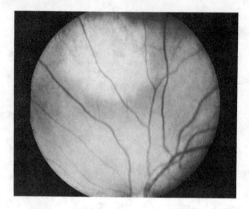 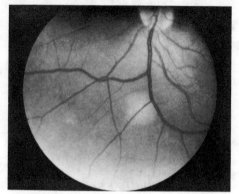

Fig. 7.32 Metastatic bronchiogenic carcinoma in a 57-year-old man whose ocular symptoms prompted discovery of his chest disease. Visual acuity was limited to finger counting at 1 meter with correction. The retina was detached inferiorly.

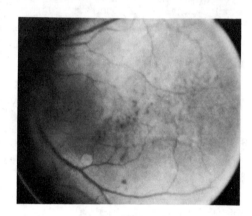

Symptoms & signs

o   Decreased vision occurs in about 80 percent of patients.

o   Pain and exophthalmos are more common in orbital metastasis, and double vision may also occur. Lid swelling is a rare complaint.

o   Field loss due to retinal detachment is common; the usual flashes described in rhegmatogenous retinal detachment are absent. Patient may describe floaters.

o   Photophobia, redness, and aching suggestive of iritis are reported in about 7 percent of patients.

o   Glaucoma occurs in about 6 percent of patients.

Other confirming findings

o   Table 7.3 lists the sites of primary tumors in 227 patients.

o   Table 7.4 lists sites of primary tumors in patients who presented with ocular symptoms before detection of the tumors.

o   Period between treatment of the primary and detection of the ocular or orbital metastasis is less than three years in 27 percent and less than five years in 38 percent. In mammary tumor, the peak ocular tumor discovery time is within two years of treatment of the primary.

o   Indirect ophthalmoscopy aids diagnosis through cloudy media.

o   Fluorescein angiography helps define the nature of suspicious lesions.

o   Ultrasonography measures elevation and tissue consistency.

o   Appropriate diagnostic studies for discovery of the primary tumor.

o   Median survival after discovery of ocular or orbital metastasis is 7.4 months.

Table 7.3

SITE OF PRIMARY TUMOR IN 227 CASES OF CARCINOMA METASTATIC TO THE EYE AND ORBIT

Site	Male Intraocular	Orbit	Female Intraocular	Orbit
Breast	—	—	78.6%	61.5%
Lung	53.8%	20.0%	11.6	7.7
Kidney	7.5	13.3	—	—
Testicle	6.5	6.7	—	—
Prostate	2.2	6.7	—	—
Pancreas	1.1	6.7	—	—
Colon	1.1	—	1.0	—
Rectum	1.1	—	1.0	—
Stomach	1.1	—	—	—
Thyroid	1.1	—	—	—
Ileum	—	6.7	—	—
Not determined	24.7	40.0	7.8	30.8
Total	100.0%	100.0%	100.0%	100.0%

Adapted from System of Ophthalmology, vol 9. Duke-Elder S, Perkins ES: St. Louis: Mosby, 1966. Used with permission.

Table 7.4

SITE OF PRIMARY TUMOR IN PATIENTS WHO PRESENTED
WITH OCULAR COMPLAINT

Primary tumor	No.
Lung	43
Breast	8
Kidney	8
Pancreas	2
Prostate	1
Testicle	1
Stomach	1
Total	64

Adapted from Ferry AP, Font RL: Carcinoma metastatic to the eye and orbit. Arch Ophthalmol 92:276, 1974. Copyright © 1974, American Medical Association. Used with permission.

o Plasma carcinoembryonic antigen (CEA) is elevated in 83 percent of metastatic tumor and 36 percent of melanoma patients. Levels are above 10 ng/ml in 58 percent of metastatic disease patients and none of melanoma patients.

o Gamma glutaryl transpeptidase (GTP) is elevated in 46 percent of patients with uveal and liver metastasis. Use of GTP and CEA is helpful in differentiating metastatic tumors from primary melanomas.

Main differential diagnosis

o Senile macular degeneration (Kuhnt-Junius disciform type)

o Amelanotic melanoma

o Localized choroidal hemangioma

o Rhegmatogenous retinal detachment

o Vitelliform macular degeneration

o Chorioretinal scars

References

Char DH, Schwartz A, Miller TR, et al: Ocular metastases from systemic melanoma. Am J Ophthalmol 90:702, 1980.

Ferry AP, Font RP: Carcinoma metastatic to the eye and orbit. Arch Ophthalmol 92:276, 1974.

Michelson JB, Felberg NT, Shields JA: Evaluation of metastatic cancer to the eye. Arch Ophthalmol 95:692, 1977.

D. OTHER CHOROIDAL TUMORS

Choroidal osteoma, neurofibromatosis, amyloidosis, and others are rare causes of choroidal elevation.

1. Amyloidosis (Fig. 7.33; see also in color section)

Amyloidosis involving the eye more commonly affects the vitreous than the choroid. A rare choroidal mass of presumed amyloid is shown. Amyloidosis is discussed in Chapter 8.

2. Choroidal osteoma (osseus choristoma of choroid) (Fig. 7.34; see also in color section)

This puzzling ossification of the choroid near the optic disc occurs only in young women. Spontaneous calcification of a choroidal hemangioma is unconfirmed, and it's considered a separate entity.

Ophthalmoscopic findings

o   Yellow-white slightly elevated tumor near or even surrounding the disc.

o   Various amounts of pigment atrophy and clumping present.

o   Multiple branching choroidal vascular networks are often visible on the orange-gray mottled tumor surface.

o   Outer margins are usually orange, with irregular sharply defined pseudopods.

o   Gradual increases in size have been reported.

Fig. 7.33 Presumed amyloidosis of the choroid in the right eye of a man with biopsy-proven amyloidosis of the orbit. The eye became blind. Several other similar shallow choroidal elevations are present in the left eye. Also shown in color section.

Fig. 7.34 Osseous choristoma of the choroid in a 47-year-old female. Visual acuity was 6/6 (20/20). Also shown in color section.

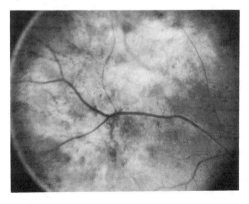

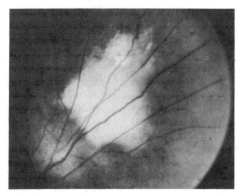

o   Subretinal hemorrhage may occur.

o   Shallow retinal detachment is uncommon.

Symptoms & signs

o   Mild blurred vision, distortions, or a blind spot are the usual complaints. Vision may deteriorate, if the macula is involved.

o   Pupil reactions are normal.

o   A scotoma is present.

Other confirming findings

o   No known hereditary pattern. All cases reported have been in young women; the oldest was 26 years old.

o   Serum calcium, phosphorous, and alkaline phosphatase are normal in reported patients.

o   Radiological examinations and computerized axial tomography show the calcification.

o   Ultrasonography confirms the dense nature of the tumor.

o   Fluorescein angiography has a characteristic appearance.

Main differential diagnosis

o   Metastatic carcinoma

o   Amelanotic melanoma

o   Chorioretinal scarring

o   Localized hemangioma

References

Gass JDM, Guerry RK, Jack RL, et al: Choroidal osteoma. Arch Ophthalmol 96:428, 1978.

Joffe L, Shields JA, Fitzgerald JR: Osseous choristoma of the choroid. Arch Ophthalmol 96:1809, 1978.

3. Neurofibroma

Choroidal neurofibromas are usually associated with evidence of von Recklinghausen's disease elsewhere in the body. The involvement of the choroid in patients with the disease must be considered (see Chapter 5: VIB, 2).

References

Cotlier E: Café-au-lait spots of the fundus in neurofibromatosis. Arch Ophthalmol 95:1990, 1977.

4. Neurilemoma

This rare tumor of peripheral ocular nerves is diagnosed by the pathologist.

E. CHOROIDAL EFFUSION (CHOROIDAL DETACHMENT, CHOROIDALS) AND ANTERIOR OR POSTERIOR SCLERITIS (EPISCLERITIS, BRAWNY SCLERITIS, NECROTIZING SCLERITIS)

(Figs. 7.35-7.37; see 7.37 also in color section)

Fluid accumulation between the sclera and choroid occurs spontaneously or in association with ocular inflammation, trauma, or surgery.

Ophthalmoscopic findings

o Dark, smooth, multilobulated elevations in the anterior part of the eye may extend to the disc. Color of elevation is the same as adjacent choroid.

o Choroidal elevations commonly go all the way around the periphery of the eye.

o Retina is usually tightly bound to the elevations, but in some patients has fine folds or retinal detachment with subretinal fluid that shifts with patient position.

o Greatest elevation is often inferior, if patient has been upright for a few hours. It may be localized to an area of scleritis.

o No to and fro motion of the choroidal elevation with eye movement.

o Vitreous is often hazy and usually without hemorrhage, unless there has been trauma or surgery.

o Disc may appear swollen with indistinct margins (see Chapter 3: VIIB, 2b).

o Pigmented lines (high water marks, concave side toward the disc) may be left by receding choroidals (see Chapter 6: VIB).

Symptoms & signs

o Vision is often surprisingly good and may be normal, unless the macula is involved by retinal detachment or vitreous is very turbid.

o Patient may describe the light as dim in the affected eye.

o Pain is common and is often referred to the brow or zygoma. There may be point tenderness and pain over a specific area of scleritis.

o Pupil reactions are often sluggish, and pupil may be dilated; patients may be taking mydriatic eye drops.

o Anterior chamber may be shallow or flat in extensive choroidals.

Fig. 7.35 Anterior and posterior scleritis (a, left) in a 52-year-old man associated with uveal effusion (b, right). The patient stated he got logwood crystals (eosin), a material used for dying wood, in his eye while sweeping them up.

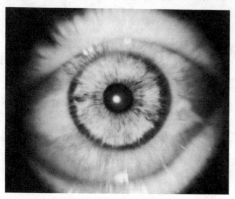 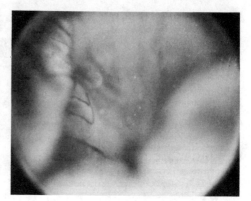

o   Intraocular pressure usually is low, perhaps zero, and upper eyelid can indent cornea.

o   Corneal striae and haziness of aqueous may be seen with a flashlight.

o   Conjunctival and episcleral injection are common.

o   Peripheral field is constricted.

Other confirming findings

o   Choroidal effusion is common in penetrating trauma or surgery, especially cataract extraction, retinal detachment, or glaucoma operations. It usually occurs in the first two weeks and is more common if a wound leak allows intraocular pressure to become very low. Late unexplained choroidals also occur years after cataract surgery. When they occur after glaucoma surgery, leaking of the surgically created filtering bleb is always a concern. Choroidals may persist for years, but are usually transient with proper treatment.

o   Choroidal effusion in nanophthalmos (small eye) may occur spontaneously or following any operative procedure. Rare effusions also occur spontaneously in full-size eyes without evidence of trauma or inflammation.

o   Scleritis, either anterior or posterior, is more common in females, especially those with rheumatoid arthritis. Recurrent episodes are common. Gout may predispose patients to choroidal effusion.

o   Indirect ophthalmoscopy offers the advantages of binocular viewing, a larger field, and better penetration of turbid media.

- Biomicroscopy of recently traumatized or operated eyes provides evidence of a wound leak (Seidel's sign).
- Transillumination confirms the fluid consistency of the choroidal effusion.
- Fluorescein angiography demonstrates vascular decompensation.
- Ultrasonography confirms position, elevation, and fluid nature of the elevation.
- Computerized axial tomography aids differential diagnosis.
- Radioactive phosphorus (^{32}P) aids in differential diagnosis (false positives have been reported in posterior scleritis).

Main differential diagnosis

- Malignant melanoma
- Metastatic choroidal tumor
- Orbital tumor
- Scleral buckle for retinal detachment
- Retinal detachment, rhegmatogenous or nonrhegmatogenous
- Vogt-Koyanagi-Harada disease
- Panuveitis (cause unknown)
- Sympathetic ophthalmia

Fig. 7.36 Choroidal effusion in a 67-year-old female following cataract surgery. No wound leak occurred. Visual acuity was eventually 6/6 (20/20).

Fig. 7.37 Choroidal effusion in a 44-year-old man with rheumatoid arthritis and localized episcleritis (arrow). The effusion is usually over the inflamed sclera. Note how the effusion has rotated the ora serrata into view (curved arrow). Also shown in color section.

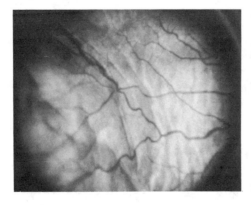

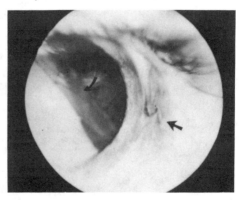

References

Benson WE, Shields JA, Tasman W, et al: Posterior scleritis: A cause of diagnostic confusion. Arch Ophthalmol 97:1482, 1979.

Brockhurst RJ: Nanophthalmos with uveal effusion: A new clinical entity. Arch Ophthalmol 93:1289, 1975.

Feldon SE, Sigelman J, Albert DM: Clinical manifestations of brawny scleritis. Am J Ophthalmol 85:781, 1977.

Gass JDM: Differential Diagnosis of Intraocular Tumors. St. Louis: Mosby, 1974.

Schepens CL, Brockhurst RJ: Uveal effusion. Arch Ophthalmol 70:189, 1963.

F. FOREIGN BODIES (Figs. 7.38-7.41; see 7.41 also in color section)

Surgical placement of foreign materials on or in the sclera to indent, or buckle, the eye is standard procedure to repair retinal detachment. The materials used for this purpose have changed over the years. Accordingly, you'll see successfully operated patients wearing various types. Some are well tolerated, others tend to gradually erode into the eye. Soft silicone materials seem tolerated best and are the most commonly used. Trauma may also introduce foreign materials into the sclera (see Fig. 7.16).

Ophthalmoscopic findings

o Height of the elevation varies considerably, but often requires adding plus lenses to clearly see the surface.

o Elevation may be localized to a single quadrant or may encircle the globe.

o Color of the foreign material may be visible.

o Various degrees of retinal pigment epithelium and choroidal atrophy from diathermy, cryotherapy, photocoagulation, or erosion may be present on the elevation.

o Persistent retinal detachment may be present, but a successfully repaired retinal detachment drapes smoothly over the elevation.

Symptoms & signs

o Visual acuity will vary from 6/6 (20/20) to hand motion, even in eyes with successful retinal repair. Vision depends on the recovery of macular function.

o Pupil responses are usually normal, if vision is good.

o Field defects may correspond with the elevated area.

o Eroding foreign materials may cause hemorrhage (floaters), pain in or around the eye — especially in infection — or redetachment of the retina.

Fig. 7.38 Elevated choroid caused by suture placed in the sclera for treatment of a retinal detachment. The knot in the suture and two additional white sutures over it are clearly visible because of atrophy of the sclera and choroid as it eroded into the eye.

Fig. 7.39 Elevated choroid caused by a poly-ethylene tube placed in the sclera for treatment of a retinal detachment. The edge of the sleeve of tubing and the dark streak of a suture in the lumen are easily visible (arrow).

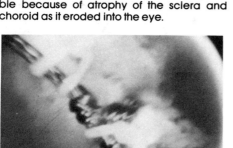

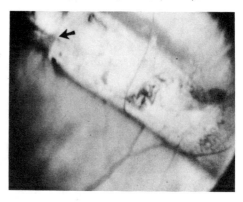

Fig. 7.40 Elevated choroid caused by a silicone band on the scleral surface for the treatment of a retinal detachment. The sclera and choroid are thin, but intact.

Fig. 7.41 Elevated choroid from a large posterior meridional silicone sponge sutured to the sclera to repair a retinal detachment. Compare with Fig. 7.27. Also shown in color section.

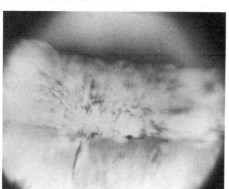

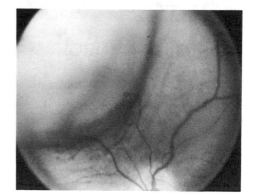

o Intraocular pressure is often lower than in the other eye.

o Anteriorly placed foreign materials can often be seen with a flashlight under the conjunctiva.

Other confirming findings

o History of surgery for trauma, retinal detachment, or diabetic retinopathy can usually be elicited.

o Indirect ophthalmoscopy confirms the location and elevation.

o Ultrasonography may be necessary, if the vitreous is very turbid.

o Computerized axial tomography demonstrates scleral indentation.

Main differential diagnosis

o Malignant melanoma

o Metastatic choroidal tumors

o Recurrent retinal detachment or nonrhegmatogenous retinal detachment

o Choroidal effusion

o Chorioretinal scarring

o Vogt-Koyanagi-Harada disease

References

Gass JDM: Stereoscopic Atlas of Macular Diseases. St. Louis: Mosby, 1977, p 148.

Havener WH, Gloeckner SL: Atlas of Diagnostic Techniques and Treatment of Intraocular Foreign Bodies. St. Louis: Mosby, 1969.

Havener WH, Gloeckner SL: Atlas of Diagnostic Techniques and Treatment of Intraocular Foreign Bodies. St. Louis: Mosby, 1969.

VII. DEPRESSED CHOROID

Weakness of the sclera from trauma, surgery, degeneration, or developmental anomaly may result in an out-pouching of the sclera by the hydraulic pressure within the eye.

A. POSTERIOR STAPHYLOMA IN MYOPIC DEGENERATION
(see Fig. 7.9)

B. COLOBOMA (see Fig. 7.6)

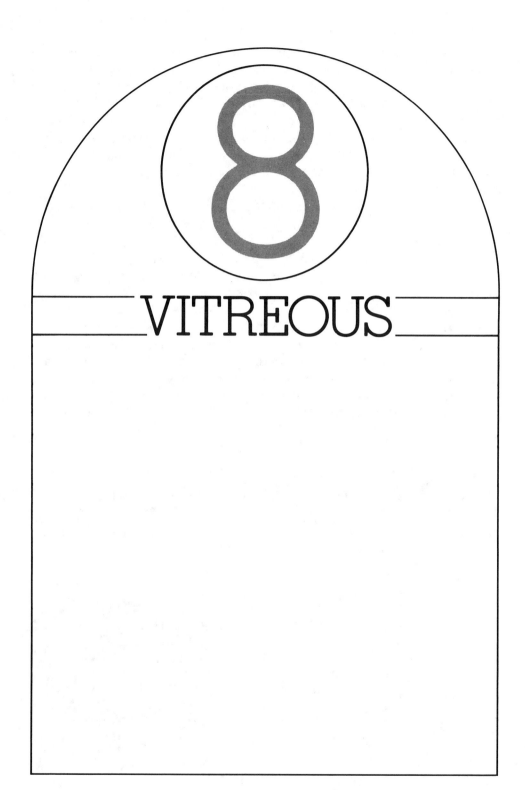

8
VITREOUS

The vitreous constitutes about two-thirds of the total volume of the eye. It is 99 percent fluid, principally water, hence its transparency. The one percent solid material is a collagen-like fibrous protein called vitrosin. It holds the components in a gel state with the aid of hyaluronic acid. Soluble albumin and globulin, ascorbic acid, sugars, sodium, potassium, chloride, bicarbonate, calcium, phosphate, lactic acid, and urea are all present in vitreous. Oxygen tension is variable at different locations. Electrolyte movement in experimental animals is found to be principally from the ciliary body toward the optic disc.

The vitreous is derived principally from the neuroectoderm of the optic cup, with a small contribution by mesoderm and surface ectoderm. Begun before the sixth week of gestation, it's near completion by the sixth month. The primary vitreous supports the hyaloid vascular system and becomes crowded into Cloquet's canal as these vessels atrophy during development. The secondary vitreous constitutes the bulk of the gel, while specialized tertiary vitreous forms the zonules that support the lens (Fig. 8.1).

A circular band of vitreous, approximately 2-3 mm wide straddling the ora serrata, is called the vitreous base. The vitreous cortex is the surface opposed to the adjacent lens, ciliary body, retina, and disc. The vitreous cells (hyalocytes) are in the cortex, mostly at the base and over the retinal vessels.

The vitreous base is firmly attached to the peripheral retina and pars plana. In children, vitreous has a strong attachment to the back of the lens,

Fig. 8.1 Rendering of the vitreous body showing the zonules to support the lens, the bulk vitreous filling the eye, and remnants of the early embryonic vitreous in the S-shaped Cloquet's canal where the hyaloid vessels once passed from the disc to the lens.

Fig. 8.2 Gross pathology specimen of an aphakic eye. The upper and lower eye have been removed to expose the vitreous; the pupil is seen from behind on the right (arrow). Vitreous is firmly attached at the pars plana, ora serrata (base), and the disc (to left). Attachments at the macula and retinal blood vessels are weaker and have pulled away in sectioning.

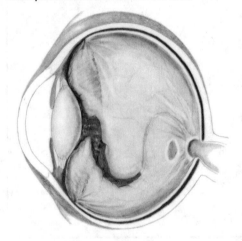

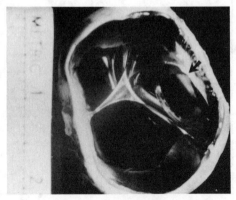

about 2 mm from its equator (Egger's line). Posteriorly, it's attached loosely at the margins of the disc, the macula, and along the retinal vessels near the equator (Fig. 8.2).

References

Eisner G: Biomicroscopy of the Peripheral Fundus. New York: Springer, 1973.

Tolentino FI, Schepens CL, Freeman HM: Vitreoretinal Disorders: Diagnosis and Management. Philadelphia: Saunders, 1976.

I. OPHTHALMOSCOPIC ANATOMY

Because of its transparency, the vitreous is the most difficult ocular tissue to examine. The slit lamp biomicroscope and contact lens, by forming an optical section, provide the best view. The ophthalmoscope is good for gross orientation and viewing. However, ophthalmoscopy shouldn't be limited to straight-in viewing; it can be used to inspect all quadrants.

We've all seen vitreous fibers. They are the fine, gelatinous, sometimes knobby threads that drift across our vision while we view a bright background, such as snow or a blue sky. These are the common muscae volitantes, or flying flies. They're visible to the persistent ophthalmoscopist who has a steady patient. Because they move with eye motion, often in an anterior-posterior direction, they constantly move in and out of focus.

Cloquet's canal, which contains the remnants of primordial vitreous, is not seen in the diffuse light of the ophthalmoscope, unless embryonic hyaloid vascular tissue has persisted. This developmental variation is quite common in health or may be part of congenital abnormalities of the eye.

In general, the transparent vitreous is invisible with the ophthalmoscope, unless congenitally abnormal, aged, or diseased. Pathology may involve the whole vitreous body, a localized area, or multiple separate sites. It may be close to the lens or retina or in the mid-vitreous space.

II. LOSS OF VITREOUS TRANSPARENCY FROM BIRTH

White pupil (leukocoria) often involves the vitreous. All known infections and parasitic, traumatic, and neoplastic diseases described in section IV, below, could appear at birth, but rarely do. This section is limited to vitreous abnormalities more commonly present at birth.

References

Peyman GA, Sanders DR, Goldberg MF: Principles and Practice of Ophthalmology. Philadelphia: Saunders, 1980.

A. HEMORRHAGE

Peripheral intraretinal hemorrhage is common in newborns and more frequent in premature infants. Intravitreal or serious intraretinal hemorrhage is rare. There is nothing specific about the appearance of hemorrhage at birth. Birth trauma is blamed for the majority of cases; however, the many other causes of intravitreal hemorrhage should not be overlooked. Transplacental anticoagulation and drug toxicity are possible causes. In cases of battered children, the eye is frequently involved, either by direct trauma or severe papilledema and hemorrhage (see Figs. 3.53-3.56).

B. RETROLENTAL FIBROPLASIA

This retinal vascular disease occurring mostly in premature infants results in vitreous bands or veils (see Chapter 4: VIIIA).

C. PERSISTENT HYPERPLASTIC PRIMARY VITREOUS (Fig. 8.3; see also in color section)

Anterior and posterior forms of this disease may occur together or separately. Either may be accompanied by persistence of the hyaloid artery (see Fig. 8.4) and other developmental anomalies, such as falciform fold.

Ophthalmoscopic findings

o   White, retrolenticular membrane obscuring a view of the retina.

o   Unilateral in 89 percent of cases.

o   Eyes are microphthalmic in one case out of two.

o   Frequently, there are other developmental anomalies of the eye.

Symptoms & signs

There's wide variation in the degree of ocular affliction. Vision may vary from normal to no light perception. Children with severe persistent hyperplastic primary vitreous have or develop the following:

o   Cataract.

o   Redness as a ciliary flush and conjunctival injection.

o   Pain or discomfort in severely affected eyes, manifested by child's rubbing or kneading the eye.

o   Shallow anterior chamber.

o   Hyphema.

o   Glaucoma and a steamy cornea.

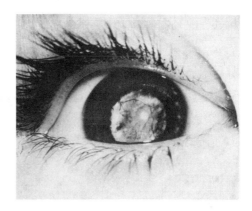

Fig. 8.3 Persistent anterior hyperplastic primary vitreous, a developmental anomaly. For posterior persistent hyperplastic primary vitreous, see Fig. 3.28. From Sugar HS: Primary hyperplastic vitreous. **Arch Ophthalmol** 75:290, 1966. Copyright © 1966, American Medical Association. Used with permission. Also shown in color section.

Fig. 8.4 Thread-like hyaloid artery remnant in Cloquet's canal from the disc to the lens in an otherwise healthy eye (a, left). Visual acuity was 6/6 (20/20). Other fine strands (arrow) may cross the vitreous unrelated to the hyaloid system (b, right).

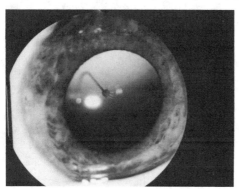 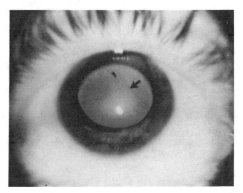

In milder forms of the disease, the child may have no symptoms but have such other signs of ocular malformation as:

o   Coloboma of iris, lens, choroid, retina, or optic disc.

o   Falciform retinal fold.

o   Persistent hyaloid artery and tunica vasculosa lentis.

o   Retinal dysplasia.

Other confirming findings

o   Family history and chromosomal studies are negative, except in rare cases; toxicologic causes are not known.

o   Other developmental anomalies of the eye are present in 31 percent of patients with persistent hyperplastic primary vitreous, and in about 11 percent of cases there are developmental anomalies in other organs.

Main differential diagnosis

o   Retinoblastoma

o   Toxocara canis

o   Coats's disease

o   Congenital cataract

o   Endophthalmitis

References

Apple DJ, Rabb MF: Clinicopathologic Correlation of Ocular Disease: A Text and Stereoscopic Atlas. St. Louis: Mosby, 1978.

Haddad R, Font RL, Reeser F: Persistent hyperplastic primary vitreous: A clinicopathologic study of 62 cases and review of the literature. Surv Ophthalmol 23:123, 1978.

Peyman GA, Sanders DR, Goldberg MF: Principles and Practice of Ophthalmology. Philadelphia: Saunders, 1980.

D. HYALOID ARTERY SYSTEM REMNANTS (Fig. 8.4)

Ophthalmoscopic findings

o   White dot on the back of the lens (Mittendorf's dot).

o   Branching diaphanous strands meet in a single strand farther back in vitreous.

o   Single strand can be traced to the vessels on the disc.

o   Often associated with other developmental anomalies, such as persistent hyperplastic primary vitreous, retinal dysplasia, falciform retinal folds, and microphthalmos.

o   In some patients, may be associated with prepapillary, intravitreal, or retrolenticular hemorrhage.

Symptoms & signs

o   This developmental anomaly often accompanies persistent hyperplastic primary vitreous and is usually asymptomatic.

o   In rare cases, prepapillary or intravitreal hemorrhage, with all of the accompanying complaints, can occur.

Other confirming findings

o   Family history and chromosomal studies are negative, except in rare cases; toxicologic causes are not known.

o Hyaloid remnants have been described in three out of 100 mature infants and in 95 percent of premature babies.

o Remnants persist throughout life.

Main differential diagnosis

o Trauma with intravitreal hemorrhage

o Persistent hyperplastic primary vitreous

o Endophthalmitis

o Toxocara canis

o Toxoplasmosis

References

Tolentino FI, Schepens CL, Freeman HM: Vitreoretinal Disorders: Diagnosis and Management. Philadelphia: Saunders, 1976, p 191.

E. VITREOUS CYSTS AND VEILS (Fig. 8.5)

These rare developmental anomalies are found in Cloquet's canal along the path of the embryonic hyaloid artery. From time to time, unexplained vitreous condensations also are found that seem to have no relationship to the common developmental anomalies of the eye. Some may be the residua of ocular inflammation.

Ophthalmoscopic findings

o Translucent; retina can be viewed through them.

o Adjacent vitreous is clear.

o May move with eye movements.

o Do not become enlarged.

o Usually unilateral.

Symptoms & signs

o Transient blurring and floaters.

o Acquired cysts may accompany toxoplasmosis, retinitis pigmentosa, or parasites, with all of their respective symptoms and signs.

Main differential diagnosis

o Juvenile retinoschisis

o Longstanding rhegmatogenous retinal detachment

Fig. 8.5 Fundus photograph, left eye, showing large oval translucent vitreous cyst (a, left). Surface is covered with numerous pigment dots. Veil just behind the lens in a 34-year-old male with an inflammation of unknown cause (b, right). An oval hole in the veil can be seen just below the light reflection on the cornea. Fig. 8.5a from Bullock JD: Developmental vitreous cysts. **Arch Ophthalmol** 91:83, 1974. Copyright ©1974, American Medical Association. Used with permission.

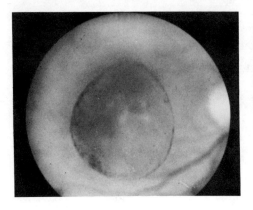 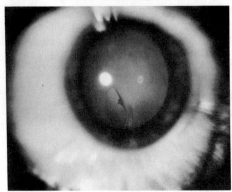

- o Hyaloid vessel remnant
- o Retrolental fibroplasia

References

Bullock JD: Developmental vitreous cysts. Arch Ophthalmol 91:83, 1974.

Tolentino FI, Schepens CL, Freeman HM: Vitreoretinal Disorders: Diagnosis and Management. Philadelphia: Saunders, 1976.

III. AGING (Fig. 8.6)

In older persons, Cloquet's canal takes a less direct course from the lens to the disc by falling inferiorly. Pockets of vitreous liquefaction (synchysis) are present, and separation of the posterior hyaloid from the retina becomes common past the age of 60 (Fig. 8.6).

Ophthalmoscopic findings

- o Cloquet's canal and lacunae of liquefaction are optically inactive, causing no reflection; red reflection is homogeneous, compared to the surrounding vitreous.
- o Partial or complete rings are seen against the red reflection by focusing up into the vitreous from the disc or macula. The elevation of the rings from the retina or disc depends on the degree of vitreous detachment and forward collapse (Fig. 8.7).

o Rings are diaphanous and move with eye movement.

o Ophthalmoscopically visible findings may be more advanced in highly myopic younger patients. Strands or cylinders of vitreous may cross the vitreous space.

o Usually mild but occasionally severe intravitreal hemorrhage occurs with vitreous separation. A small hemorrhage may be found at the disc margin or along a major retinal vessel. The association of posterior vitreous detachment with retinal tears and detachment is common, and the peripheral retina has to be searched carefully. Avulsed retinal vessels associated with posterior vitreous detachment are usually found posterior to the equator of the globe. The presence of diabetic retinopathy does not rule out the possiblility of either a retinal tear or an avulsed retinal vessel.

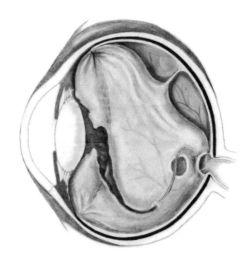

Fig. 8.6 Rendering of change in vitreous consistency and position with aging. Note the liquefaction (synchisis) over the macula and that Cloquet's canal has descended, leaving a ring of glial tissue where vitreous used to be attached to the disc. Compare with Fig. 8.1.

Fig. 8.7 Separation of the vitreous from around the disc margin leaves a defect in the posterior vitreous surface. This ring may be far forward if collapse of the vitreous collagen is present (a, left), or still close to the disc (arrow) if only partial separation has occurred (b, right).

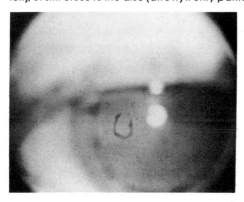 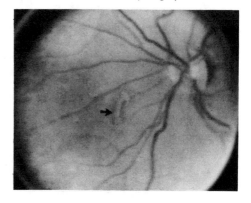

Symptoms & signs

Some patients, particularly those who are myopic, may, with age, notice an increase in density and number of vitreous floaters. Most have no symptoms attributable to vitreous aging alone, unless posterior vitreous separation occurs. Vitreous separation occurs in nearly all elderly people, is eventually bilateral, and afflicts men and women equally. It's a common cause of complaint. On the other hand, many patients have asymptomatic separation, judging from the high rate of discovery on routine examination. The symptoms and signs in posterior vitreous detachment are:

o Sudden onset.

o May be described as a net, sometimes with one or two round or oval, and sometimes incomplete, rings that drift in front of the patient's vision.

o May be associated with mild and/or occasionally severe intravitreal hemorrhage that patients describe as showers of black specks. Because the blood is mostly in the liquid vitreous posteriorly, it often clears quickly with ocular quiet and with the head elevated.

o Patient may describe flashes of light in the peripheral field of vision. The flashes are white or yellow, more noticeable in a dark area, and may be aggravated by head or eye movement. This phenomenon contrasts with the aura described by migrainous patients and the central colored lights seen by some patients with macular degeneration.

Other confirming findings

o By age 70, six out of 10 patients have at least partial vitreous separation in both eyes. These percentages are greater in aphakic and highly myopic eyes.

Other signs of ocular aging and the patient's general health should be compared with the vitreous findings. Some ocular aging changes visible with the ophthalmoscope, the biomicroscope, and fluorescein angiography include:

o Arcus senilis of the cornea.

o Decreasing endothelial cell population of cornea (seen with biomicroscope).

o Nuclear sclerosis of the lens.

o Retinal vessel arteriosclerosis.

o Thinning of retina (judged by shadow casting).

o Increasing diameter of the capillary-free zone at the fovea (seen with fluorescein angiography).

Main differential diagnosis

o   Retinal tear or avulsed retinal blood vessel

o   Retinal detachment

o   Old branch artery and vein occlusion with neovascularization

o   Diabetic retinopathy

References

Eisner G: Biomicroscopy of the Peripheral Fundus. New York: Springer, 1973.

Foos RY: Posterior vitreous detachment. Trans Am Acad Ophthalmol Otolaryngol 76:480, 1972.

Tolentino FI, Schepens CL, Freeman HM: Vitreoretinal Disorders: Diagnosis and Management. Philadelphia: Saunders, 1976, p 112.

IV. ACQUIRED LOSS OF VITREOUS TRANSPARENCY

Loss of transparency of the vitreous may result from trauma, inflammation, and neoplastic and degenerative diseases. The vitreous has no blood vessels of its own, yet it can be the site of blood-borne disease.

Loss of transparency may involve the whole vitreous body or only a small part of it, depending upon duration, severity, type, and patient resistance. The disease may be one primarily affecting the vitreous, such as asteroid hyalosis, or may be a sign of systemic disease, such as intravitreal hemorrhage in diabetes mellitus.

Light transmission of the vitreous, principally over the macula, affects the patient's visual acuity. Dense opacities, if they cover only the peripheral retina, may not be a significant factor in loss of vision.

A. HEMORRHAGE (Fig. 8.8; see Figs. 4.17, 4.79)

The vitreous does not contain blood vessels and therefore cannot bleed. All hemorrhage into the vitreous originates in adjacent tissues, and intravitreal hemorrhage is a sign of abnormality in the iris, ciliary body, retina, or choroid.

Ophthalmoscopic findings

o   Vitreous transparency may vary from a totally black (eight-ball) appearance to a fine dispersion of red blood cells just clouding the view. The blood may appear red in the ophthalmoscope's light, or yellow-orange, if hemolysis has begun.

o Intravitreal blood often does not clot and settles inferiorly when the patient stays upright. The speed of this positional change is enhanced by posterior vitreous separation and liquefaction (synchysis). You improve your view through the ophthalmoscope by having the patient change positions.

o The ophthalmoscope's light may seem dim; disc and retina have a rosy color.

o Strands of red blood may cross the vitreous cavity.

o Vitreous opacities often move freely with ocular motion. Ophthalmoscopy of the vitreous should be done with the patient taking different positions. Opacities in cornea, anterior chamber, and lens don't drift as vitreous opacities usually do.

Symptoms & signs

o Almost invariably a sudden onset.

o May be so severe that the patient perceives only light, or so mild that the patient describes myriad of fine dots but has no visual loss; dots appear black, not red, to patient.

o Vision may be intermittently obscured if vitreous is liquid. Blood swirls with eye movements and settles down with ocular quiet; vision may be better on awakening in the morning.

o Blood may form "strings" before the patient's vision.

o Bleeding may be recurrent, especially in patients with neovascularization.

o If accompanied by stimulation of the retina from vitreous traction, the patient may describe flashes of light, usually in the temporal field.

o Field loss may vary from none to total. Intravitreal blood tends to settle into the inferior vitreous and obstructs the upper field for some time after a severe hemorrhage, even though central vision has returned.

Other confirming findings

o A complete list of the causes of intravitreal bleeding is so long as to be useless. Some of the more common causes include diabetes mellitus of 10 years duration or more in a juvenile and two years or more in an adult, retinal tears, ocular trauma, compensatory neovascularization of the retina following retinal vascular occlusion from arteriosclerosis or embolism. A patient and family history consistent with these and other diseases should be sought in a general review of systems.

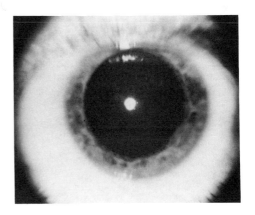

Fig. 8.8 Intravitreal blood turns an ochre color as it hemolyzes. The patient had diabetic retinopathy. Visual acuity reduced to perception of hand motion.

o Physical findings associated with history of hemorrhagic diseases — anemia, splenomegaly, easy bruising, telangiectasis, and the like — should be sought.

o Indirect ophthalmoscopy greatly aids examination of the interior of the eye in presence of cloudy vitreous.

o Laboratory and radiologic investigation for diabetes mellitus, leukemia, hypercholesterolemia, bleeding tendencies, and other such conditions as indicated by medical history and findings from physical and ocular examinations.

o Fluorescein angiography helps identify abnormal or leaking vasculature.

o Ultrasonography provides gross study of retinal and vitreal anatomy.

Main differential diagnosis

o Corneal epithelial disturbance, such as traumatic, chemical, viral

o Aqueous turbidity, as with iritis

o Cataract

o Inflammatory cells and protein

References

Morse PH, Aminlari A, Scheie HG: Spontaneous vitreous hemorrhage. Arch Ophthalmol 92:297, 1974.

Tolentino FI, Schepens CL, Freeman HM: Vitreoretinal Disorders: Diagnosis and Management. Philadelphia: Saunders, 1976, p 413.

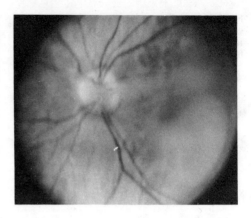

Fig. 8.9 Peripheral uveitis (pars planitis) in a 10-year-old female. This disease of unknown etiology is invariably worse in the lower part of the eye. Note that the cloudy vitreous obscures the inferior retina. The cloud may follow Cloquet's canal back to the disc. Also shown in color section.

B. INFLAMMATORY CELLS AND PROTEIN (Fig. 8.9; see also in color section; see also Figs. 5.34, 5.43)

The ophthalmoscope allows identification of cloudy vitreous for association with other evidence of inflammation.

Ophthalmoscopic findings

o   Retinal blood vessels on the disc cannot be clearly focused.

o   Ophthalmoscope's light seems dim.

o   On focusing into the vitreous with plus lenses, clumps of cells may be seen against the background of the disc and retina.

o   May be unilateral or bilateral.

o   Loss of vitreous transparency is often worse over a specific inflammatory lesion.

o   Strands or sheets of cells may cross the vitreous cavity.

o   White clumps of cells around foreign material or foci of inflammation give the appearance of dense clouds with a hazy halo.

Symptoms & signs

o   Acute onset may be associated with pain, if iritis is also present.

o   Clouding may be so severe as to allow the patient only light perception, but visual acuity is usually better than this. With extremely poor vision, involvement of the macular retina by the inflammation must be considered.

- o In chronic inflammation, patient may complain of dim vision and/or floaters. Onset may be so gradual that patient is aware only of vision loss.
- o Position change rarely affects vision, as in patients with preretinal hemorrhage.
- o Field loss rarely occurs from vitreous inflammatory cells alone; if field loss is present, retinal function is usually disrupted.

Other confirming findings

- o A system review includes exposure to infectious and parasitic disease as well as collagen and autoimmune diseases. Trauma, especially foreign-body penetration, should be considered. Endophthalmitis may follow sepsis or any ophthalmic surgical procedure, but is most common after cataract or trauma surgery. Filtering operations for glaucoma leave an open fistula into the eye, and minor conjunctivitis may later result in infection within the eye.
- o Evidence of inflammation at other body sites should be investigated. Toxoplasmosis is transmitted transplacentally and may be acquired from eating raw meat. Intracranial calcifications may be demonstrated on roentgenogram. Hematologic titer and enzyme-linked immunoserum assay (ELISA) test provide laboratory confirmation.
- o Indirect ophthalmoscopy provides a better view.
- o Slit lamp biomicroscopy confirms the nature of the vitreous opacity.
- o Ultrasonography gives a gross anatomic study.
- o Fluorescein angiography, if possible through the hazy vitreous, aids diagnosis.
- o The removal of vitreous is becoming more commonplace; biopsy for diagnostic purposes is feasible in difficult diagnostic problems of the vitreous. In infestation by larval parasites, excisional biopsy may be sight-saving.

Main differential diagnosis

See Table 8.1.

References

Tasman W: Retinal Diseases in Children. New York: Harper & Row, 1971.

Tolentino FI, Schepens CL, Freeman HM: Vitreoretinal Disorders: Diagnosis and Management. Philadelphia: Saunders, 1976, p 155.

Table 8.1

CAUSES OF VITREOUS TURBIDITY, PARTIAL LIST

Infants
Hemorrhage from birth trauma
Hemorrhage from trauma (battered child)
Posterior hyperplastic primary vitreous
    and other developmental anomalies
Retrolental fibroplasia
Toxoplasmosis

Children
Coats's disease
Hemorrhage from trauma (battered child)
Pars planitis
Retinal detachment
Retinoblastoma
Toxocara canis and other parasites
Toxoplasmosis

Young adults
Chorioretinitis (unknown cause)
Hemorrhage from trauma, diabetes,
    vascular abnormality, e.g. Coats's disease
Intraocular foreign body or penetrating injury
Pars planitis
Sepsis with endophthalmitis

Older adults
Amyloidosis
Asteroid hyalitis
Choroidal tumor: choroidal melanoma,
    metastasis from breast or lung tumor
Hemorrhage from diabetes mellitus, retinal
    tear, retinal detachment, retinal vascular
    occlusion
Leukemia
Postoperative infection, endophthalmitis
Reticulum cell sarcoma
Sepsis with endophthalmitis, bacterial
    or fungal

PHYSICIANS' GUIDE TO OCULOSYSTEMIC DISEASES

C. DEPOSITED MATERIAL

1. Suspended yellow particles (asteroid hyalosis, asteroid hyalitis, Benson's disease) (Fig. 8.10; see also in color section)

Deposit of magnesium and calcium soaps in the vitreous in adults may be more common in diabetes and those with peripheral retinal degeneration. The cause is unknown, but it is a common finding.

Ophthalmoscopic findings

o   Glistening, golden yellow, round or oval dots may be so numerous that they hinder your view of the disc.

o   Particles may involve only part of the vitreous; they may be more numerous in one eye than the other.

o   Bilateral in three cases out of four.

o   There usually are more particles inferiorly, especially after vitreous collapse (posterior vitreous separation).

Symptoms & signs

o   Usually no symptoms; patient's visual acuity is better than your view would indicate.

o   In some patients, decreased vision occurs if posterior vitreous detachment condenses the asteroid particles over macula.

o   Flashes, floaters, and field loss suggest retinal detachment.

Fig. 8.10 Asteroid hyalosis of the vitreous. The patient's vision is better than the ophthalmoscopic view suggests.

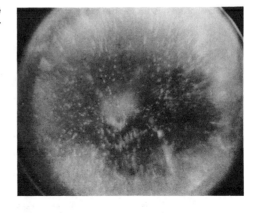

Other confirming findings

o The history and ocular findings are nearly always diagnostic, requiring no additional confirmation.

o Diabetes mellitus may be present.

o Incidence of retinal detachment may be higher in patients with asteroid hyalosis.

Main differential diagnosis

o Intravitreal hemorrhage and synchysis scintillans

o Amyloidosis

o Reticulum cell sarcoma

o Acute leukemia

References

Rodman HI, Johnson FB, Zimmerman LE: New histopathological and histochemical observations concerning asteroid hyalitis. Arch Ophthalmol 66:552, 1961.

Smith JL: Asteroid hyalitis and diabetes mellitus. Trans Am Acad Ophthalmol Otolaryngol 69:269, 1965.

Tolentino FI, Schepens CL, Freeman HM: Vitreoretinal Disorders: Diagnosis and Management. Philadelphia: Saunders, 1976.

2. Amyloidosis (Fig. 8.11; see also in color section)

This uncommon disease may involve the vitreous. Despite its rarity, it shouldn't be ignored, because it may cause severe visual loss that is correctable.

Ophthalmoscopic findings

o Wavy sheets of "glass wool," consisting of dull, yellow-white particles and stringy colored fibrils.

o May involve the central vitreous more than the periphery.

o Usually bilateral.

Symptoms & signs

o Black floating spots and veils in front of vision.

o Gradual visual loss.

o Field loss determined by location and density of vitreous opacity.

Fig. 8.11 Suspected amyloidosis of the vitreous in an 84-year-old female. Opacities had been increasing in both eyes gradually for several years in an otherwise healthy woman. Also shown in color section.

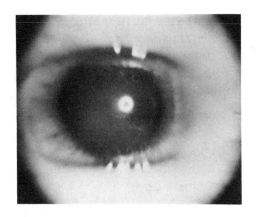

Other confirming findings

o Amyloid vitreous disease is usually associated with primary familial systemic amyloidosis with an incidence probably higher than reported 8 percent. The disease may occur sporadically and without systemic involvement.

o Indirect ophthalmoscopy.

o Biomicroscopy.

o Multisystem involvement, including heart, lung, spleen, liver, kidney, and adrenal and thyroid glands.

o Diagnosis best made by biopsy, and this may include vitrectomy, if vitreous is severely involved.

Main differential diagnosis

o Intravitreal hemorrhage
o Asteroid hyalosis
o Reticulum cell sarcoma
o Acute leukemia
o Endophthalmitis
o Uveitis

References

Ferry AP, Lieberman TW: Bilateral amyloidosis of the vitreous body. Arch Ophthalmol 94:982, 1976.

3. Synchysis scintillans (cholesterosis)

This rare but striking vitreous abnormality has been found principally after severe intravitreal hemorrhage.

Ophthalmoscopic findings

o Sharp-pointed iridescent particles that swirl up with eye movement or positioning, then settle inferiorly. They are multicolored and disappear in ultraviolet light.

Symptoms & signs

o Patient may note swirls of fine opacities with activity or on arising.

o Eyes with synchysis scintillans are often blind or have poor vision from severity of disease or trauma.

Other confirming findings

o History of severe trauma or intraocular hemorrhage usually precedes findings by several years.

o Indirect ophthalmoscopy.

o Ultrasonography.

Main differential diagnosis

o Intravitreal hemorrhage

o Asteroid hyalosis

o Amyloidosis

References

Berliner H: Biomicroscopy of the Eye, vol 2. New York: Hoeber, 1949.

Tolentino FI, Schepens CL, Freeman HM: Vitreoretinal Disorders: Diagnosis and Management. Philadelphia: Saunders, 1976, p 163.

4. Retinoblastoma (Fig. 8.12; see also in color section; see Chapter 5: VIB, 1)

5. Reticulum cell sarcoma and acute leukemic vitreous infiltration
(Fig. 8.13; see 8.13b also in color section)

Reticulum cell sarcoma (histiocytic lymphoma) may involve the vitreous and must enter the differential diagnosis in older patients with uveitis. Reticulum cells are normally present in the retina and choroid, but it's still

Fig. 8.12 Retinoblastoma in the vitreous, or "seeding." This complication is associated with a poor prognosis. Courtesy of Robert Ellsworth, M.D., New York. See also in color section.

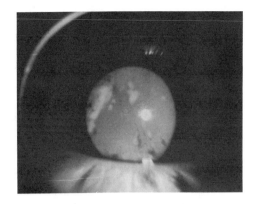

Fig. 8.13 Reticulum cell sarcoma at the base of the brain in a 56-year-old woman was associated with yellow retinal lesions (a, left) and cloudy vitreous (b, right). Sarcoma cells were found on vitrectomy. Fig. 8.13b also shown in color section.

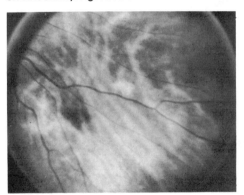 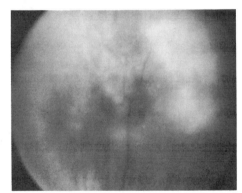

unknown whether the disease originates in the eye or the vitreous is secondarily involved. Acute lymphoblastic leukemia cells have been found in the vitreous.

Ophthalmoscopic findings

o   Cells and clumps of grayish debris in vitreous.

o   May be severe enough to cause opaque sheets or strands crossing the vitreous cavity and obscuring any view of retina.

o   Retina and optic disc, if seen, usually appear normal, although multiple areas of pigment atrophy and small gray lesions with pigment proliferation have been seen.

o   Both eyes are often involved.

Symptoms & signs

o   Photophobia, mild discomfort, and floaters are frequent complaints.

o   Patients may have been treated for anterior and posterior uveitis.

o   Vision reduced often to hand motion.

o   Neurological symptoms may include confusion, dysarthria, facial and ocular muscle palsy, abnormal reflexes, speech difficulty.

Other confirming findings

o   All patients with reticulum cell sarcoma reported to date have been older than age 40 and most older than 60 at onset of the disease. Acute leukemia patients were younger.

o   Thorough medical evaluation is indicated.

o   Bone marrow and cerebrospinal fluid analysis occasionally aid in diagnosis.

o   Computerized axial tomography may be needed.

o   Ultrasonography of eye defines vitreous disease when ophthalmoscopy is impossible.

o   Fluorescein angiography helps define retinal lesions.

o   Tissue biopsy is the best method of diagnosis, and this may require vitrectomy, if other studies are equivocal and vision is deteriorating.

Main differential diagnosis

o   Uveitis and other inflammatory disease

o   Intravitreal hemorrhage

o   Asteroid hyalosis

o   Amyloidosis

o   Endophthalmitis

References

Michels RG, Knox DL, Erozan YS, et al: Intraocular reticulum cell sarcoma: Diagnosis by pars plana vitrectomy. Arch Ophthalmol 93:1331, 1975.

Neault RW, VanScoy RE, Okazaki H, et al: Uveitis associated with isolated reticulum cell sarcoma of the brain. Am J Ophthalmol 73:431, 1972.

Parver LM, Font RL: Malignant lymphoma of the retina and brain. Arch Ophthalmol 97:1505, 1979.

Swartz M, Schumann GB: Acute leukemic infiltration of the vitreous diagnosed by pars plana aspiration. Am J Ophthalmol 90:326, 1980.

6. Foreign bodies (Figs. 8.14-8.16; see 8.14a and 8.15a also in color section; see also Figs. 5.39, 7.36)

Foreign material may forcefully enter the eye from an explosion or any source propelling a high-velocity projectile. One of the most common is a metal chip from pounding metal against metal. Foreign bodies less than 1.5 mm in diameter (1 disc diameter) rarely have the mass and velocity to penetrate the eye very far, and therefore smaller particles are more likely to be suspended in the vitreous. Slowly eroding surgically placed materials may also enter the vitreous.

Ophthalmoscopic findings

- o   Various materials of all colors, shapes, and sizes have been found.
- o   A metallic foreign body may have a sparkling gray side, the side that was attached to original object.
- o   Circular glistening oil droplets, air, or wax carried in with the foreign body may form a track through the vitreous.
- o   The foreign body may not penetrate the eye itself, but drive ahead of it objects in its path, such as glass, eyelashes (see Fig. 5.22).
- o   Sutures, polyethylene, or silicone used for retinal reattachment or other surgery may cross the vitreous space.
- o   Vitreous may be discolored by blood initially or later by rust (siderosis) or copper (chalcosis). The latter gives a green tint.
- o   Inflammatory cells and protein make the vitreous turbid.
- o   Suspended foreign bodies drift with ocular movement. Liquefaction of the vitreous eventually causes them to fall into the lower part of the eye.

Symptoms & signs

- o   Most adult patients are aware of sudden penetrating injury. In small children, injury may be overlooked as benign when the foreign body is small.
- o   Often there's immediate loss of vision from hemorrhage; however, small objects slowed by the cornea or lens may not reach the retina to cause hemorrhage, but remain suspended in the vitreous. Patients may note only temporary distortion of vision and slight pain.
- o   Blood in the anterior chamber, a distorted pupil, or transillumination of light (red reflex) through the iris (see Fig. 2.29) indicate penetration.
- o   Slowly penetrating or eroding foreign materials are usually asymptomatic, unless hemorrhage or retinal detachment occurs.

Fig. 8.14 Foreign body suspended in the vitreous of a 28-year-old male injured by a particle from a chainsaw (a, left). Fine metallic foreign bodies on the surface of the retina following vitrectomy (b, right). Presumably they originated from the moving parts of the vitrectomy instrument. Fig. 8.14a also shown in color section.

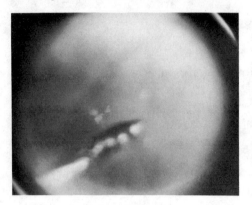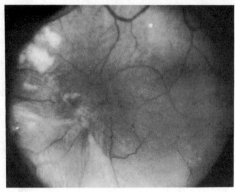

Fig. 8.15 Air bubble carried into the eye by a penetrating foreign body (a, left). Hemorrhage streams inferiorly from the impact site in the retina. Courtesy of Philip Lempert, M.D., Ithaca, New York. Air bubble introduced at the time of retinal surgery (top of photograph) to aid in tamponading retina against the buckle (b, right). Fig. 8.15a also shown in color section.

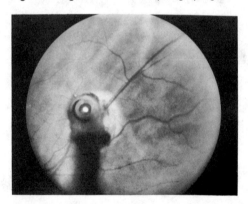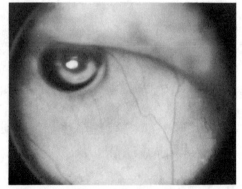

Fig. 8.16 Dacron suture used for repair of a retinal detachment has eroded through the sclera, choroid, and retina and passes through the vitreous. The white sclera is seen to the right of the suture.

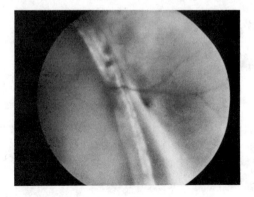

Fig. 8.17 Dislocated lens in the posterior vitreous of a 60-year-old woman struck in the eye (a, left). Similar dislocation in an 18-year-old male injured by an exploding cartridge (b, right). The patient also has chalcosis (copper deposits) in the macula. Fig. 8.17b also shown in color section.

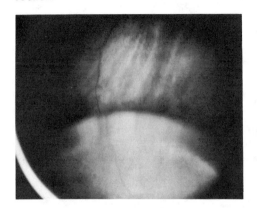 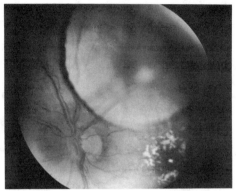

o   Some foreign bodies are very destructive and cause severe inflammatory reaction; nickel, copper, wood, and iron are the worst. Plastic and glass may be well tolerated. Alloys tend to be more inert than pure metals.

o   Infection often complicates ocular penetration, compounding the symptoms and signs of the trauma.

Other confirming findings

o   History and ocular findings of penetrating trauma are nearly always diagnostic. Surgical procedures using foreign materials should be reviewed.

o   Indirect ophthalmoscopy and biomicroscopy are indispensable. Movement of a metallic foreign body when a magnet is brought near the eye is confirmatory evidence.

o   Radiologic study and computerized tomography are helpful, especially with metallic foreign bodies; they aid also in localization.

o   Ultrasonography may be helpful.

Main differential diagnosis

o   Intravitreal hemorrhage from multiple causes

o   Toxocara canis or other parasites

o   Retinoblastoma with vitreous seeding

o   Toxoplasmosis

o   Displaced ocular tissue, such as the lens

References

Havener WH, Gloeckner SL: Atlas of Diagnostic Techniques and Treatment of Intraocular Foreign Bodies. St. Louis: Mosby, 1969.

D. DISPLACED OCULAR TISSUE (Fig. 8.17; see 8.17b also in color

The lens may be dislocated into the vitreous by trauma or surgery. Rarely, free-floating cysts of ciliary epithelium are found in the vitreous (see Chapter 2: VIC and Chapter 5: VD).

E. LARVA (Fig. 8.18; see also in color section)

Multiple larval parasites invade the eye. Individual worms have been observed crossing the vitreous and causing no ill effect, while others incite a severe inflammatory reaction (see Chapter 6: IIID, 7c).

F. BLOOD VESSELS (Fig. 8.19)

Vessel proliferation from the retina or disc may extend far forward with the vitreous as a scaffolding. Abnormal, and even normal, retinal vessels may be avulsed from their location by vitreous traction (see Chapter 4: VA, VIA, VIIA, and VIIIE).

Fig. 8.18 Intravitreal cysticercus worms overlying the optic disc. Courtesy of Keith Zinn, M.D., New York. Also shown in color section.

Fig. 8.19 Blood vessels in the vitreous of a 73-year-old woman with advanced proliferative diabetic retinopathy. Note they are in focus well above the retinal plane and equal to normal retinal vessels in caliber.

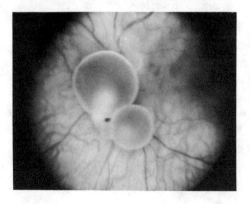

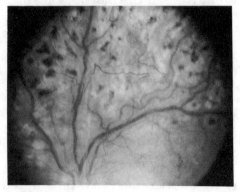

Fig. 8.20 Vitreous membranes in proliferative diabetic retinopathy may be subtle (a), very highly elevated and vascular (b), or remain as white preretinal tissue in spontaneous remission (c). Peripheral remnants of a dense vitreous hemorrhage removed by vitrectomy obscure the retina in some patients (d). Fig. 8.20c and 8.20d also shown in color section.

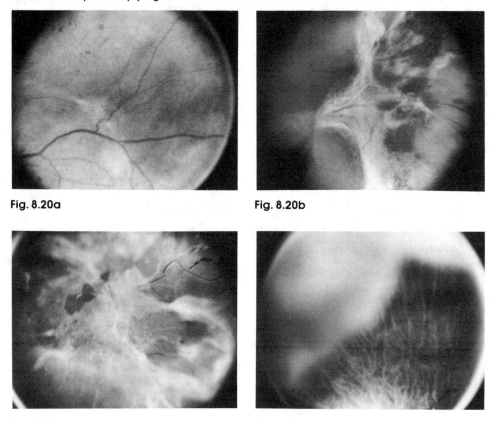

Fig. 8.20a　　　　　　　**Fig. 8.20b**

Fig. 8.20c　　　　　　　**Fig. 8.20d**

G. VEILS, BANDS, AND MEMBRANES WITH RETINAL DISEASE

1. Proliferative diabetic retinopathy (Fig. 8.20; see 8.20c and 8.20d also in color section)

Metabolism of the vitreous is intimately related to that of the retina. In diabetic retinopathy, the vitreous is affected, and bands, veils, and sheets of opacification accompany the retinal vascular disease.

Ophthalmoscopic findings

o Abnormalities vary from fine, barely discernible preretinal opacities, faintly hiding the retina, to dense, white, avascular sheets that obscure retinal detail.

o Vitreous often turbid or hemorrhagic.

o Veils and bands are attached and often distort retinal vessels.

Symptoms & signs

o Poor vision is common because of the advanced state of retinopathy; however, extensive vitreous disease away from the macula may still allow normal vision and an asymptomatic patient.

o Symptoms suggestive of intravitreal hemorrhage or retinal detachment may occur.

Other confirming findings

o Slit lamp biomicroscopic evidence of depigmentation and vascularization of the iris and cataracts is essential.

o Fluorescein angiography demonstrates retinal and iris neovascular disease.

o Kidney function needs to be assessed in all proliferative diabetic retinopathy patients. Proliferative diabetic retinopathy and Kimmelstiel-Wilson syndrome often go together.

o Hypertensive, cardiovascular, and peripheral vascular disease are common in proliferative diabetic retinopathy patients.

Main differential diagnosis

o Uveitis

o Endophthalmitis

o Amyloidosis

o Reticulum cell sarcoma

o Retinal tear or detachment

References

Tolentino FI, Lee P-F, Schepens CL: Biomicroscopic study of vitreous cavity in diabetic retinopathy. Arch Ophthalmol 75:238, 1966.

2. Other retinal vascular diseases

These are discussed in Chapter 4.

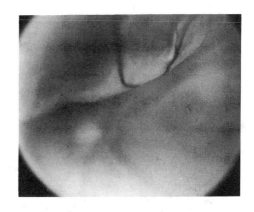

Fig. 8.21 Retinal detachment. The retina has moved so far into the vitreous it can be seen right behind the lens. Note the retinal vessels are visible in the elevated retina, while the disc is out of focus. Also shown in color section.

H. RETINAL DETACHMENT (Fig. 8.21)

If the vitreous is liquified from age or disease, a retinal hole or tear may result in the separation of the neurosensory retina from the retinal pigment epithelium, shifting forward as fluid accumulates between the layers (see Chapter 5: IIIB).

V. VITREORETINAL DEGENERATIONS (SEE APPROPRIATE SECTIONS OF CHAPTER 5: VI)

INDEX

Herpes zoster
  cornea, 27
  retinopathy, **379**
Histoplasmosis syndrome, **352**
Holes, retinal. See Missing retina
Homocystinuria, 48-49
Hooft's hypolipidemia syndrome, 372
Hurler's disease, 27
Hyaloid artery, persistent, **74, 468**
Hydroxychloroquine.
      See Drug-induced disease
Hyperparathyroidism, 27
Hypertension, malignant,
      retinal detachment and, **243**
Hypertensive retinopathy, **163,** 170
  clinical classification, 162
Hyperviscosity states, **179**
Hypoplasia, optic nerve, **62**
Hypopyon, 30

I
Ichthyosis, 27
Incontinentia pigmenti, **205,** 206
Indomethacin, 27.
      See also Drug-induced disease
Infantile amaurotic idiocy, 331
Influenza, **379**
Injections, loss of vision and, 170
Injury, loss of vision and, 170
Intestinal lipodystrophy.
      See Whipple's disease
Intracerebral vascular calcification, 372
Intraocular lens, 31
Iodates. See Drug-induced disease
Iris
  red reflection and, **32**
  skin, hair, and eye pigment disease,
    308
Iron deposits, 27. See also Siderosis
Ischemic atrophy of the retinal
      pigment epithelium, **320**
Ischemic optic neuritis.
      See Ischemic optic neuropathy
Ischemic optic neuropathy, **98**

J
Juvenile GM$_2$ gangliosidosis, 331
Juvenile macular degeneration, **327**
Juvenile mucolipidosis.
      See Ganglion cell storage disease
Juvenile rheumatoid arthritis, 27
Juxtapapillary scarring, **68**

K
Kandori, fleck retina of, **384**
Kayser-Fleischer ring.
      See Copper deposits, cornea
Kearns-Sayre syndrome.
      See Ophthalmoplegia,
      progessive external
Klinefelter's syndrome, 372
Kuhnt-Junius degeneration.
      See Disciform degeneration,
      retinal pigment epithelium

L
Larva, **389, 488**
Laser burn, retina
  accidental, **365**
  treatment, **362,** 194
Lattice degeneration, retina, **297**
Leber's congenital amaurosis.
      See Retinitis pigmentosa
Leber's miliary aneurysm.
      See Coats's disease
Leber's optic neuropathy, **103**
Lens
  cataract, **39,** 43
  deposits on, **44**
  foreign bodies, 45
  pigment, 45
  pseudoexfoliation, 45
  subluxation and dislocation,
    23, 30, **46,** 48-49
Leprosy, 27
Leukemia, **179**
  myelogenous, 207
Lipemia retinalis, **218**
Lymphoma, orbit, 101

M
Macroglobulinemia, **179,** 207
Macular disease, inherited, 257
Macular fibrosis, preretinal
  acquired. See Surface wrinkling
      retinopathy
  congenital, **258**
Malaria, 170, 207
Malignant melanoma.
      See Melanoma, choroid
Marfan's syndrome, 48-49, 372
Measles, **378**
Melanocytoma, disc, **80**
Melanoma, choroid, 257, **445**
Melanosarcoma, choroid.

Osseous choristoma, choroid.
    See Osteoma, choroid
Osteogenesis imperfecta, 372
Osteoma, choroid, **455**
Osteoporosis, 372
Oxalosis, 373, **386**

P

Paget's disease of bone, 372
Pale disc, **115**
Papilledema
    acute, **108**
    chronic, **112**
    drusen and, **105**
    false, **89**
    resolving, **113**
Pars planitis, **278**
Paving stone degeneration, **303**
Pelizaeus-Merzbacher disease, 372
Pemphigus, 27
Periarteritis nodosa, **379**
Peripheral uveitis. See Pars planitis
Photocoagulation, 207, **362.**
        See also Laser burn
Pigment fallout, **361**
Pigment hyperplasia, **319**
Pigmentation
    choroidal effusion and, **380**
    retinal detachment and, **380**
    retinoschisis and, **380**
Pipecolic acidemia, 372
Poikiloderma, **162**
Poliomyelitis, **379**
Polycythemia vera, **179,** 207
Polymyalgia rheumatica.
        See Giant cell arteritis
Porphyria cutanea tarda, 372
Posterior hyperplastic primary vitreous.
    See Falciform fold
Pseudopapilledema. See Drusen, disc
Pseudophakos. See Intraocular lens
Pseudoretinitis pigmentosa, **374, 379**
Pseudotumor cerebri. See Papilledema
Psoriasis and retinitis pigmentosa, 373

Q

Quinine optochin.
        See Drug-induced disease

R

Radiation retinopathy, 207
Refsum's disease, 27, 373
Renoretinal dysplasia, 373
Respiratory distress, **179**
Reticular dystrophy, **329**
Reticulum cell sarcoma, **482**
Retinal artery occlusion, **167**
    causes of, 170
Retinal detachment
    cystoid macular edema and, 257
    nonrhegmatogenous, **240**
    rhegmatogenous, **236**
Retinal dysplasia. See Falciform fold
Retinitis pigmentosa, **368**
    associated conditions, 372-373
    cystoid macular edema and, 257
Retinitis pigmentosa sine pigmento.
        See Retinitis pigmentosa
Retinitis punctata albescens.
        See Retinitis pigmentosa;
        Fundus albipunctatus
Retinoblastoma, 51, 87, **281**
Retinoschisis
    juvenile, **252,** 257
    senile, **249**
    sex-linked. See Juvenile retinoschisis
Retrolental fibroplasia, 207, **209**
Rheumatic heart disease,
        retinal arterial occlusion and, 170
Rheumatoid arthritis, juvenile, 27
Rickettsial infection.
        See Rocky Mountain spotted fever;
        Hyperviscosity states
Rocky Mountain spotted fever, **271**
Rod-cone dystrophy.
        See Retinitis pigmentosa
Rosacea, 27
Rothmund-Thomson syndrome, **162**
Rubella retinopathy, **376**
Rubeola retinopathy, 170.
        See also Measles
Rubeosis irides.
        See Neovascularization, retinal, iris
Rud's syndrome, 373

S

San Joaquin valley fever.
        See Coccidioidomycosis
Sandhoff's disease.

Other Titles of Related Interest
From Medical Economics Books

Color Atlas of Anterior Segment Eye Diseases
Ira A. Abrahamson Jr., M.D.
ISBN 0-87489-055-1

Manual for Eye Exam and Diagnosis, Second Edition
Mark W. Leitman, M.D.
Samuel Gartner, M.D.
Paul Henkind, M.D.
ISBN 0-87489-227-9

A Singular View: The Art of Seeing With One Eye, Second Edition
Frank B. Brady
ISBN 0-87489-224-4

Human Disease in Color
Chandler Smith, M.D.
ISBN 0-87489-188-4

Physicians' Guide to Diseases of the Oral Cavity
Harriet Goldman, D.D.S., M.P.H.
Michael Z. Marder, D.D.S.
ISBN 0-87489-240-6

Patient Care FlowCharts
Editors of Patient Care Magazine
ISBN 0-87489-295-3

Core Pathology
Chandler Smith, M.D.
ISBN 0-87489-239-2

Physicians' Guide to Etiology and Treatment of Diarrhea
Horacio Jinich, M.D.
Teodoro Hersh, M.D.
ISBN 0-87489-268-6

Clinical Aspects of Malpractice
Robert Seymour Pollack, A.B., M.D.
ISBN 0-87489-230-9

Outline Guide to Antimicrobial Therapy
John E. McGowan, M.D.
ISBN 0-87489-249-X

For information, write to:
Medical Economics Books
680 Kinderkamack Road
Oradell, New Jersey 07649